THE COMPLETE GUIDE TO

SPORTS NUTRITION

8TH EDITION

Anita Bean

B L O O M S B U R Y

LONDON · OXFORD · NEW YORK · NEW DELHI · SYDNEY

Bloomsbury Sport
An imprint of Bloomsbury Publishing Plc

50 Bedford Square   1385 Broadway
London   New York
WC1B 3DP   NY 10018
UK   USA

www.bloomsbury.com

British Library Cataloguing-in-Publication Data
A catalogue record for this book is available from the
British Library.

Library of Congress Cataloguing-in-Publication data
has been applied for.

ISBN: Print: 978-1-4729-2420-9
        ePDF: 978-1-4729-2422-3
        ePub: 978-1-4729-2421-6

4 6 8 10 9 7 5

Typeset in ITC Galliard by seagulls.net

Printed and bound in China by Toppan Leefung Printing

To find out more about our authors and books visit
www.bloomsbury.com. Here you will find extracts,
author interviews, details of forthcoming events and the
option to sign up for our newsletters.

// CONTENTS

ACKNOWLEDGEMENTS

I would like to thank Simon, my husband, for his patience during the writing of this book, and for putting up with my many hours of working at the computer. I am so very grateful to Chloe and Lucy, my two beautiful (and sporty) daughters for providing me with inspiration, joy and fulfilment. This book would not have been written without the vision, support and talent of the wonderful editorial team at Bloomsbury, especially Charlotte Croft and Sarah Skipper. Many other people have contributed directly and indirectly to this book. These include the many athletes, coaches and scientists whom I have had the privilege to meet and work with over the years. They have provided me with inspiration, knowledge and precious insights into sport. I value their suggestions, comments and honesty.

FOREWORD

I know from first-hand experience just how important good nutrition is for sports performance. It's always been a crucial part of my training strategy and has, undoubtedly, helped me achieve the success I've enjoyed. I've learned over the years that I have to fuel my body properly, otherwise I wouldn't have the energy or the strength to push my body through gruelling workouts and races.

My biggest nutritional challenge has always been eating enough food. In training, I burn 5000–6000 calories a day, which is a vast amount of food! And definitely not easy to fit in around training and everything else. I've worked out – often through trial and error – how much I have to eat, the right times to eat and which are the best foods for fast recovery.

There are so many things to think about before a big race but, for me, nutrition is right up there near the top. I have to plan what I'm going to eat and drink beforehand and make sure I have the right amounts of carbohydrates, protein and fats. It's not always easy, especially when I'm travelling or competing in other countries – I have to check beforehand that I'll be able to get *all* the food and drink I need.

That's why this book is such a useful resource to me. It explains clearly and concisely the science of nutrition for sport. It's helped me with my training and competitions. And it's answered loads of questions I've had about my diet. Anita has managed to make a complex subject accessible and exciting.

Her advice is accurate and, importantly, it's also realistic and achievable. So it's hardly surprising that, since it was first published in 1993, *The Complete Guide to Sports Nutrition* has become the top-selling book on sports nutrition in the UK. I would thoroughly recommend it to anyone who wants to get more out of their sport. I've learned a lot from this book and I'm confident it will help you, whether you're just training for fitness or getting ready for the next Olympics.

James Cracknell OBE, MSc,
British international rowing double
Olympic champion and world record holder.

PREFACE TO THE EIGHTH EDITION

This book was first published in 1993, when the science of sports nutrition was in its infancy and there was little reliable nutrition information available to athletes. Since then, our knowledge of how nutrition influences sport and exercise performance has grown, new guidelines have evolved and high quality research continues to be published. There is now overwhelming evidence that diet significantly influences athletic performance. Having advised hundreds of athletes over the past 25 years, I have seen first-hand how important diet is in supporting any training programme and helping athletes reach their goals.

The aim of this book has always been to translate the science of nutrition into practical information that athletes can understand and use. It provides evidence-based facts and recommendations in an easy-to-digest format, not opinions or anecdotes. All the information is backed with scientific references, which are listed at the back of the book. I am happy to say that, over the years, this book has remained a trusted reference and practical handbook for many athletes, trainers, coaches and sports professionals.

So what's new? This eighth edition brings together the latest research and information on sport and exercise nutrition. It includes the current consensus recommendations of leading sports organisations: the International Olympic Committee, the American College of Sports Medicine, the Academy of Nutrition and Dietetics and Dietitians of Canada, as well as the findings from hundreds of sports nutrition studies around the world.

Since the publication of the seventh edition, research in sports nutrition has focused on new topics such as nutrition periodisation, 'training low', protein timing, energy availability and optimisation of body composition. There has been a trend toward higher fat intakes and a move away from very low fat diets once believed beneficial for athletes. However, the controversy surrounding low carbohydrate diets is ongoing and new research is beginning to provide some interesting insights into the effects of strategic periods of carbohydrate restriction on training adaptations, body composition and performance.

Guidelines for energy, carbohydrate and protein are now expressed in grams per kg body weight, instead of as a percentage of total energy. This is more accurate as it takes account of body size. There have been new recommendations on the optimal amount of protein to be consumed after exercise as well as the timing and type of protein. New concepts such as metabolic efficiency and flexibility have evolved.

It is clear that when it comes to optimal performance, one size doesn't fit all. Athletes should follow a personalised nutrition and hydration plan that takes account of the specific physiological demands of their event, their training and performance goals, practical considerations, food preferences and individual circumstances.

Scientists have also made progress in the quest for giving elite athletes the edge in long-duration competitions, with the development of sports drinks containing 'multiple transportable carbohydrates' that allow the body to absorb higher amounts of carbohydrate per hour. Other changes include the abolition of advice to drink ahead of thirst and a warning against overhydration during long events. There are no longer hard and fast guidelines on fluid intake and, in practice, athletes have to find a compromise between preventing dehydration and ensuring they don't overhydrate.

I have always taken a 'food first' approach when it comes to optimising nutrition for performance, despite the enormous array of expensive engineered supplements out there! Pills, powders and gels cannot replicate the complex matrix of nutrients and phytochemicals provided by natural food. What's more, food tastes so much nicer and provides a lot more pleasure than any supplement. If it can improve recovery and performance, then this has to be great news for every athlete.

I've watched with equal fascination and scepticism as more and more sports supplements appear on the market. Science continues to disprove the claims of most, which I am happy to report in this book. However, there is some sound evidence on the benefits of a small handful of supplements, which I have outlined in chapter 6.

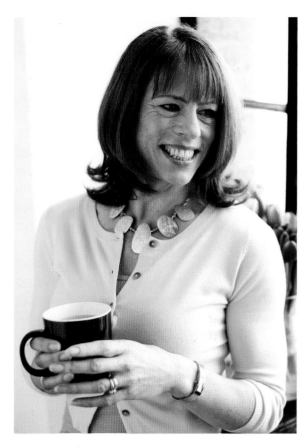

In this book, I have attempted to condense decades of sports nutrition research into practical guidelines and, ultimately, a step-by-step guide to developing a personalised nutrition plan. I hope you will find the information useful and that it will help you reach your sporting potential.

Anita Bean

An overview of sports nutrition

There is universal scientific consensus that diet affects health, performance and recovery. A well-planned eating strategy will help support any training programme, whether you are training for fitness or for competition; promote efficient recovery between workouts; reduce the risk of illness or overtraining; and help you to achieve your potential in sport.

Of course, everyone has different nutritional needs and there is no single diet that suits all. Some athletes require more calories, protein or vitamins than others; and each sport has its unique nutritional demands. But it is possible to find broad scientific agreement as to what constitutes a healthy diet for sport generally. The following guidelines are based on the Joint Position Statement on Nutrition and Athletic Performance from the American College of Sports Medicine, Academy of Nutrition and Dietetics and Dietitians of Canada (ACSM/AND/DC, 2016) and the International Olympic Committee Consensus Conference on Sports Nutrition (IOC, 2011).

These organisations highlight the importance of nutrition strategies in optimising elite performance. They recognise the advances in sports nutrition research in recent years, including the need for nutrition periodisation, individualisation of nutrition plans to take into account the specificity and uniqueness of the event and performance goals, the new concepts of metabolic efficiency and flexibility, and energy availability (energy intake minus the energy cost of exercise); the importance of nutrient timing and optimising the intakes of protein after training to aid long-term maintenance or gain of muscle; greater intakes of carbohydrate (90 g/hr) for exercise over 3 hours; the importance of vitamin D for performance; and the need for a personalised hydration plan to prevent dehydration as well as hyponatraemia. They recommend that the requirement for energy, carbohydrate and protein should be expressed using guidelines per kg body weight to take account of a range of body sizes.

The process leading to publication was extremely thorough and drew on the combined expertise of many of the world's leading sports nutrition experts. Of course, these guidelines are only intended to give you an overview of the evidence linking nutrition and performance. Everyone is different and some people respond better or worse to various dietary strategies. So it is important to experiment and find out what works best for you. But, being based on high quality research, these guidelines are a great place to start.

1. Energy

It is crucial that athletes meet their energy (calorie) needs during hard periods of training in order to achieve improvements in performance and maintain good health. Failure to consume sufficient energy can result in muscle loss, reduced performance, slow recovery, disruption of hormonal function (in females) and increased risk of fatigue, injury and illness. Researchers have recently identified the concept of energy availability (EA), defined as dietary intake minus exercise energy expenditure, or the amount of energy available to the body to perform all other functions after exercise training expenditure is subtracted. In healthy adults, a value of 45 kcal/kg fat-free mass (FFM)/day equates with energy balance and optimum health. It has been suggested that 30 kcal/kg FFM/day should be the lower threshold of energy availability in females. (Fat-free mass includes muscles, organs, fluid and bones.) A low EA may compromise athletic performance in the short and long term. It may occur when energy intake is too low, energy expenditure is too high or a combination of both. The term 'Relative Energy Deficiency in Sport (RED-S)' refers to the impaired physiological function, including metabolic rate, menstrual function, bone health, immunity, protein synthesis and cardiovascular health, caused by relative energy deficiency or low EA in male and female athletes. It more accurately describes the clinical syndrome previously known as the Female Athlete Triad.

Your daily calorie needs will depend on your genetic make-up, age, weight, body composition,

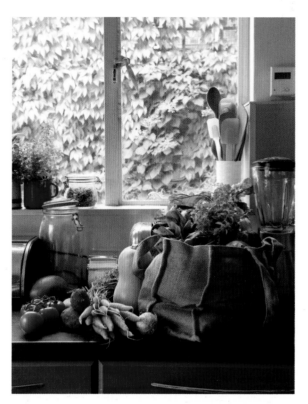

your daily activity and your training programme. It is possible to estimate the number of calories you need daily from your body weight (BW) and your level of daily physical activity.

STEP 1: ESTIMATE YOUR RESTING METABOLIC RATE (RMR)

Your RMR is an estimate of how many calories you would burn if you were to do nothing but rest for 24 hours. It represents the minimum amount of energy needed to keep your body functioning, including breathing and keeping your heart beating. It can be estimated using the Mifflin-St Jeor equation, which utilises age, weight and height, and is considered more accurate than the more commonly used Harris-Benedict equation.

Men

$(10 \times \text{weight (kg)}) + (6.25 \times \text{height (cm)})$
$- (5 \times \text{age (y)}) + 5$

Women

$(10 \times \text{weight (kg)}) + (6.25 \times \text{height (cm)})$
$- (5 \times \text{age (y)}) - 161$

STEP 2: WORK OUT YOUR PHYSICAL ACTIVITY LEVEL (PAL)

This is the ratio of your overall daily energy expenditure to your RMR – a rough measure of your lifestyle activity.

- Mostly inactive or sedentary (mainly sitting): 1.2
- Fairly active (include walking and exercise 1–2 × week): 1.3
- Moderately active (exercise 2–3 × weekly): 1.4
- Active (exercise hard more than 3 × weekly): 1.5
- Very active (exercise hard daily): 1.7

STEP 3: MULTIPLY YOUR RMR BY YOUR PAL TO WORK OUT YOUR DAILY CALORIE NEEDS

Daily calorie needs = RMR × PAL

This figure gives you a rough idea of your daily calorie requirement to maintain your weight. If you eat fewer calories, you will lose weight; if you eat more then you will gain weight.

2. Body composition

There is no single or 'optimal' body composition for a particular event or sport. Each individual athlete has an optimal fat range at which their

Resting Metabolic Rate

The Resting Metabolic Rate (RMR) is the amount of energy required to maintain the body's normal metabolic activity, such as respiration, maintenance of body temperature and digestion. Specifically, it is the amount of energy required at rest with no additional activity. The energy consumed is sufficient only for the functioning of the vital organs. It is closely related to the basal metabolic rate (BMR), which can only be measured in an awake, but totally rested and post-absorptive state, and in a neutrally temperate environment. It is quite restrictive and only used in clinical or laboratory settings. RMR accounts for 60–75% of the calories you burn daily. Generally, men have a higher RMR than women.

Physical activity includes all activities from doing the housework to walking and working out in the gym. The number of calories you burn in any activity depends on your weight, the type of activity and the duration of that activity.

performance improves yet their health does not suffer. However, this should not be achieved at the expense of continual low energy availability, otherwise performance and health are likely to be impaired. Instead, weight and body composition should be periodised in line with the training programme, accepting fluctuations throughout the year. Excessive weight gain should be avoided in the off-season and rapid weight loss strategies avoided in the competition season. The best time to lose weight is in the base training phase or well out from competition to minimise loss of performance. A modest energy deficit of 250–500 kcal/day to achieve a slow rate of weight loss (<1% per week) is recommended along with increasing protein intake to 1.8–2.7 g/kg body weight/day to preserve muscle mass.

3. Carbohydrate

Carbohydrate is an important fuel for the brain and central nervous system as well as for muscular work. It is stored as glycogen in your liver and muscles. The size of the body's carbohydrate stores is relatively limited. Approximately 100 g glycogen (equivalent to 400 kilocalories) may be stored in the liver, and up to 400 g glycogen (equivalent to 1600 kilocalories) in muscle cells. The purpose of liver glycogen is to maintain blood sugar levels. When blood glucose dips, glycogen in the liver breaks down to release glucose into the bloodstream. The purpose of muscle glycogen is to fuel physical activity. Carbohydrate offers advantages over fat as a fuel since it provides more adenosine triphosphate (ATP) per volume of oxygen and is therefore considered a more efficient fuel. There is significant evidence that performance of prolonged, sustained or intermittent high intensity exercise is enhanced by strategies that maintain high carbohydrate availability (i.e. matching glycogen stores and blood glucose to the fuel demands of exercise).

When it is important to train hard or with high intensity, daily carbohydrate intakes should match the fuel needs of training and glycogen replenishment. General guidelines for carbohydrate intake to provide high carbohydrate availability are based on body weight (a proxy for the volume of muscle) and exercise load. These are shown in Table 1.1. The more active you are and the greater your muscle mass, the higher your carbohydrate needs. While guidelines for carbohydrate intake have been provided in terms of percentage contribution to total dietary energy intake in the past, experts now recommend expressing carbohydrate requirements in terms of grams per kg body weight. Guidelines for daily intakes are 3–5 g to 5–7 g per kg of body weight (BW) per day for low and moderate intensity daily training lasting up to 1 hour respectively. Depending on the fuel cost of the training schedule, an endurance

Table 1.1	GUIDELINES FOR DAILY CARBOHYDRATE INTAKE
Activity level	**Recommended carbohydrate intake**
Very light training (low intensity or skill-based exercise)	3–5 g/kg BW daily
Moderate intensity training (approx 1 h daily)	5–7 g/kg BW daily
Moderate–high intensity training (1–3 h daily)	6–10 g/kg BW daily
Very high intensity training (> 4 h daily)	8–12 g/kg BW daily

Source: Burke *et al.*, 2011.

athlete may need to consume 8–12 g of carbohydrate per kg body weight each day (560–840 g per day for a 70 kg athlete) to ensure adequate glycogen stores.

To promote rapid post-exercise recovery, experts recommend consuming 1.0–1.2 g carbohydrate per kg BW per hour for the first 4 hours after exercise. If you plan to train again within 8 hours, it is important to begin refuelling as soon as possible after exercise. Moderate and high glycaemic index (GI) carbohydrates (*see* p. 50) will promote faster recovery during this period. When carbohydrate intake is sub-optimal for refuelling, adding protein to a meal/snack will enhance glycogen storage. However, for recovery periods of 24 hours or longer, the type and timing of carbohydrate intake is less critical, although you should choose nutrient-dense sources wherever possible.

It is recommended that the pre-exercise meal provides 1–4 g carbohydrate per kg body weight, depending on exercise intensity and duration, and that this should be consumed between 1 and 4 hours before exercise.

During exercise lasting less than 45 minutes, there is no performance advantage to be gained by consuming additional carbohydrates. For intense exercise lasting between 45 and 75 minutes, simply swilling (not swallowing) a carbohydrate drink in your mouth ('mouth rinsing') can improve performance. The carbohydrates stimulate oral sensors that act on the central nervous system (brain) to mask fatigue and reduce perceived exertion, thus allowing you to maintain exercise intensity for longer. But for exercise lasting longer than about 1 hour, consuming between 30 and 60 g carbohydrate helps maintain your blood glucose level, spare muscle glycogen stores, delay fatigue and increase your endurance. The amount depends on the intensity and duration of exercise, and is unrelated to body size.

The longer and the more intense your workout or event, the greater your carbohydrate needs. Previously, it was thought that the body could absorb only a maximum of 60 g carbohydrate per hour. However, recent research suggests that it may be higher – as much as 90 g, a level that

Table 1.2	RECOMMENDATIONS FOR PRE- AND POST-EXERCISE CARBOHYDRATE INTAKE	
Dietary strategy	**When**	**Recommended carbohydrate intake**
Pre-exercise fuelling	Before exercise > 60 min	1–4 g/kg BW consumed 1–4 h before exercise
Post-exercise rapid refuelling	< 8 h recovery between two sessions	1.0–1.2 g · kg^{-1} · h^{-1} for first 4 h then resume daily fuel needs
Carbohydrate loading	For events > 90 min of sustained/intermittent exercise	36–48 h of 10–12 g/kg BW/24 h

Source: Burke *et al.*, 2011.

would be appropriate during intense exercise lasting more than 3 hours. Studies have shown that consuming multiple transportable carbohydrates (e.g. glucose and fructose) increases the rate of carbohydrate uptake and oxidation during exercise compared with glucose alone. A 2:1 mixture of glucose + fructose is generally associated with minimal GI distress. Choose high GI carbohydrates (e.g. sports drinks, energy gels and energy bars, bananas, fruit bars, cereal or breakfast bars), according to your personal preference and tolerance.

However, recent research has shown that training in a glycogen-depleted state can enhance the adaptive responses to exercise stimulus and increase exercise capacity. The concept of 'training low but competing high' as well as 'carbohydrate periodisation' (integrating short periods of 'training low' into the training programme) has become very popular among elite endurance athletes. Strategies include occasional fasted training, training following an overnight fast, and not replenishing carbohydrate stores after the first of two training sessions of the day. These have been shown to increase muscle adaptation to training by altering signalling and upregulating the metabolic response to exercise. However, it is important to undertake high intensity training sessions with high carbohydrate stores. Whether implementing these strategies ultimately improves performance is unclear.

4. Protein

Amino acids from proteins form the building blocks for new tissues and the repair of body cells. They are also used for making enzymes, hormones and antibodies. Protein also provides a (small) fuel source for exercising muscles.

Athletes have higher protein requirements than non-active people. Extra protein is needed to compensate for the increased muscle breakdown that occurs during and after intense exercise, as well as to build new muscle cells. The ACSM/AND/DC consensus statement recommends between 1.2 and 2.0 g protein/kg BW/day for athletes, which equates to 84–140 g daily for a 70 kg person, considerably more than for a sedentary person, who requires 0.75 g protein/kg BW daily. These recommendations encompass a range of training programmes and allow for adjustment according to individual needs, training goals and experience. The timing as well as the amount of protein is crucial when it comes to promoting muscle repair and growth. It is best to distribute protein intake throughout the day rather than consuming it in just one or two meals. Experts recommend consuming 0.25 g protein/kg BW or 15–25 g protein with each main meal as well as immediately after exercise.

Several studies have found that eating carbohydrate and protein together immediately after exercise enhances recovery and promotes muscle building. The types of protein eaten after exercise are important – high quality proteins, particularly fast-absorbed proteins that contain leucine (such as whey), are considered optimal for recovery. Leucine is both a substrate and a trigger for muscle protein synthesis (MPS). An intake of 2–3 g leucine has been shown to stimulate maximum MPS.

Some athletes eat high protein diets in the belief that extra protein leads to increased strength and muscle mass, but this isn't true – it is stimulation of muscle tissue through exercise plus adequate – not *extra* – protein that leads to muscle growth. As protein is found in so many foods, most people – including athletes – eat a little more protein than they need. This isn't harmful – the excess is broken down into urea (which is excreted) and fuel, which is either used for energy or stored as fat if your calorie intake exceeds your output.

5. Fat

Some fat is essential – it makes up part of the structure of all cell membranes, your brain tissue, nerve sheaths and bone marrow and it cushions your organs. Fat in food also provides essential fatty acids and the fat-soluble vitamins A, D and E, and is an important source of energy for exercise. The ACSM/AND/DC position statement currently makes no specific recommendation for fat intake. The focus should be on meeting carbohydrate and protein goals with fat making up the calorie balance. It is recommended that athletes' fat intakes are consistent with public health guidelines for fat intake, less than 35% of daily energy intake. The exact amount depends on individual training and body composition goals. However, it is recommended that athletes should consume a minimum of 20% energy from fat, otherwise they risk deficient intakes of fat-soluble vitamins and essential fatty acids (ACSM/AND/DC, 2016).

The Department of Health recommends that the proportion of energy from saturated fatty acids be less than 11%, with the majority coming from unsaturated fatty acids. Omega-3s may be particularly beneficial for athletes, as they help increase the delivery of oxygen to muscles, improve endurance and may speed recovery and reduce inflammation and joint stiffness.

6. Hydration

You should ensure you are hydrated before starting training or competition by consuming 5–10 ml/kg body weight in the 2–4 hours prior to exercise, and aim to minimise dehydration during exercise. Severe dehydration can result in reduced endurance and strength, and heat-related illness. The IOC and the ACSM/AND/DC advise matching your fluid intake to your fluid losses as closely as possible and limiting dehydration to no more than 2–3% loss of body weight (e.g. a body weight loss of no more than 1.5 kg for a 75 kg person). Routinely weigh yourself before and after exercise, accounting for fluid consumed and urine lost, to estimate your sweat loss during exercise. A loss of 1 kg body weight equates to 1 litre of sweat lost.

Additionally, experts caution against over-hydrating yourself before and during exercise, particularly in events lasting longer than 4 hours. Drinking too much water may dilute your blood so that your sodium levels fall. Although this is quite rare, it is potentially fatal. The American College of Sports Medicine advises drinking when you're thirsty or drinking only to the point at which you're maintaining your weight, not gaining weight.

Sports drinks containing sodium are advantageous when sweat losses are high (more than 1.2 litres/h) – for example, during intense exercise lasting more than 2 hours – because their sodium content will promote water retention and prevent hyponatraemia.

After exercise, both water and sodium need to be replaced to re-establish normal hydration. This can be achieved by normal eating and drinking practices if there is no urgent need for recovery. But for rapid recovery, or if you are severely

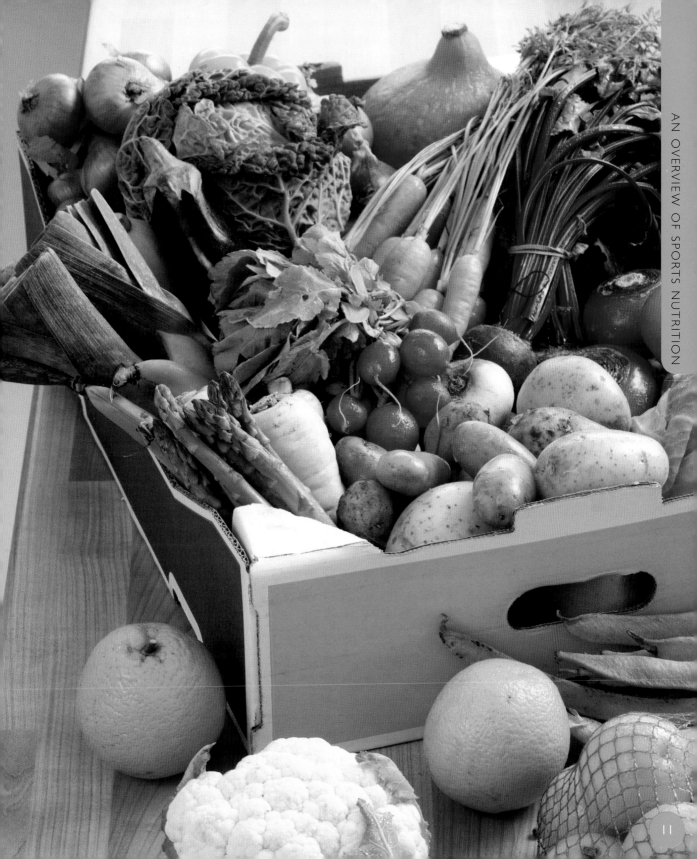

dehydrated, it is recommended you drink 25–50% more fluid than lost in sweat. You can replace fluid and sodium losses with rehydration drinks or water plus salty foods.

7. Vitamins and minerals

While intense exercise increases the requirement for several vitamins and minerals, there is no need for supplementation provided you are eating a balanced diet and consuming adequate energy to maintain body weight. The IOC, IAAF and ACSM/AND/DC believe most athletes are well able to meet their needs from food rather than supplements. There's scant proof that vitamin and mineral supplements improve performance, although supplementation may be warranted in athletes eating a restricted diet or when food intake or choices are limited – for example, due to travel. However, athletes should be particularly aware of their needs for calcium, iron and vitamin D, as low intakes are relatively common among female athletes. The role of vitamin D in muscle structure and function, and the risk of deficiency, has been highlighted by the IOC and ASCM/AND/DC. Those who have low vitamin D intakes and get little exposure to the sun may need to take vitamin D supplements.

Similarly, there is insufficient evidence to recommend antioxidant supplementation for athletes. Caution against antioxidant supplements is currently advised during training, as oxidative stress may be beneficial to the muscles' adaptation to exercise. The IOC also cautions against the indiscriminate use of supplements and warns of the risk of contamination with banned substances. Only a few have any performance benefit; these include creatine, caffeine, nitrate (as found in beet-root juice), beta-alanine and sodium bicarbonate, along with sports drinks, gels and bars and protein supplements. For the majority, there is little evidence to support their use as ergogenic aids.

8. Competition nutrition

PRE-EVENT
Performance in endurance events lasting longer than 90 minutes may benefit from carbohydrate-loading in the 36–48 hours prior to the event (10–12 g carbohydrate/kg body weight/24 hours). During the 1–4 hours prior to a race, consume 1–4 g of carbohydrate per kg of body weight. Food choices should be high in carbohydrate and moderate in protein, while low in fat and fibre to reduce risk of gastrointestinal problems.

DURING THE EVENT
In events lasting less than 75 minutes, additional carbohydrate will not benefit performance but rinsing the mouth with a carbohydrate drink may reduce perception of fatigue via the central nervous system. In events lasting 1–2.5 hours, consuming 30–60 g carbohydrate/h will help maintain blood glucose and liver glycogen, and increase endurance. In events lasting more than 2.5 hours, it may be beneficial to increase carbohydrate intake to up to 90 g per hour. This may be in the form of dual energy source drinks or gels, containing a mixture of glucose/maltodextrin and fructose to achieve faster carbohydrate absorption.

AFTER THE EVENT
Replenish glycogen by consuming 1–1.2 g of carbohydrate/kg body weight in the first 4–6 hours after finishing. Consuming protein (in 15–25 g servings) in the recovery period also

promotes glycogen recovery and enhances muscle protein resynthesis. Rehydrate with 25–50% more fluid than that lost in sweat.

How to plan your training diet

A balanced diet is one that provides enough energy, carbohydrate, protein, fat, fibre, vitamins and minerals to meet your needs. These nutrients should come from a wide variety of foods. In the UK, the Department of Health has produced a guide describing a balanced diet centred around the five main food groups (*see* Figure 1.1). It shows the proportions in which different types of foods are needed to have a balanced diet. This applies to your food intake over a day or week, not necessarily each meal. Although this does not take into account the specific requirements of athletes, you can use it as a base for developing your daily training diet. The main differences between the diet of an athlete and that of a sedentary person are the greater amounts of energy and nutrients required. Table 1.3 gives a practical guide to estimating food portions.

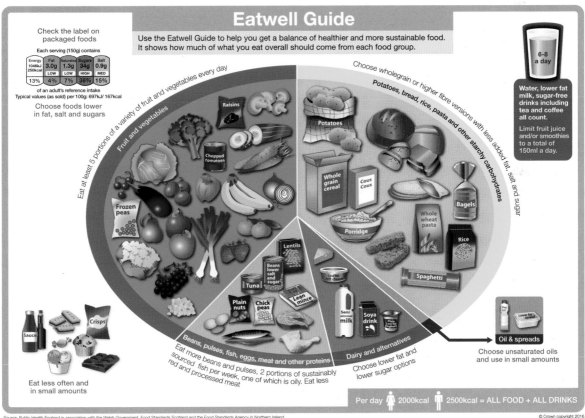

Figure 1.1 The Eatwell Guide

Table 1.3	ESTIMATING FOOD PORTIONS		
Food Group	**Number of portions per day**	**Food**	**Portion size**
Vegetables	3–5	*1 portion = 80 g*	*The amount you can hold in your hand (2 tbsp)*
		Broccoli	3 florets
		Carrots	1 medium carrot
Fruit	2–4	*1 portion = 80 g*	*The size of a tennis ball*
		Apple, pear, banana	1 medium fruit
		Plum, kiwi, satsuma	2 small fruit
Carbohydrate-rich foods	4–6 +	*1 portion = 50 g carbs*	*The size of your clenched fist*
		Potato (250 g)	Size of tennis ball
		Bread	3 slices
		Pasta, rice	3 handfuls (uncooked, 75 g) Size of 3 tennis balls (cooked, 225 g)
		Oats/cereal (50 g)	2 sachets porridge
Calcium-rich foods	2–4	Milk *1 portion = approx. 250 mg calcium*	1 cup (200 ml)
		Cheese	Size of matchbox (40 g)
		Yoghurt	1 pot (150 ml)
Protein-rich foods	4	*1 portion = approx. 20 g protein*	
		Meat, poultry, fish	Size of pack of cards (70 g meat)
		Eggs	3
		Lentils/beans	1 tin/5 tbsp (250 g)
		Tofu	Half a cup (120 g)
Healthy fats and oils	2–3	Nuts and seeds	2 tbsp (25 g)
		Olive/rapeseed oil/ peanut butter/butter	1 tbsp (15 ml)
		Oily fish	1 fillet (140 g)/week

FRUIT AND VEGETABLES
5–9 portions a day
Fruit and vegetables contain vitamins, minerals, fibre, antioxidants and other phytonutrients, which are vital for health, immunity and optimum performance.

CARBOHYDRATE-RICH FOODS
4–6 portions a day
A diet rich in wholegrain foods – bread, breakfast cereals, rice, pasta, porridge oats – and beans, lentils and potatoes maintains high glycogen (stored carbohydrate) levels, needed to fuel hard training. Aim for at least half of all grains eaten to be whole grains.

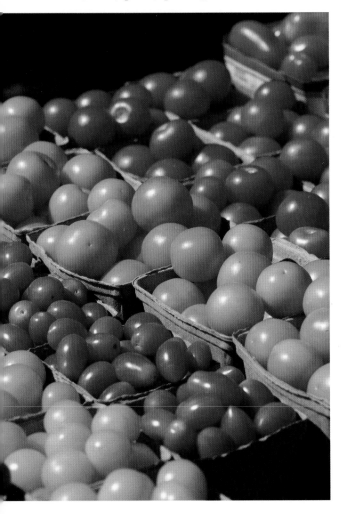

CALCIUM-RICH FOODS
2–4 portions a day
Including dairy products, nuts, pulses and tinned fish in your daily diet is the easiest way to get calcium, which is needed for strong bones.

PROTEIN-RICH FOODS
4 portions a day
Regular exercisers need more protein than inactive people, so include lean meat, poultry, fish, eggs, soya or Quorn in your daily diet. Beans, lentils, dairy foods and protein supplements can also be counted towards your daily target.

HEALTHY FATS AND OILS
2–3 portions a day
The oils found in nuts, seeds, rapeseed oil, olive oil, flaxseed oil and oily fish may improve endurance and recovery as well as protect against heart disease.

DISCRETIONARY CALORIES
These are the calories that you have left after you have eaten all the fruit, vegetables, grains, protein-rich foods, calcium-rich foods and healthy fats recommended for the day. The more active you are, the more discretionary calories are allowed. For most regular exercisers this is likely to be around 200–300 calories worth of treats such as biscuits, cakes, puddings, alcoholic drinks, chocolate or crisps, but these extra calories also need to account for any added sugar in sports drinks and energy bars, or the jam you spread on your toast, or sugar you add to coffee or tea.

Energy for
// exercise

When you exercise, your body must start producing energy much faster than it does when it is at rest. The muscles start to contract more strenuously, the heart beats faster to pump blood around the body more rapidly, and the lungs work harder. All these processes require extra energy. Where does it come from, and how can you make sure you have enough to last through a training session?

Before we can fully answer such questions, it is important to understand how the body produces energy, and what happens to it. This chapter looks at what takes place in the body when you exercise, where extra energy comes from, and how the fuel mixture used differs according to the type of exercise. It explains why fatigue occurs, how it can be delayed, and how you can get more out of training by changing your diet.

WHAT IS ENERGY?

Although we cannot actually see energy, we can see and feel its effects in terms of heat and physical work. But what exactly is it?

Energy is produced by the splitting of a chemical bond in a substance called adenosine triphosphate (ATP). This is often referred to as the body's 'energy currency'. It is produced in every cell of the body from the breakdown of carbohydrate, fat, protein and alcohol – four fuels that are transported and transformed by various biochemical processes into the same end product.

WHAT IS ATP?

ATP is a small molecule consisting of an adenosine 'backbone' with three phosphate groups attached (Fig 2.1).

Energy is released when one of the phosphate groups splits off. When ATP loses one of its phosphate groups it becomes adenosine diphosphate, or ADP. Some energy is used to carry out work

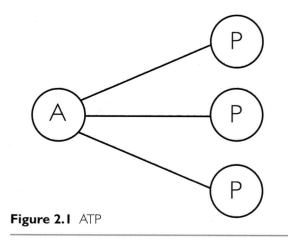

Figure 2.1 ATP

(such as muscle contractions), but most (around three-quarters) is given off as heat. This is why you feel warmer when you exercise. Once this has happened, ADP is converted back into ATP. A continual cycle takes place, in which ATP forms ADP and then becomes ATP again (Fig 2.2).

THE INTER-CONVERSION OF ATP AND ADP

The body stores only very small amounts of ATP at any one time. There is just enough to keep up basic energy requirements while you are at rest – sufficient to keep the body ticking over. When you start exercising, energy demand suddenly increases, and the supply of ATP is used up within a few seconds. As more ATP must be produced to continue exercising, more fuel must be broken down.

WHERE DOES ENERGY COME FROM?

There are four components in food and drink that are capable of producing energy:

- carbohydrate
- protein
- fat
- alcohol

When you eat a meal or have a drink, these components are broken down in the digestive system into their various constituents or building blocks. Then they are absorbed into the bloodstream. Carbohydrates are broken down into small, single sugar units: glucose (the most common unit), fructose and galactose. Fats are broken down into fatty acids, and proteins into amino acids. Alcohol is mostly absorbed directly into the blood.

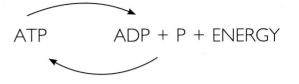

Figure 2.2 The relationship between ATP and ADP

The ultimate fate of all of these components is energy production, although carbohydrates, proteins and fats also have other important functions.

Carbohydrates and alcohol are used mainly for energy in the short term, while fats are used as a long-term energy store. Proteins can be used to produce energy either in 'emergencies' (for instance, when carbohydrates are in short supply) or when they have reached the end of their useful life. Sooner or later, all food and drink components are broken down to release energy. But the body is not very efficient in converting this energy into power. For example, during cycling, only 20% of the energy produced is converted into power. The rest becomes heat.

HOW IS ENERGY MEASURED?

Energy is measured in calories or joules. In scientific terms, one calorie is defined as the amount of heat required to increase the temperature of 1 gram (or 1 ml) of water by 1 degree centigrade (°C) (from 14.5 to 15.5 °C). The SI (International Unit System) unit for energy is the joule (J). One joule is defined as the work required to exert a force of one Newton for a distance of 1 metre.

As the calorie and the joule represent very small amounts of energy, kilocalories (kcal or Cal) and kilojoules (kJ) are more often used. As their names suggest, a kilocalorie is 1000 calories and a kilojoule 1000 joules. You have probably seen these units on food labels. When we mention calories in the everyday sense, we are really talking about Calories with a capital C, or kilocalories. So, food containing 100 kcal has enough energy potential to raise the temperature of 100 litres of water by 1 °C.

To convert kilocalories into kilojoules, simply multiply by 4.2. For example:

- 1 kcal = 4.2 kJ
- 10 kcal = 42 kJ

Metabolism

Metabolism is the sum of all the biochemical processes that occur in the body. There are two aspects: anabolism is the formation of larger molecules; catabolism is the breakdown of larger molecules into smaller molecules. Aerobic metabolism includes oxygen in the processes; anaerobic metabolism takes place without oxygen. A metabolite is a product of metabolism. That means that anything made in the body is a metabolite.

The body's rate of energy expenditure is called the metabolic rate. Your basal metabolic rate (BMR) is the number of calories expended to maintain essential processes such as breathing and organ function during sleep. However, most methods measure the resting metabolic rate (RMR), which is the number of calories burned over 24 hours while lying down but not sleeping.

To convert kilojoules into kilocalories, divide by 4.2. For example, if 100 g of food provides 400 kJ, and you wish to know how many kilocalories that is, divide 400 by 4.2 to find the equivalent number of kilocalories:

- 400 kJ ÷ 4.2 = 95 kcal

WHY DO DIFFERENT FOODS PROVIDE DIFFERENT AMOUNTS OF ENERGY?

Foods are made of different amounts of carbohydrates, fats, proteins and alcohol. Each of these nutrients provides a certain quantity of energy when it is broken down in the body. For instance, 1 g of carbohydrate or protein releases about 4 kcal of energy, while 1 g of fat releases 9 kcal, and 1 g of alcohol releases 7 kcal.

THE ENERGY VALUE OF DIFFERENT FOOD COMPONENTS

1 g provides:

- carbohydrate 4 kcal (17 kJ)
- fat 9 kcal (38 kJ)
- protein 4 kcal (17 kJ)
- alcohol 7 kcal (29 kJ)

Fat is the most concentrated form of energy, providing the body with more than twice as much energy as carbohydrate or protein, and also more than alcohol. However, it is not necessarily the 'best' form of energy for exercise.

All foods contain a mixture of nutrients, and the energy value of a particular food depends on the amount of carbohydrate, fat and protein it contains. For example, one slice of wholemeal bread provides roughly the same amount of energy as one pat (7 g) of butter. However,

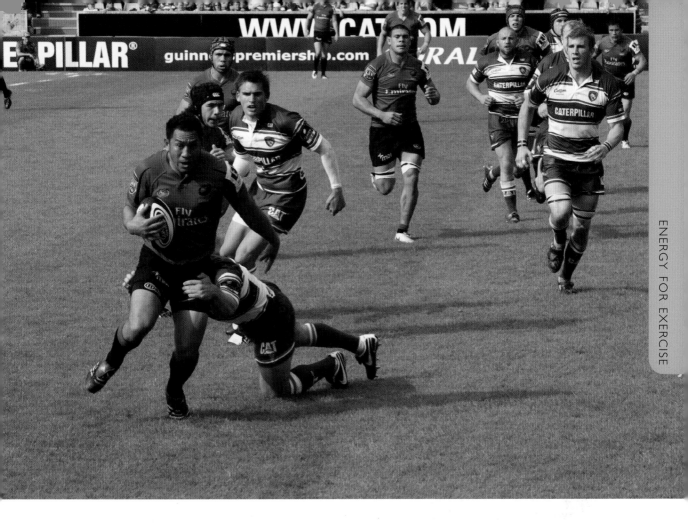

their composition is very different. In bread, most energy (75%) comes from carbohydrate, while in butter, virtually all (99.7%) comes from fat.

HOW DOES MY BODY STORE CARBOHYDRATE?

Carbohydrate is stored as *glycogen* in the muscles and liver, along with about three times its own weight of water. Altogether there is about three times more glycogen stored in the muscles than in the liver. Glycogen is a large molecule, similar to starch, made up of many glucose units joined together. However, the body can store only a relatively small amount of glycogen – there is no endless supply! Like the petrol tank in a car, the body can hold only a certain amount.

The total store of glycogen in the average body amounts to about 500 g, with approximately 400 g in the muscles and 100 g in the liver. This store is equivalent to about 2000 kcal – enough to last one day if you were to eat nothing. This is why a low carbohydrate diet tends to make people lose quite a lot of weight in the first few days. The weight loss is almost entirely due to loss of glycogen and water. Endurance athletes have higher muscle glycogen concentrations compared with sedentary people. Increasing your muscle mass will also increase your storage capacity for glycogen.

The purpose of liver glycogen is to maintain blood glucose levels both at rest and during prolonged exercise.

Small amounts of glucose are present in the blood (approximately 15 g, which is equivalent to 60 kcal) and in the brain (about 2 g or 8 kcal) and their concentrations are kept within a very narrow range, both at rest and during exercise. This allows normal body functions to continue.

HOW DOES MY BODY STORE FAT?

Fat is stored as *adipose* (fat) tissue in almost every region of the body. A small amount of fat, about 300–400 g, is stored in muscles – this is called intramuscular fat – but the majority is stored around the organs and beneath the skin. The amount stored in different parts of the body depends on genetic make-up and individual hormone balance. The average 70 kg person stores 10–15 kg fat. Interestingly, people who store fat mostly around their abdomen (the classic potbelly shape) have a higher risk of heart disease than those who store fat mostly around their hips and thighs (the classic pear shape).

Unfortunately, there is little you can do to change the way that your body distributes fat. But you can definitely change the *amount* of fat that is stored, as you will see in Chapter 8.

You will probably find that your basic shape is similar to that of one or both of your parents. Males usually take after their father, and females after their mother. Female hormones tend to favour fat storage around the hips and thighs, while male hormones encourage fat storage around the middle. This is why, in general, women are 'pear shaped' and men are 'apple shaped'.

HOW DOES MY BODY STORE PROTEIN?

Protein is not stored in the same way as carbohydrate and fat. It forms muscle and organ tissue, so it is mainly used as a building material rather than an energy store. However, proteins *can* be broken down to release energy if need be, so muscles and organs represent a large source of potential energy.

WHICH FUELS ARE MOST IMPORTANT FOR EXERCISE?

Carbohydrates, fats and proteins are all capable of providing energy for exercise; they can all be transported to, and broken down in, muscle cells. Alcohol, however, cannot be used directly by muscles for energy during exercise, no matter how strenuously they may be working. Only the liver has the specific enzymes needed to break down alcohol. You cannot break down alcohol faster by exercising harder, either – the liver carries out its job at a fixed speed. Do not think you can work off a few drinks by going for a jog, or by drinking a cup of black coffee!

Table 2.1	FUEL RESERVES IN A PERSON WEIGHING 70 KG		
Fuel stores	**Potential energy available (kcal)**		
	Glycogen	Fat	Protein
Liver	400	450	400
Adipose tissue (fat)	0	135,000	0
Muscle	1600	350	24,000

Source: Cahill, 1976.

Proteins do not make a substantial contribution to the fuel mixture. It is only during very prolonged or very intense bouts of exercise that proteins play a more important role in giving the body energy.

The production of ATP during most forms of exercise comes mainly from broken down carbohydrates and fats.

Table 2.1 illustrates the potential energy available from the different types of fuel that are stored in the body.

WHEN IS PROTEIN USED FOR ENERGY?

Protein is not usually a major source of energy, but it may play a more important role during the latter stages of very strenuous or prolonged exercise as glycogen stores become depleted. For example, during the last stages of a marathon or a long-distance cycle race, when glycogen stores are exhausted, the proteins in muscles (and organs) may make up around 10% of the body's fuel mixture.

During a period of semi-starvation, or if a person follows a low carbohydrate diet, glycogen would be in short supply, so more proteins would be broken down to provide the body with fuel. Up to half of the weight lost by someone following a low calorie or low carbohydrate diet comes from protein (muscle) loss. Some people think that if they deplete their glycogen stores by following a low carbohydrate diet, they will force their body to break down more fat and lose weight. This is not the case: you risk losing muscle as well as fat, and there are many other disadvantages, too. These are discussed in Chapter 9.

How is energy produced?

The body has three main energy systems it can use for different types of physical activity. These are called:

1. the ATP–PC (phosphagen) system;
2. the anaerobic glycolytic, or lactic acid, system;
3. the aerobic system – comprising the glycolytic (carbohydrate) and lipolytic (fat) systems.

At rest, muscle cells contain only a very small amount of ATP, enough to maintain basic energy needs and allow you to exercise at maximal intensity for about 1 second. To continue exercising, ATP must be regenerated from one of the three energy systems, each of which has a very different biochemical pathway and rate at which it produces ATP.

HOW DOES THE ATP–PC SYSTEM WORK?

This system uses ATP and phosphocreatine (PC) that is stored within the muscle cells, to generate energy for maximal bursts of strength and speed that last for up to 6 seconds. The ATP–PC system would be used, for example, during a 20-metre sprint, a near-maximal lift in the gym, or a single jump. Phosphocreatine is a high energy compound formed when the protein, creatine, is linked to a phosphate molecule (*see* box 'What is creatine?' on p. 22). The PC system can be thought of as a back-up to ATP. The job of PC is to regenerate ATP rapidly (*see* Fig. 2.3 on p. 22). PC breaks down into creatine and phosphate, and the free phosphate bond transfers to a molecule of ADP forming a new ATP molecule. The ATP–PC system can release energy

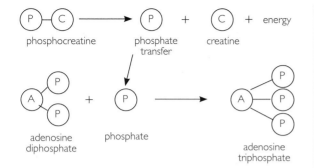

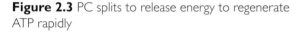

Figure 2.3 PC splits to release energy to regenerate ATP rapidly

very quickly, but, unfortunately, it is in very limited supply and can provide only 3–4 kcal. After this the amount of energy produced by the ATP–PC system falls dramatically, and ATP must be produced from other fuels, such as glycogen or fat. When this happens, other systems take over.

HOW DOES THE ANAEROBIC GLYCOLYTIC SYSTEM WORK?

This system is activated as soon as you begin high intensity activity. It dominates in events lasting up to 90 seconds, such as a weight training set in the gym or a 400–800 m sprint. In order to meet sudden, large demands for energy, glucose bypasses the energy producing pathways that would normally use oxygen, and follows a different route that does not use oxygen. This saves a good deal of time. After 30 seconds of high intensity exercise this system contributes up to 60% of your energy output; after 2 minutes its contribution falls to only 35%.

The anaerobic glycolytic system uses carbohydrate in the form of muscle glycogen or glucose as fuel. Glycogen is broken down to glucose, which rapidly breaks down in the absence of

What is creatine?

Creatine is a compound that's made naturally in our bodies to supply energy. It is mainly produced in the liver from the amino acids glycine, arginine and methionine. From the liver it is transported in the blood to the muscle cells where it is combined with phosphate to make phosphocreatine (PC).

The muscle cells turn over about 2–3 g of creatine a day. Once PC is broken down into ATP (energy), it can be recycled into PC or converted into another substance called creatinine, which is then removed via the kidneys in the urine.

Creatine can be obtained in the diet from fish (tuna, salmon, cod), beef and pork (approx. 3–5 g creatine/kg uncooked fish or meat). That means vegetarians have no dietary sources. However, to have a performance-boosting effect, creatine has to be taken in large doses. This is higher than you could reasonably expect to get from food. You would need to eat at least 2 kg of raw steak a day to load your muscles with creatine.

The average-sized person stores about 120 g creatine, almost all in skeletal muscles (higher levels in fast-twitch muscle fibres, see p. 24). Of this amount, 60–70% is stored as PC, 30–40% as free creatine.

oxygen to form ATP and lactic acid (*see* Fig. 2.4). Each glucose molecule produces only two ATP molecules under anaerobic conditions, making it a very inefficient system. The body's glycogen stores dwindle quickly, proving that the benefits

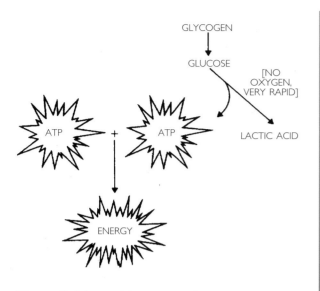

GLYCOGEN

GLUCOSE

[NO OXYGEN, VERY RAPID]

ATP + ATP

LACTIC ACID

ENERGY

Figure 2.4 Anaerobic energy system

of a fast delivery service come at a price. The gradual build-up of lactic acid will eventually cause fatigue and prevent further muscle contractions. (Contrary to popular belief, it is not lactic acid but the build-up of hydrogen ions and acidity that causes the 'burning' feeling during or immediately after maximal exercise)

HOW DOES THE AEROBIC SYSTEM WORK?

The aerobic system can generate ATP from the breakdown of carbohydrates (by glycolysis) and fat (by lipolysis) in the presence of oxygen (*see* Fig. 2.5 on p. 24). Although the aerobic system cannot produce ATP as rapidly as can the other two anaerobic systems, it can produce larger amounts. When you start to exercise, you initially use the ATP–PC and anaerobic glycolytic systems, but after a few minutes your energy supply gradually switches to the aerobic system.

What happens to the lactic acid?

Lactic acid produced by the muscles is not a wasted by-product. It constitutes a valuable fuel. When the exercise intensity is reduced or you stop exercising, lactic acid has two possible fates. Some may be converted into another substance called pyruvic acid, which can then be broken down in the presence of oxygen into ATP. In other words, lactic acid produces ATP and constitutes a valuable fuel for aerobic exercise. Alternatively, lactic acid may be carried away from the muscle in the bloodstream to the liver where it can be converted back into glucose, released back into the bloodstream or stored as glycogen in the liver (a process called gluconeogenesis). This mechanism for removing lactic acid from the muscles is called the lactic acid shuttle.

This explains why the muscle soreness and stiffness experienced after hard training is not due to lactic acid accumulation. In fact, the lactic acid is usually cleared within 15 minutes of exercise.

Most of the carbohydrate that fuels aerobic glycolysis comes from muscle glycogen. Additional glucose from the bloodstream becomes more important as exercise continues for longer than 1 hour and muscle glycogen concentration dwindles. Typically, after 2 hours of high intensity exercise (greater than 70% VO_2max), almost all of your muscle glycogen will be depleted. Glucose delivered from the bloodstream is then used to fuel your muscles, along with increasing amounts of fat (lipolytic glycolysis). Glucose from the bloodstream may be derived from the breakdown of liver glycogen or from carbohydrate consumed during exercise.

In aerobic exercise, the demand for energy is slower and smaller than in an anaerobic activity, so there is more time to transport sufficient oxygen from the lungs to the muscles and for glucose to generate ATP with the help of the oxygen. Under these circumstances, one molecule of glucose can create up to 38 molecules of ATP. Thus, aerobic energy production is about 20 times more efficient than anaerobic energy production.

Anaerobic exercise uses only glycogen, whereas aerobic exercise uses both glycogen and fat, so it can be kept up for longer. The disadvantage, though, is that it produces energy more slowly.

Fats can also be used to produce energy in the aerobic system. One fatty acid can produce between 80 and 200 ATP molecules, depending on its type (*see* Fig. 2.5). Fats are therefore an even more efficient energy source than carbohydrates. However, they can only be broken

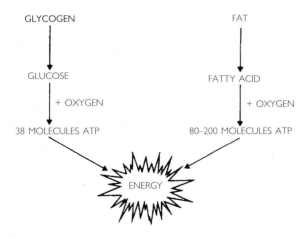

Figure 2.5 Aerobic energy system

down into ATP under aerobic conditions when energy demands are relatively low, and so energy production is slower.

MUSCLE FIBRE TYPES AND ENERGY PRODUCTION

The body has several different muscle fibre types, which can be broadly classified into fast-twitch (FT) or type II, and slow-twitch (ST) or type I (endurance) fibres. Both muscle fibre types use all three energy systems to produce ATP, but the FT fibres use mainly the ATP–PC and anaerobic glycolytic systems, while the ST fibres use mainly the aerobic system.

Everyone is born with a specific distribution of muscle fibre types; the proportion of FT fibres to ST fibres can vary quite considerably between individuals. The proportion of each muscle fibre type you have has implications for sport. For example, top sprinters have a greater proportion of FT fibres than average and thus can generate explosive power and speed. Distance runners, on the other hand, have proportionally more ST fibres and are better able to develop aerobic power and endurance.

HOW DO MY MUSCLES DECIDE WHETHER TO USE CARBOHYDRATE OR FAT DURING AEROBIC EXERCISE?

During aerobic exercise, the use of carbohydrate relative to fat varies according to a number of factors. The most important are:

1. the intensity of exercise;
2. the duration of exercise;
3. your fitness level;
4. your pre-exercise diet.

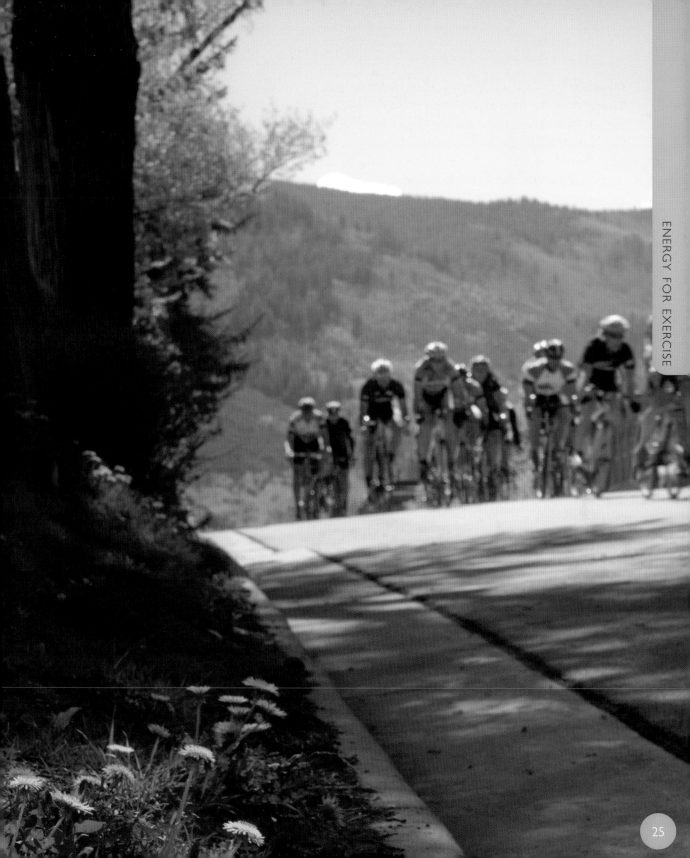

Intensity

The higher the intensity of your exercise, the greater the reliance on muscle glycogen (*see* Fig. 2.6). During anaerobic exercise, energy is produced by the ATP–PC and anaerobic glyco-lytic systems. So, for example, during sprints, heavy-weight training and intermittent maximal bursts during sports like football and rugby, muscle glycogen, rather than fat, is the major fuel.

During aerobic exercise you will use a mixture of muscle glycogen and fat for energy. Exercise at a low intensity (less than 50% of VO_2max) is fuelled mainly by fat. As you increase your exercise intensity – for example, as you increase your running speed – you will use a higher proportion of glycogen than fat. During moderate intensity exercise (50–70% VO_2max), muscle glycogen supplies around half your energy needs; the rest comes from fat. When your exercise intensity exceeds 70% VO_2max, fat cannot be broken down and transported fast enough to meet energy demands, so muscle glycogen provides at least 75% of your energy needs.

Duration

Muscle glycogen is unable to provide energy indefinitely because it is stored in relatively small quantities. As you continue exercising, your muscle glycogen stores become progressively lower (*see* Fig. 2.7). Thus, as muscle glycogen concentration drops, the contribution that blood glucose makes to your energy needs increases. The proportion of fat used for energy also increases but it can never be burned without the presence of carbohydrate.

On average, you have enough muscle glycogen to fuel 90–180 minutes of endurance activity; the higher the intensity, the faster your muscle

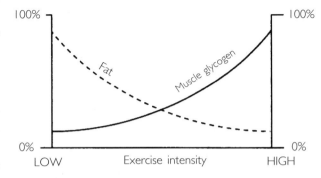

Figure 2.6 Fuel mixture/exercise intensity
Source: Costill, 1986.

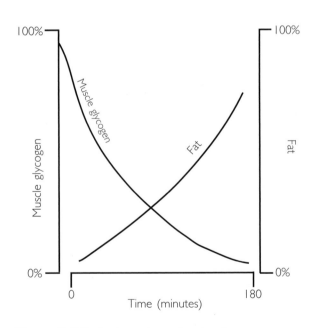

Figure 2.7 Fuel mixture/exercise duration

glycogen stores will be depleted. During interval training, i.e. a mixture of endurance and anaerobic activity, muscle glycogen stores will become depleted after 45–90 minutes. During mainly anaerobic activities, muscle glycogen will deplete within 30–45 minutes.

Once muscle glycogen stores are depleted, protein makes an increasing contribution to energy needs. Muscle proteins break down to provide amino acids for energy production and to maintain normal blood glucose levels.

Fitness level

As a result of aerobic training, your muscles make a number of adaptations to improve your performance, and your body's ability to use fat as a fuel improves. Aerobic training increases the numbers of key fat-oxidising enzymes, such as hormone-sensitive lipase, which means your body becomes more efficient in breaking down fat into fatty acids. The number of blood capillaries serving the muscle increases so you can transport the fatty acids to the muscle cells. The number of mitochondria (the sites of fatty acid

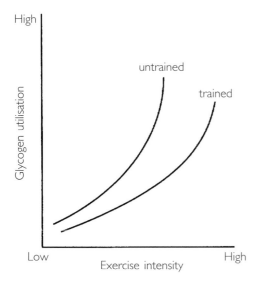

Figure 2.8 Trained people use less glycogen and more fat

oxidation) also increases, which means you have a greater capacity to burn fatty acids in each muscle cell. Thus, improved aerobic fitness enables you to break down fat at a faster rate at any given intensity, thus allowing you to spare glycogen (*see* Fig. 2.8). This is important because glycogen is in much shorter supply than fat. By using proportionally more fat, you will be able to exercise for longer before muscle glycogen is depleted and fatigue sets in.

Pre-exercise diet

A low carbohydrate diet will result in low muscle and liver glycogen stores. Many studies have shown that initial muscle glycogen concentration is critical to your performance and that low muscle glycogen can reduce your ability to sustain exercise at 70% VO_2max for longer than 1 hour (Bergstrom *et al.*, 1967). It also affects your ability to perform during shorter periods of maximal power output.

When your muscle glycogen stores are low, your body will rely heavily on fat and protein. However, this is not a recommended strategy for fat loss, as you will lose lean tissue. (*See* Chapter 9 for appropriate ways of reducing body fat.)

Which energy systems do I use in my sport?

Virtually every activity uses all three energy systems to a greater or lesser extent. No single energy system is used exclusively and at any given time energy is being derived from each of the three systems (*see* Fig. 2.9 on p. 28). In every activity, ATP is always used and is replaced by PC. Anaerobic glycolysis and aerobic energy production depend on exercise intensity.

For example, during explosive strength and power activities lasting up to 5 seconds, such as a sprint start, the existing store of ATP is the primary energy source. For activities involving high power and speed lasting 5–30 seconds, such as 100–200 m sprints, the ATP–PC system is the primary energy source, together with some muscle glycogen broken down through anaerobic glycolysis. During power endurance activities such as 400–800 m events, muscle glycogen is the primary energy source and produces ATP via both anaerobic and aerobic glycolysis. In aerobic power activities, such as running

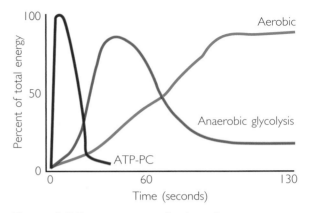

Figure 2.9 Percentage contribution of energy systems during exercise of different durations

Table 2.2	THE MAIN ENERGY SYSTEMS USED DURING DIFFERENT TYPES OF EXERCISE	
Type of exercise	**Main energy system**	**Major storage fuels used**
Maximal short bursts lasting less than 6 sec	ATP–PC (phosphagen)	ATP and PC
High intensity lasting up to 30 sec	ATP–PC Anaerobic glycolytic	ATP and PC Muscle glycogen
High intensity lasting up to 15 min	Anaerobic glycolytic Aerobic	Muscle glycogen
Moderate–high intensity lasting 15–60 min	Aerobic	Muscle glycogen Adipose tissue
Moderate–high intensity lasting 60–90 min	Aerobic	Muscle glycogen Liver glycogen Blood glucose Intramuscular fat Adipose tissue
Moderate intensity lasting longer than 90 min	Aerobic	Muscle glycogen Liver glycogen Blood glucose Intramuscular fat Adipose tissue

5–10 km, muscle glycogen is the primary energy source producing ATP via aerobic glycolysis. During aerobic events lasting 2 hours or more, such as half- and full marathons, muscle glycogen, liver glycogen, intramuscular fat and fat from adipose tissue are the main fuels used. The energy systems and fuels used for various types of activities are summarised in Table 2.2.

WHAT HAPPENS IN MY BODY WHEN I START EXERCISING?

When you begin to exercise, energy is produced without oxygen for at least the first few seconds, before your breathing rate and heart can catch up with energy demands. Therefore, a build-up of lactic acid takes place. As the heart and lungs work harder, getting more oxygen into your body, carbohydrates and fats can be broken down aerobically. If you are exercising fairly gently (i.e. your oxygen supply keeps up with your energy demands), any lactic acid that accumulated earlier can be removed easily since there is now enough oxygen around.

If you continue to exercise aerobically, more oxygen is delivered around the body and more fat starts to be broken down into fatty acids. They are taken to muscle cells via the bloodstream and then broken down with oxygen to produce energy.

In effect, the anaerobic system 'buys time' in the first few minutes of an exercise, before the body's slower aerobic system can start to function.

For the first 5–15 minutes of exercise (depending on your aerobic fitness level) the main fuel is carbohydrate (glycogen). As time goes on, however, more oxygen is delivered to the muscles, and you will use proportionally less carbohydrate and more fat.

On the other hand, if you begin exercising very strenuously (e.g. by running fast), lactic acid quickly builds up in the muscles. The delivery of oxygen cannot keep pace with the huge energy demand, so lactic acid continues to accumulate and very soon you will feel fatigue. You must then either slow down and run more slowly, or stop. Nobody can maintain a fast run for very long.

If you start a distance race or training run too fast, you will suffer from fatigue early on and be forced to reduce your pace considerably. A head start will not necessarily give any benefit at all. Warm up *before* the start of a race (by walking, slow jogging, or performing gentle mobility exercises), so that the heart and lungs can start to work a little harder, and oxygen delivery to the muscles can increase. Start the race at a moderate pace, gradually building up to an optimal speed. This will prevent a large 'oxygen debt' and avoid an early depletion of glycogen. In this way, your optimal pace can be sustained for longer.

The anaerobic system can also 'cut in' to help energy production, for instance when the demand for energy temporarily exceeds the body's oxygen supply. If you run uphill at the same pace as on the flat, your energy demand increases. The body will generate extra energy by breaking down glycogen/glucose anaerobically. However, this can be kept up for only a short period of time, because there will be a gradual build-up of lactic acid. The lactic acid can be removed aerobically afterwards, by running back down the hill, for example.

The same principle applies during fast bursts of activity in interval training, when energy is produced anaerobically. Lactic acid accumulates and is then removed during the rest interval.

What is fatigue?

In scientific terms, fatigue is an inability to sustain a given power output or speed. It is a mismatch between the demand for energy by the exercising muscles and the supply of energy in the form of ATP. Runners experience fatigue when they are no longer able to maintain their speed; footballers are slower to sprint for the ball and their technical ability falters; in the gym, you can no longer lift the weight; in an aerobics class, you will be unable to maintain the pace and intensity. Subjectively, you will find that exercise feels much harder to perform, your legs may feel hollow and it becomes increasingly hard to push yourself.

WHY DOES FATIGUE DEVELOP DURING ANAEROBIC EXERCISE?

During explosive activities involving maximal power output, fatigue develops due to ATP and PC depletion. In other words, the demand for ATP exceeds the readily available supply.

During activities lasting between 30 seconds and 30 minutes, fatigue is caused by a different

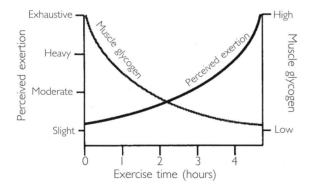

Figure 2.10 The increase in perceived exertion as glycogen stores become depleted
Source: Costill, 1986.

mechanism. The rate of lactic acid removal in the bloodstream cannot keep pace with the rate of lactic acid production. This means that during high intensity exercise lasting up to half an hour there is a gradual increase in muscle acidity, which reduces the ability of the muscles to maintain intense contractions. It is not possible to continue high intensity exercise indefinitely because the acute acid environment in your muscles would inhibit further contractions and cause cell death. The burning feeling you experience when a high concentration of lactic acid develops is a kind of safety mechanism, preventing the muscle cells from destruction.

Reducing your exercise intensity will lower the rate of lactic acid production, reduce the build-up, and enable the muscles to switch to the aerobic energy system, thus enabling you to continue exercising.

WHY DOES FATIGUE DEVELOP DURING AEROBIC EXERCISE?

Fatigue during moderate and high intensity aerobic exercise lasting longer than 1 hour occurs when muscle glycogen stores are depleted. It's like running out of petrol in your car. Muscle glycogen is in short supply compared with the body's fat stores. Liver glycogen can help maintain blood glucose levels and a supply of carbohydrate to the exercising muscles, but stores are also very limited and eventually fatigue will develop as a result of both muscle and liver glycogen depletion and hypoglycaemia (*see* Fig. 2.10).

During low to moderate intensity exercise lasting more than 3 hours, fatigue is caused by additional factors. Once glycogen stores have been exhausted, the body switches to the aerobic lipolytic system where fat is able to supply most (not all) of the fuel for low intensity exercise. However, despite having relatively large fat reserves, you will not be able to continue exercise indefinitely because fat cannot be converted to energy fast enough to keep up with the demand by exercising muscles. Even if you slowed your pace to enable the energy supplied by fat to meet the energy demand, other factors will cause you to fatigue. These include a rise in the concentration of the brain chemical serotonin, which results in an overall feeling of tiredness, acute muscle damage, and fatigue due to lack of sleep.

HOW CAN I DELAY FATIGUE?

Glycogen is used during virtually every type of activity. Therefore the amount of glycogen stored in your muscles and, in certain events, your liver, before you begin exercise will have a direct effect on your performance. The greater your pre-exercise muscle glycogen store, the longer you will be able to maintain your exercise intensity and delay the onset of fatigue. Conversely, sub-optimal muscle glycogen stores can cause earlier fatigue, reduce your endurance, reduce your intensity level and result in smaller training gains.

You may also delay fatigue by reducing the rate at which you use up muscle glycogen. You can do this by pacing yourself, gradually building up to your optimal intensity.

Summary of key points

- The body uses three energy systems: (1) the ATP–PC, or phosphagen, system; (2) the anaerobic glycolytic, or lactic acid, system; (3) the aerobic system, which comprises both glycolytic (carbohydrate) and lipolytic (fat) systems.

- The ATP–PC system fuels maximal bursts of activity lasting up to 6 seconds.

- Anaerobic glycolysis provides energy for short duration, high intensity exercise lasting from 30 seconds to several minutes. Muscle glycogen is the main fuel.

- The lactic acid produced during anaerobic glycolysis is a valuable fuel for further energy production when exercise intensity is reduced.

- The aerobic system provides energy from the breakdown of carbohydrate and fat for sub-maximal intensity, prolonged exercise.

- Factors that influence the type of energy system and fuel usage are exercise intensity and duration, your fitness level and your pre-exercise diet.

- The proportion of muscle glycogen used for energy increases with exercise intensity and decreases with exercise duration.

- For most activities lasting longer than 30 seconds, all three energy systems are used to a greater or lesser extent; however, one system usually dominates.

- The main cause of fatigue during anaerobic activities lasting less than 6 seconds is ATP and PC depletion; during activities lasting between 30 seconds and 30 minutes, it is lactic acid accumulation and muscle cell acidity.

- Fatigue during moderate and high intensity exercise lasting longer than 1 hour is usually due to muscle glycogen depletion. For events lasting longer than 2 hours, fatigue is associated with low liver glycogen and low blood sugar levels.

- For most activities, performance is limited by the amount of glycogen in the muscles. Low pre-exercise glycogen stores lead to early fatigue, reduced exercise intensity and reduced training gains.

Carbohydrate //and performance

Carbohydrate is needed to fuel almost every type of activity and the amount of glycogen stored in your muscles and liver has a direct effect on your exercise performance. A high muscle-glycogen concentration will allow you to train at your optimal intensity and achieve a greater training effect. A low muscle-glycogen concentration, on the other hand, will lead to early fatigue, reduced training intensity and suboptimal performance.

Clearly, then, glycogen is the most important and most valuable fuel for any type of exercise. This chapter explains the link between carbohydrate availability and athletic performance. It shows you how to calculate your carbohydrate requirements and considers the latest research on training with low carbohydrate availability and carbohydrate periodisation, as well as the optimal timing of carbohydrate intake in relation to training.

Each different carbohydrate produces a different response in the body, so this chapter gives advice on which types of carbohydrate foods to eat. It presents comprehensive information on the glycaemic index (GI), a key part of every athlete's nutritional tool box. Finally, it considers the current thinking on carbohydrate loading before a competition.

THE RELATIONSHIP BETWEEN MUSCLE GLYCOGEN AND PERFORMANCE

The importance of carbohydrates in relation to exercise performance was first demonstrated in 1939 by Christensen and Hansen, who found that a high carbohydrate diet significantly increased endurance (Christensen & Hansen, 1939). However, it wasn't until the 1960s that scientists discovered that the capacity for endurance exercise is related to pre-exercise glycogen stores and that a high-carbohydrate diet increases glycogen stores.

In a pioneering study, three groups of athletes were given a low carbohydrate diet, a high carbohydrate diet or moderate carbohydrate diet (Bergstrom et al., 1967). Researchers measured the concentration of glycogen in their leg muscles and found that those athletes eating the high-carbohydrate diet stored twice as much glycogen as those on the moderate carbohydrate diet and seven times as much as those eating the low carbohydrate diet. Afterwards, the athletes were instructed to cycle to exhaustion on a stationary bicycle at 75% of VO_2max. Those on the high-carbohydrate diet managed to cycle for 170 minutes, considerably longer than those on the moderate carbohydrate diet (115 minutes) or the low carbohydrate diet (60 minutes) (*see* Fig 3.1).

How much carbohydrate should I eat per day?

For most athletes, scientists recommend consuming a high-carbohydrate diet to replenish muscle glycogen stores and promote optimal adaptation to regular training. There is plentiful evidence that exercising with 'high carbohydrate availability' (i.e. high levels of glycogen and consumption of carbohydrate during exercise) enhances endurance and performance for exercise lasting longer than 90 minutes or intermittent high intensity exercise (Hargreaves *et al.*, 2004; Coyle, 2004; Burke *et al.*, 2004; ACSM/ADA/DC, 2016; Burke *et al.*, 2011).

This recommendation is based on the fact that carbohydrate availability is a limiting factor for endurance exercise since carbohydrate stores – as muscle and liver glycogen – are limited. Depletion of these stores ('low carbohydrate availability') results in fatigue and reduced perfor-

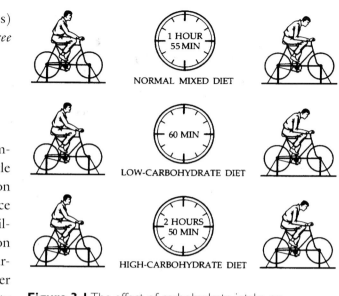

Figure 3.1 The effect of carbohydrate intake on performance

mance. This can easily happen if your pre-exercise glycogen stores are low. In order to get the most out of your training session when exercising for longer than 90 minutes or doing high intensity intermittent exercise, you should ensure your daily carbohydrate intake matches the fuel needs

Table 3.1	GUIDELINES FOR DAILY CARBOHYDRATE INTAKE
Activity level	**Recommended carbohydrate intake**
Very light training (low intensity or skill-based exercise)	3–5 g/kg BW daily
Moderate intensity training (approx 1 h daily)	5–7 g/kg BW daily
Moderate–high intensity training (1–3 h daily)	6–10 g/kg BW daily
Very high intensity training (> 4 h daily)	8–12 g/kg BW daily

Source: Burke et al., 2011.

of your training and that pre-exercise glycogen stores are high. This will help to improve your endurance, delay exhaustion and help you exercise longer and harder (Coyle, 1988; Costill & Hargreaves, 1992).

Previously, researchers recommended a diet providing 60–70% energy from carbohydrate based on the consensus statement from the International Conference on Foods, Nutrition & Performance in 1991 (Williams & Devlin, 1992).

However, this method is not very user-friendly and can be misleading, as it assumes an optimal energy (calorie) intake. It does not provide optimal carbohydrate for those with very high or low energy intakes. For example, for an athlete consuming 4000–5000 calories daily, 60% energy from carbohydrate (i.e. 600 g +) would exceed their glycogen storage capacity (Coyle, 1995). Conversely, for athletes consuming 2000 calories daily, a diet providing 60% energy from carbohydrate (i.e. 300 g) would not contain enough carbohydrate to maintain muscle glycogen stores.

Scientists recommend calculating your carbohydrate requirement from your body weight and also your training volume (Burke *et al.*, 2011; IOC, 2011; ACSM/AND/DC, 2016; IAAF, 2007; Burke *et al.*, 2004; Burke, 2001; Schokman, 1999), since your glycogen storage capacity is roughly proportional to your muscle mass and body weight – i.e. the heavier you are, the greater your muscle mass and the greater your glycogen storage capacity. The greater your training volume, the more carbohydrate you need to fuel your muscles. It is more flexible because it takes account of different training requirements and can be calculated independently of calorie intake.

Is a high carbohydrate diet practical?

For athletes with very high energy needs, eating a high carbohydrate diet can be difficult. Many carbohydrate-rich foods, such as bread, potatoes and pasta, are quite bulky and filling, particularly if wholegrain and high fibre foods make up most of your carbohydrate intake. Several surveys have found that endurance athletes often fail to consume the recommended carbohydrate levels (Frentsos & Baer, 1997). This may be partly due to the large number of calories needed and therefore the bulk of their diet, and partly due to lack of awareness of the benefits of a higher carbohydrate intake. It is interesting that most of the studies upon which the carbohydrate recommendations were made used liquid carbohydrates (i.e. drinks) to supplement meals. Tour de France cyclists and ultra-distance athletes, who require more than 5,000 calories a day, often consume up to one-third of their carbohydrate in liquid form. If you are finding a high carbohydrate diet impractical, try eating smaller, more frequent meals and supplementing your food with liquid forms of carbohydrate such as meal replacement products and carbohydrate drinks (see p. 155).

Table 3.1 indicates the amount of carbohydrate per kg of body weight needed per day according to your activity level (Burke, 2011). Most athletes training for up to 1 hour daily require about 5–7 g/kg body weight, but during periods of heavy training requirements may increase to 6–10 g/kg BW.

For example, for a 70 kg athlete who trains for 1 hour a day:

- Carbohydrate intake = 5–7 g/kg of body weight
- Daily carbohydrate intake = $(70 \times 5) - (70 \times 7) = 350$–490 g

Low carbohydrate diets and sports performance

Although it is generally accepted that optimal adaptation to repeated days of endurance training requires a high carbohydrate diet to replenish muscle glycogen stores, there is also much debate about the possible benefits of consuming a low carbohydrate, high fat (LCHF) diet.

The thinking behind this strategy is that since fat is a major fuel during prolonged endurance exercise, then training with low carbohydrate availability or 'training low' (i.e. with low muscle glycogen stores and no additional carbohydrate consumed during exercise) will enhance endurance training adaptations and 'train' the muscles to burn more fat during exercise, conserving precious glycogen and giving muscles greater access to a more plentiful supply of energy in the body. In other words, training low may improve your ability to burn fat for fuel and, ultimately, increase performance during endurance exercise lasting longer than 90 minutes.

This innovative approach to training is, of course, in contrast to the traditional advice that every training session should always be done with high carbohydrate availability (i.e. high glycogen levels and carbohydrates consumed during training).

WHAT ARE THE BENEFITS OF LOW CARBOHYDRATE DIETS?

A number of studies have considered whether a LCHF diet might enhance the muscles' ability to burn fat and, in turn, increase endurance capacity. One of the first of such studies was carried out in 1983 at the University of Connecticut (Phinney *et al.*, 1983). Here, researchers found that athletes who consumed an LCHF diet for 4 weeks managed to exercise for an average of 4 minutes longer before reaching exhaustion. However, this was a poor quality study and the average result is somewhat misleading. First, the study involved just five subjects (a very small number), two of whom experienced a significant *drop* in endurance. Two subjects had only a small increase but one subject had a large increase in time to exhaustion, thus skewing the overall study result. Second, exercise was performed at a relatively low intensity ($64\% \, VO_2 max$), not a race-level effort, which makes the findings irrelevant to the majority of competitive athletes.

Since then, a number of studies have shown that consuming an LCHF diet enhances the storage and burning of intramuscular fat as well as improving the ability of the muscles to take up fat from the bloodstream during exercise (Muoio *et al.*, 1994; Helge *et al.*, 2001; Lambert *et al.*, 1994).

Further studies have found that 'training low' enhances metabolic adaptations in muscles: increased levels of several enzymes involved in mitochondrial biogenesis (formation of new mitochondria), increased number of mitochondria and increased levels of fat-oxidising enzymes in the muscles (Bartlett *et al.*, 2015; Lane *et al.*, 2015; Hansen *et al.*, 2005; Yeo *et al.*, 2008; Hawley *et al.*, 2011). Thus, by training with low carbohydrate availability, training adaptations may be amplified and the muscles' ability to use fat as an energy source may be increased.

In 2005, Danish researchers measured increased endurance adaptation and performance in a group of novices when half of the training sessions were undertaken in a muscle glycogen depleted state (training twice per day, so the second session was glycogen depleted), compared with every session done in a glycogen loaded state (Hansen *et al.*, 2005). A 2008 study at RMIT University, Australia, found that

cyclists who performed some of their sessions with low glycogen availability had higher levels of fat-burning mitochondrial enzymes (Yeo *et al.*, 2008). And a 2010 study at the University of Birmingham found that fat oxidation during steady-state cycling was higher in cyclists when they 'trained low' than when they trained with high glycogen levels (Hulston et al, 2010).

Perhaps one of the easiest ways to 'train low' is to perform a sub-maximal workout first thing in the morning following an overnight fast. Belgian researchers found that this protocol resulted in higher levels of fat oxidising enzymes in cyclists compared with non-fasted training (i.e. with high carbohydrate availability) (Van Proeyen *et al.*, 2011).

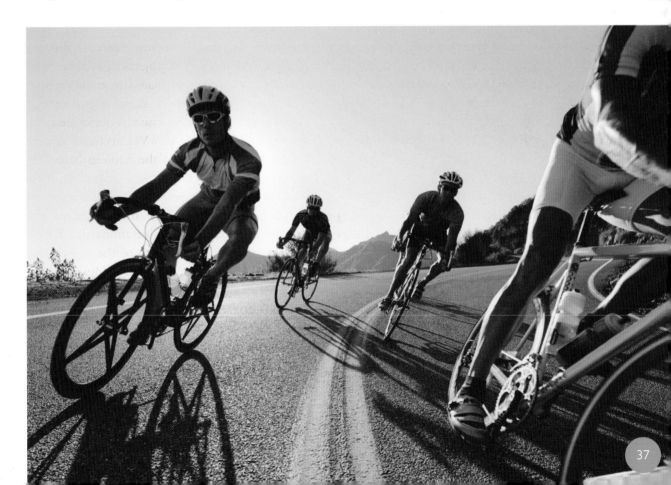

More recently, a 2015 study by Australian, Swedish and Malaysian researchers found that cyclists who did a fasted 2-hour low intensity workout in the morning following a high intensity workout the previous evening ('trained high, slept low', *see* opposite) had lower muscle glycogen and increased transcription for metabolically adaptive genes than those who performed the same workouts with high glycogen stores (Lane *et al.*, 2015). In other words, periodically training with low carbohydrate stores might have some benefits in terms of stimulating greater training adaptations.

However, despite increases in markers of muscle adaptation, there was no improvement in performance. In the cycling studies, 'training low' hampered the cyclists' ability to do high intensity training: their power output was significantly lower. This is clearly a disadvantage for competitive athletes.

Interestingly, these effects are observed only

'Training low' in a nutshell

Restricting carbohydrate intake and training in a glycogen-depleted state, i.e. 'training low', changes your overall resting fuel metabolism and patterns of fuel utilisation during exercise. It triggers acute regulatory processes underlying enzyme and gene expression, which regulate the adaptive response to exercise. This results in increased maximal mitochondrial enzyme activities, increased mitochondrial content, an increased capacity to oxidise fat and a reduced reliance on glucose as a preferred substrate.

in elite or well-conditioned athletes – and the performance advantage suggested in some of the studies only applies at relatively low exercise intensities below about 65% of VO_2max, i.e. moderate, conversational pace. At higher exercise intensities, carbohydrate becomes the principal fuel source. This is sometimes referred to as the 'crossover point' – that intensity at which you start to burn more carbohydrate than fat. Therefore, for less conditioned athletes or untrained individuals, or those exercising above 65% VO_2max, chronically training on an LCHF diet would have no performance advantage (Burke *et al.*, 2004).

Nevertheless, there are a few scenarios where LCHF diets may benefit performance or at least not be detrimental. LCHF diets may suit those who do mostly low to moderate intensity training (such as ultra-endurance runners), as well as those wanting to lose weight or athletes with type 2 diabetes or insulin resistance (when your cells are less sensitive to insulin so cannot process carbohydrate into fuel efficiently). Some studies suggest that LCHF diets may promote greater weight loss than conventional low fat diets, but the consensus of evidence from large-scale meta-analyses suggests that they are no more effective in reducing body weight and insulin resistance (Pagoto & Appelhans, 2013; Hu *et al.*, 2012; Johnston *et al.*, 2006). What matters most when it comes to weight loss is achieving a calorie deficit and then being able to sustain the diet long term.

DO LOW CARBOHYDRATE DIETS IMPROVE PERFORMANCE?

Despite increasing the muscles' ability to use fat as an energy source, there is no clear evidence

'Train low' protocols

There are a number of ways to 'train low'. These include:

A chronically low carbohydrate diet

This involves consuming a low carbohydrate diet (i.e. less carbohydrate than you need for fuelling training) and 'training low' for all training sessions. This method may improve fat adaptation but will result in a reduced capacity for high intensity exercise. It may also reduce immune function and increase the risk of illness.

Training after an overnight fast

This is perhaps the most popular 'train low' protocol and the easiest to adopt. Training is performed in the morning before breakfast following an overnight fast and without consuming carbohydrate during the workout (Van Proeyen et al., 2011).

Train high, sleep low

A high intensity training session is performed in the evening to deplete muscle glycogen, followed by an overnight fast so muscle glycogen stores are not replenished. The next morning a light training session is carried out on an empty stomach (i.e. 'train low'). After this, glycogen stores are replenished by consuming normal meals for the rest of the day. Thus, high intensity sessions are done with high carbohydrate availability and low intensity sessions are done with low carbohydrate availability (Lane et al., 2015).

Training twice a day

When training twice a day, the first (high intensity) session is performed with high carbohydrate availability and the second (low intensity) with low carbohydrate availability (Yeo et al., 2008). This is achieved by limiting carbohydrate consumption after the first session and then consuming a high carbohydrate meal after the second session.

Prolonged training without consuming carbohydrate

During a long training session lasting more than 90 minutes, no carbohydrate is consumed. This means the latter stages of the session will be performed with low muscle glycogen stores (Morton et al., 2009).

No carbohydrate during recovery

By avoiding carbohydrate for 1–2 hours after exercise, it may be possible to achieve greater training adaptations (Pilegaard et al., 2005). However, post-exercise recovery may take longer.

to date that chronically eating an LCHF diet or training with low carbohydrate availability spares glycogen, improves training capacity or enhances performance (Hawley & Leckey, 2015; Maughan & Shirreffs, 2012; Hawley *et al.*, 2011; Morton *et al.*, 2009). Quite the opposite: a comprehensive analysis of studies concluded that chronically training with low glycogen stores can hamper the muscles' ability to store and use carbohydrate during high intensity exercise (Burke, 2010).

In a landmark study at the University of Guelph, Canada, researchers found that cyclists who consumed an LCHF diet for 5 days followed by 1 day of high carbohydrate diet were better able to utilise fat for fuel during aerobic exercise (they burned 45% more fat and 30% less carbohydrate during a 20-minute ride at 70% VO_2max) but they had a reduced ability to use carbohydrate for fuel during a high intensity time trial even though they had full glycogen stores prior to the trial (Stellingwerff *et al.*, 2006). The researchers concluded that an LCHF diet results in down-regulation of carbohydrate-burning enzymes. This is clearly a disadvantage for many athletes since most competitive events involve high intensity efforts, sprints or tactical changes in pace.

An analysis of 20 studies by researchers at Kansas State University, US, concluded that LCHF diets provide no performance advantage for non-elite athletes but all athletes (especially non-elite) benefited from a high carbohydrate diet (Erlenbusch *et al.*, 2005).

Numerous studies have demonstrated that carbohydrates, not fats, are the main fuel used for high intensity endurance exercise and that carbohydrate availability is a limiting factor for performance (Hawley & Leckey, 2015). In a joint Australian and UK study, runners consumed a pre-exercise meal with different nutritional values prior to a treadmill run at 95% of their half-marathon pace (Leckey *et al.*, 2016). Participants in trials one and two were fed carbohydrates in the form of jelly. Participants in trials three and four fasted overnight and were given a calorie-free placebo jelly. In order to test whether blocking the use of fat as fuel hampered run performance, participants in trials two and four were given nicotinic acid, which prevented the use of fat stores during the test runs. The study found that there was no difference in running distance (20–21 km) or time to exhaustion (approx. 85 min) between the four trials, which suggests that even when you suppress lipolysis (fat breakdown) you do not hamper exercise capacity. In other words, carbohydrate is the primary fuel (83–91%) used during high intensity exercise (approx. 80% VO_2max) and fat plays only a minimal role.

What are the drawbacks of low carbohydrate diets?

The main drawback of training with low glycogen stores is that it reduces your capacity for high intensity exercise, exercise feels harder, and power output and speed drop. You simply cannot train so hard. Athletes training in a glycogen depleted state tend to choose a lower workload or intensity because the exercise feels harder.

A study at the University of Cape Town found that an LCHF diet resulted in impaired performance during the sprint stages of a 100 km cycling time trial (Havemann *et al.*, 2006). Cyclists who consumed an LCHF diet for 6 days followed by 1 day of carbohydrate loading were not able to generate as much power during the sprint stages of a 100 km time trial compared with those cyclists who consumed a high carbohydrate diet for 7 days. Similarly, a study at the University of Birmingham, UK, with well-trained cyclists found that there was no difference in 1-hour time trial performance between those training low and those training with high carbohydrate availability (Hulston *et al.*, 2010). However, power output during high intensity interval training was significantly lower in those training low. More recently, a study with competitive mountain bikers found those who followed an LCHF diet experienced a drop in power and performance at high exercise intensities (Zajac *et al.*, 2014).

Another disadvantage of repeatedly 'training low' is the risk of illness, injury and over-reaching (short-term overtraining). The main symptoms of over-reaching are decreased performance, high fatigue rating at rest and during exercise, and altered mood state. A study at the University of Birmingham, UK, found that when runners consumed a high carbohydrate diet (8.5 g/kg/day) they performed better, experienced less fatigue and maintained a better mood state (i.e. showed fewer symptoms of over-reaching) than training on a 'normal' carbohydrate diet (5.4 g/kg/day) during an 11-day period of intense

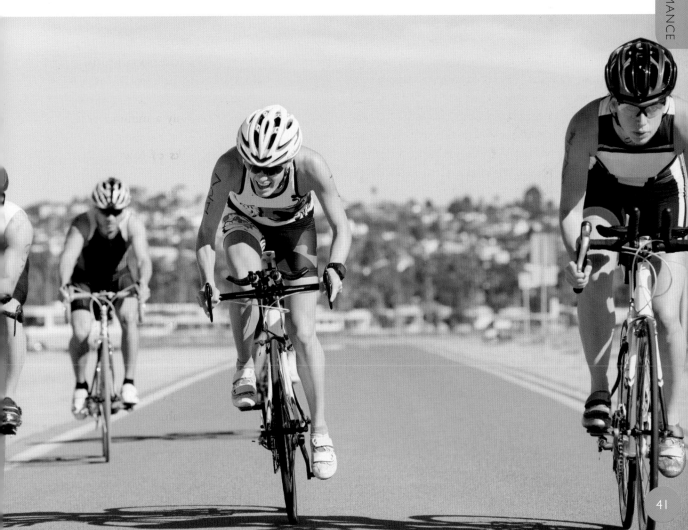

training (Achten *et al.*, 2004). All athletes experienced a drop in performance with successive days of hard training but those on the high carbohydrate diet fared significantly better. It is difficult to see how the athletes could have coped with the training load on a low carbohydrate diet. The authors speculate that the training quality would have decreased further because even a normal carbohydrate intake resulted in a bigger performance drop.

You can partially overcome the reduction in exercise capacity by consuming caffeine (1–3 mg/kg body weight, equivalent to 70–210 mg for a 70 kg athlete) before or during exercise. In one study, glycogen depleted cyclists who consumed caffeine prior to a 4 km cycling time trial performed better than those who did not consume caffeine but the same as those who were not glycogen depleted (Silva-Cavalcante *et al.*, 2013). Australian researchers also showed that caffeine consumed 1 hour before a high intensity interval training session improved power output in glycogen depleted cyclists (Lane *et al.*, 2013). However, power output was still lower than when they performed the same training session with normal glycogen stores. Caffeine is known to reduce perceived exertion and fatigue during exercise (*see* p. 117).

Alternatively, you can practise 'carbohydrate mouth-rinsing' (*see* p. 61) during your training session to help you maintain your training intensity (or at least avoid too big a reduction) and prevent muscle protein breakdown (Bartlett *et al.*, 2015). Carbohydrate mouth-rinsing (swilling a carbohydrate drink around your mouth before spitting it out) acts on the central nervous system (brain) to mask fatigue and reduce perceived exertion, thus allowing

Train low, compete high?

The concept of 'training low but competing high' has become very popular among elite athletes. The strategy involves training with low carbohydrate availability followed by a high carbohydrate diet prior to competition (Hawley & Burke, 2010). The idea is that 'training low' forces the muscles to adapt to using fat as a fuel instead of carbohydrate and increases muscle adaptation to training, while competing with high carbohydrate availability should provide a performance advantage during competition lasting more than 90 minutes. However, research has shown that long-term fuelling from fat can actually impair the body's ability to use glycogen and studies have failed to show any significant performance advantage to date. For most events, carbohydrate is the preferred fuel.

you to keep going longer. Rinsing and spitting stimulates oral sensors that tell the brain that carbohydrates are on the way. While it may be more beneficial to swallow the drink and thus make use of the calories it contains, it's a useful strategy for those athletes who want to 'train low' or who struggle to keep anything down during high intensity exercise. Combining the two methods will give you bigger performance benefits. A 2015 study at Liverpool John Moores University found that athletes who 'trained low' with a carbohydrate mouth rinse plus caffeine during a high intensity interval set were able to keep going 13 minutes longer than those who just had a mouth rinse but not caffeine, and

29 minutes longer than those who did neither (placebo) (Kasper *et al.*, 2015).

Exactly why training low does not translate into performance benefits is not known but researchers suggest this may be because studies have been too short to measure an improvement, that performance is not linked to the markers that have been measured, or that researchers have been unable to measure performance well enough to detect changes that would be significant in real-life competitive events (Burke, 2010). It is also possible that the drawbacks of 'training low' (namely, a reduction in the volume and intensity of training) counteracts the potential benefits (Hawley & Burke, 2010). In other words, instead of being glycogen sparing, 'training low' may in fact be glycogen impairing (Stellingwerff *et al.*, 2006).

It's worth noting that the world's top endurance athletes from Kenya and Ethiopia consume a high carbohydrate diet containing 9–10 g/kg, well within current ISSN and ACSM recommendations and contrary to the LCHF diet principles (Onywera *et al.*, 2004; Beis *et al.*, 2011).

Carbohydrate periodisation

Research in this area is ongoing and some elite athletes are experimenting with a newer strategy called 'carbohydrate periodisation', which involves strategically planning short periods of 'training low' into their training programme.

Many endurance athletes follow a periodised programme of training and it makes sense to adjust carbohydrate intake to reflect the different training demands of each training cycle. Incorporating 'training low' protocols is most suitable during lower intensity sessions or at the beginning of a training cycle. Conversely, 'quality' sessions, done at higher intensities or later in the training cycle when an athlete is preparing to peak for competition, are best undertaken with high carbohydrate availability.

Essentially, low intensity sessions are performed with low glycogen stores, and high intensity sessions with high glycogen stores. The idea is that matching your carbohydrate intake to your training sessions improves 'metabolic flexibility', i.e. your muscles' ability to switch between burning fat and carbohydrate, as well as your body composition and performance. The advantage of this approach is that you get the dual benefits of 'training low' – namely fat adaptation – as well as the performance benefits of high intensity training.

The **downside** to training low, though, is that high intensity exercise feels much harder. As mentioned previously, athletes find that they cannot maintain a high power as long as usual. You can get around this, at least partly, by taking caffeine before and during your 'train low' sessions and/or practising carbohydrate mouth-rinsing during your session (*see* p. 42).

The exact balance between training low and training high depends on many factors, including training goals, frequency and intensity of training, lifestyle and individual make-up. Clearly, everyone responds differently to diet and training regimes and there is no single approach that suits everyone. However, by incorporating both glycogen depleted and glycogen loaded training sessions in your programme, you can improve your fuel efficiency.

WHAT IS THE EVIDENCE FOR CARBOHYDRATE PERIODISATION?

This method looks more promising in terms of performance improvement. A multicentre study by French, Australian and UK researchers found that triathletes who employed a carbohydrate periodisation strategy (doing high intensity evening sessions with high carbohydrate availability, and low intensity fasted morning sessions with low carbohydrate availability: 'train high, sleep low') for 3 weeks improved their cycling efficiency (power output per calorie) by 11%, 10 km running performance by 2.9%, time to exhaustion during high intensity exercise by 12.5%, and also cut their body fat (1%) compared with those who did all their training with high carbohydrate availability (Marquet *et al.*, 2016). A follow-up study with cyclists by the same team found that using a 'sleeping low' strategy for just six days resulted in a 3.2 per cent improvement in a 20 km time trial.

More recently, a study at the Australian Institute of Sport compared the performance effects of a high-carbohydrate diet (60–65% carbohydrate), a periodised carbohydrate diet (same macronutrients but periodised within or between days) and a LCHF diet (<50g carbohydrate) in a group of 21 elite race-walkers. After 3 weeks on each diet, all athletes improved their aerobic fitness (VO2 max) but only those on the high carbohydrate or periodised carbohydrate diet improved their 10 km race performance. The athletes on the LCHF diet did not make any improvement. Although they were burning a higher proportion of fat during exercise, their muscles became less efficient at producing energy, requiring more oxygen at any given speed.

These results suggest that periodisation of carbohydrate around selected training sessions (i.e. doing your low intensity sessions with low carbohydrate availability) can not only lead to favourable enhanced metabolic adaptations but can also result in improved performance and body composition.

HOW DO YOU PERIODISE YOUR CARBOHYDRATE INTAKE?

'Periodisation' in simple terms means splitting your training year into 'cycles' of shorter, more manageable chunks, where you work on specific elements of fitness (e.g. aerobic endurance, speed, strength, power) before moving on to the next 'cycle'. The longest cycle is called a macrocycle and usually spans a year. The year is then broken down into 2–6 shorter training cycles – mesocycles – each spanning several weeks. Each mesocycle emphasises a particular training goal, such as aerobic endurance, strength or speed, and involves a gradual increase in intensity. Each mesocycle is then divided into week-long microcycles, around which you plan your day-to-day training sessions.

Base training phase

This is when you do your longer, low intensity rides. The goal of this phase is to build endurance fitness and develop metabolic flexibility. You won't need as much carbohydrate as in your subsequent 'build' phase so this is the training phase when you can 'train low' in some of your sessions. Also, if you need to achieve body composition goals (drop body fat or increase muscle), then this is the time to do it.

There are a number of different ways you can 'train low'. You may choose to eat a low carbohydrate, high fat diet full time, which means you'll be training low for all sessions. This method may improve fat adaptation but the downside is that you'll struggle with high intensity sessions. At exercise intensities above about 65% VO_2max, carbohydrate becomes the principal fuel source. Low carbohydrate eating alongside a heavy training schedule may also reduce immune function and increase the risk of illness.

The most practical protocol is to train after an overnight fast and before breakfast. However, this should be a low intensity session. Alternatively, if you want to train low in the evening, cut carbohydrates at lunchtime (keeping to mainly high protein foods and vegetables) and then eat carbohydrates after your evening session and also at breakfast.

Some cyclists use a 'train high, sleep low' protocol. A high intensity training session is performed in the evening to deplete muscle glycogen, followed by an overnight fast so muscle glycogen stores are not replenished. The next morning, a light training session is carried out on an empty stomach (i.e. 'train low'). After this, glycogen stores are replenished by consuming normal meals for the rest of the day. Thus, high intensity sessions are done with high carbohydrate availability and low intensity sessions are done with low carbohydrate availability.

Alternatively, when training twice a day, you can do your first (high intensity) session with high carbohydrate availability (i.e. high glycogen levels and consuming carbohydrates during training) and the second (low intensity) session with low carbohydrate availability. Cut carbohydrates after the first session and then eat a high carbohydrate meal after the second session.

Build (pre-competition) phase

This is where the intensity ramps up and you switch from long aerobic rides to shorter, harder

Sample diet plan for a microcycle

This sample diet shows you how to tailor your eating to your training sessions in a 48-hour period.

Day 1 (high intensity training session)
Breakfast: Porridge, bananas, honey
Snack: Fruit, nuts
Lunch: Rice, chicken, vegetables
Snack: Fruit, toast, honey
Evening training (high intensity intervals): Sports drink, bananas, gels or dried fruit
Post-training: Protein drink
Dinner: Grilled fish, salad

Day 2 (low intensity session)
Breakfast (optional): Eggs
Morning training (long, low intensity ride): Water
Post-training: Carbohydrate and protein recovery drink
Snack: Toast, honey, yoghurt, fruit
Lunch: Pasta, fish, salad
Snack: Fruit, nuts, granola bar
Dinner: Sweet potato, chicken, vegetables

sessions, usually targeting speed and power. As carbohydrates are the main fuel for high intensity exercise, make sure you're well fuelled up with carbohydrates before important training sessions. You'll need to eat bigger portions of porridge, pasta and potatoes and add sugars (like bananas, dried fruit, sports drinks, energy bars and gels) before, during and immediately after your session. A lack of carbohydrates before tackling a big hill or a sprint interval session means you won't be able to generate the power and speed you want. However, you can still include a few 'train low' sessions in your microcycle (*see* p. 45). Essentially, this phase is all about having enough energy to get the most out of your training.

Competition phase

In the lead-up to an important race, there's usually a taper period where you do less volume and more short, higher intensity sessions. You'll be burning fewer calories overall so you'll need to adjust your food intake if you want to avoid weight gain. If you'll be racing for longer than 90 minutes, you'll probably benefit from some form of carbohydrate loading, which involves upping carbohydrates (10–12 g/kg/day) and cutting fat for the last 36–48 hours before the race. On race days, carbohydrate is the most important fuel and numerous studies have shown that performance is significantly improved when you consume carbohydrates during high intensity exercise. Carbohydrates are also periodised during multi-stage races such as the Tour de France; riders consume more carbohydrate during long, hard stages than during the less intense stages. They also consume more carbohydrate post-race to refuel properly before the next stage.

Rest/off-season

When racing is over and you're taking a well-earned rest from training, periodisation is still important. You'll be burning considerably fewer calories so you'll need to adjust carbohydrates (as well as keeping a check on fat and alcohol) if you want to avoid excessive weight gain. Some coaches advise gaining no more than 5–8% of your competition weight during the off-season.

Nutrition for the microcycle

In any training week, there will be harder and easier sessions so your nutrition intake should reflect this. By eating an appropriate amount of carbohydrates before high intensity sessions you'll be able to train harder and maximise your performance in those sessions. Conversely, rest days and lighter sessions won't require the same intake, so you can reduce carbohydrates and total calories on these days. This is especially useful if you're trying to drop a few pounds while still having enough energy to train on harder days.

Training and immunity

During periods of intense training or immediately following endurance race events, many athletes find that they become more susceptible to minor respiratory illness, such as colds and sore throats. While moderate training boosts your immune system, intense training over a prolonged period appears to depress immune cell functions. Such changes create an 'open window' of decreased protection, during which viruses and bacteria can gain a foothold, increasing the risk of developing an infection. It is thought that the increased levels of stress hormones, such as adrenaline and cortisol, associated with intense exercise, inhibit the immune system. Other factors such as stress, lack of sleep and poor nutrition can also depress immunity.

A healthy diet that meets your energy needs and provides adequate micronutrients required for immune cell function (iron, zinc, magnesium, manganese, vitamins A, C, D, E, B_6, B_{12} and folic acid) is important for maintaining immune defences. Even short-term dieting during periods of hard training can result in a loss of immune function and make you more prone to infections.

Here are some practical ways of combating exercise-related suppression of immunity:

- Match your calorie intake and expenditure – under-eating will increase cortisol levels.
- Ensure you're consuming plenty of foods rich in immunity-boosting nutrients – vitamins A, C and E, vitamin B_6, zinc, iron and magnesium. Best sources are fresh fruit, vegetables, whole grains, beans, lentils, nuts and seeds.
- Avoid low carbohydrate diets. Low glycogen stores are associated with bigger increases in cortisol levels and bigger suppression of your immune cells.
- Consume a sports drink (approximately 6 g carbohydrate/100 ml, providing 30–60 g

What is 'metabolic efficiency'?

The concept of metabolic efficiency (ME) was first coined by sports dietitian and exercise physiologist Bob Seebohar (Seebohar, 2014), and refers to the body's ability to utilise its carbohydrate and fat stores at different exercise intensities. The theory is that by improving your ME, you should be able to preserve your limited glycogen stores, and increase your fat-burning capacity. ME training focuses on low intensity aerobic training, often incorporating strategic 'train low' sessions (see p. 39), and a 'moderate' carbohydrate intake. It is a popular training method among endurance and ultra-endurance athletes for improving performance as well as body composition (fat loss). As no carbohydrates are consumed during training, it may be also be suitable for athletes who are prone to gastrointestinal problems during races (see p. 285) and struggle to take on board carbohydrates.

For athletes following a periodised training programme, ME training is best done during the base training phase when you are doing mostly low intensity aerobic exercise and minimal high intensity training. Adaptation typically takes 4 to 10 weeks. The main nutrition strategy is outlined below.

Blood glucose control

This can be achieved by eating low GI meals – a balanced combination of carbohydrate, protein and fat, with a focus on high fibre foods (such as whole grains, fruit and vegetables). Seebohar advises 'moderate' rather than low intakes of carbohydrate and periodising carbohydrate intake to match the fuel needs for exercise.

Nutrient timing

Seebohar recommends a low GI meal 2–4 hours before long, low intensity sessions, and avoiding consuming additional carbohydrates (such as sports drinks, bars, gels and dried fruit) during (low intensity) training sessions. You may refuel with a meal or snack comprising protein and carbohydrate.

carbohydrate per hour) during intense exercise lasting longer than 1 hour. This can reduce stress hormone levels and the associated drop in immunity following exercise (Bishop, 2002).

- Drink plenty of fluid. This increases your saliva production, which contains antibacterial proteins that can fight off airborne germs.

- A modest antioxidant supplement or a vitamin C supplement may help to reduce the risk of upper respiratory tract infection during periods of intense training (Gleeson, 2011). In one study of ultra-marathon runners, those who took daily vitamin C supplements (1500 mg) 7 days prior to a race had lower levels of stress hormones following the race, which suggests greater protection against infection (Peters *et al.*, 2001).

- Glutamine supplements may reduce the risk of infections. Glutamine levels can fall by up to 20% following intense exercise (Antonio, 1999), putting the immune system under greater strain.

- Echinacea taken for up to 4 weeks during a period of hard training may boost immunity and reduce the risk of catching a cold by stimulating the body's own production of immune cells (Karsch–Völk et al, 2014).

- Quercetin supplements (1000 mg/day) taken during periods of intense training may reduce the risk of upper respiratory illness (Nieman *et al.*, 2007).

- Probiotic supplements may help reduce the severity and duration of respiratory illness and benefit immunity (Gleeson, 2008).

- Sucking zinc acetate lozenges regularly throughout the day (equivalent to a daily dose of >75mg zinc) has been shown to reduce the duration of the common cold by 44% (Hermila, 2011). However, there is no evidence for taking zinc tablets.

Which carbohydrates are best?

Carbohydrates are traditionally classified according to their chemical structure. The most simplistic method divides them into two categories: *simple* (sugars) and *complex* (starches and fibres). These terms simply refer to the number of sugar units in the molecule.

Simple carbohydrates are very small molecules consisting of 1 or 2 sugar units. They comprise the *monosaccharides* (1-sugar units): glucose (dextrose), fructose (fruit sugar) and galactose; and the *disaccharides* (2-sugar units): sucrose (table sugar, which comprises a glucose and fructose molecule joined together) and lactose (milk sugar, which comprises a glucose and galactose molecule joined together).

Complex carbohydrates are much larger molecules, consisting of between usually hundreds or thousands of sugar units (mostly glucose) joined together. They include the starches, amylose and amylopectin, and the non-starch polysaccharides (dietary fibre), such as cellulose, pectin and hemicellulose.

In between simple and complex carbohydrates are glucose polymers and maltodextrin, which comprise between 3- and 10-sugar units. They are made from the partial breakdown of corn starch in food processing, and are widely used as bulking and thickening agents in processed foods, such as sauces, dairy desserts, baby food, puddings and soft drinks. They are popular ingredients in sports drinks and engineered meal-replacement products, owing to their low sweetness and high energy density relative to sucrose.

In practice, many foods contain a mixture of both simple and complex carbohydrates, making the traditional classification of foods into 'simple' and 'complex' very confusing. For example, biscuits and cakes contain flour (complex) and sugar (simple), and bananas contain a mixture of sugars and starches depending on their degree of ripeness.

IS SUGAR HARMFUL FOR ATHLETES?

Sugar is a carbohydrate, which means it is an energy source for the body. Despite the negative press surrounding it, small amounts of sugar are unlikely to cause harm and, provided you time your sugar intake around exercise, it may even aid your performance. During high intensity exercise lasting longer than an hour, consuming sugar either in the form of solid food (e.g. bananas, dried fruit, gels or energy bars) or drinks can help maintain blood glucose concentration, spare glycogen and increase endurance. Sugar may also be beneficial for promoting rapid glycogen refuelling during the 2-hour period after prolonged intense exercise.

However, one of the main problems with sugar is its ability to cause dental caries. Studies have shown that athletes who consume lots of sports drinks, bars and gels experience significant tooth decay and erosion (Needleman *et al.*, 2015). These products are high in sugar and as they are usually consumed at frequent intervals during exercise, they are particularly damaging to the teeth.

Another problem with sugar is that it has no real nutritional value (apart from providing energy). It makes food and drink more palatable and therefore easy to over-consume. Although sugar is not uniquely fattening, it can contribute towards an over-consumption of calories, especially when combined with lots of fat in the form of cakes, chocolates, biscuits and snacks. Rather than satisfy hunger, sugar can sometimes make us want to eat more! Although high intakes have been linked with obesity and type 2 diabetes, the main contributor to these diseases is excess calories rather than sugar itself.

Some scientists believe that high sugar intakes can result in insulin resistance, where the body cells become less responsive to insulin (the hormone responsible for shunting glucose from the bloodstream to the muscles) and more prone to store fat. However, regular exercise blunts the negative effects of sugar, which means the body produces less insulin after consuming sugar. This is one of the many ways the body adapts to exercise: it becomes more sensitive to insulin (Hawley

How much sugar?

There is no specific recommendation for sugar for athletes. The Scientific Advisory Committee on Nutrition (SACN) in the UK recommends a maximum of 5% daily calories from 'free' (added) sugars for the general population, which equates to about 25 g for the average person consuming 2000 calories a day (SACN, 2015). 'Free sugars' has superseded the term 'added sugars', and is used to describe the sugars added to foods plus those naturally present in honey, syrups and fruit juices. It excludes sugars in milk and sugars contained within the cellular structure of foods such as fruit and vegetables. Current average intakes are 68 g for males and 49 g for females aged 19–64 (Bates *et al.*, 2014). The recommendation is designed to reduce the risk of obesity and improve dental health.

& Lessard, 2008). In other words, you need less insulin to do the same job and your body learns to handle sugar more efficiently.

Much of the negative health effect of sugar is thought to be due to fructose (which makes up half of the sucrose molecule). High fructose intakes can increase blood triglycerides (fats), which increase cardiovascular disease risk. However, doing regular exercise prevents this because the body increases its production of lipoprotein lipase, an enzyme that removes fats circulating in the blood and converts them into energy (Seip & Semenkovich, 1998). In a study at the University of Lausanne, Switzerland, when volunteers consumed a high fructose diet (30% fructose) their blood fats concentration increased but when they combined this diet with moderate aerobic exercise there was no increase in blood fat concentration (Egli *et al.*, 2013). In other words, exercise prevents the rise in blood fats caused by a high fructose intake.

On balance, athletes don't need to worry unduly about sugar as it does not have the same effect on blood insulin and blood fats as it does in sedentary people. It may improve endurance during prolonged high intensity exercise although it would be prudent to mitigate damage to the teeth by, for example, directing sports drinks to the back of the mouth, rather than swishing around the mouth, and rinsing with water afterwards.

NOT ALL CARBOHYDRATES ARE EQUAL

It's tempting to think that simple carbohydrates, due to their smaller molecular size, are absorbed more quickly than complex carbohydrates, and produce a large and rapid rise in blood sugar.

Unfortunately, it's not that straightforward. For example, apples (containing simple carbohydrates) produce a small and prolonged rise in blood sugar, despite being high in simple carbohydrates. Many starchy foods (complex carbohydrates), such as potatoes and bread, are digested and absorbed very quickly and give a rapid rise in blood sugar. So the old notion about simple carbohydrates giving fast-released energy and complex carbohydrates giving slow-released energy is incorrect and misleading.

What is more important as far as sports performance is concerned is how rapidly the carbohydrate is absorbed from the small intestine into your bloodstream. The faster this transfer, the more rapidly the carbohydrate can be taken up by muscle cells (or other cells of the body) and make a difference to your training and recovery.

The glycaemic index

To describe more accurately the effect different foods have on your blood sugar levels, scientists developed the glycaemic index (GI). While the GI concept was originally developed to help diabetics control their blood sugar levels, it can benefit regular exercisers and athletes too. It is a ranking of foods from 0 to 100 based on their immediate effect on blood sugar levels, a measure of the speed at which you digest food and convert it into glucose. The faster the rise in blood glucose, the higher the rating on the index. To make a fair comparison, all foods are compared with a reference food, such as glucose, and are tested in equivalent carbohydrate amounts. The GI of foods is very useful to know because it tells you how the body responds to them. If you need to get carbohydrates into your bloodstream and muscle cells rapidly – for example, immediately after exercise to kick-start glycogen replenishment – you would choose high GI foods. In 1997 the World Health Organization (WHO) and Food and Agriculture Organization (FOA) of the United Nations endorsed the use of the GI for classifying foods, and recommended that GI values should be used to guide people's food choices.

HOW IS THE GI WORKED OUT?

The GI value of food is measured by feeding 10 or more healthy people a portion of food containing 50 g carbohydrate. For example, to test baked potatoes, you would eat 250 g potatoes, which contain 50 g of carbohydrate. Over the next 2 hours, a sample of blood is taken every 15 minutes and the blood sugar level measured. The blood sugar level is plotted on a graph and the area under the curve calculated using a computer program (*see* Fig. 3.2). On another occasion, the same 10 people consume a 50 g portion of glucose (the reference food). Their response to the test food (e.g. potato) is compared with their blood sugar response to 50 g glucose (the reference food). The GI is given as a percentage,

which is calculated by dividing the area under the curve after you've eaten potatoes by the area under the curve after you've eaten the glucose. The final GI value for the test food is the average GI value for the 10 people. So, the GI of baked potatoes is 85, which means that eating baked potato produces a rise in blood sugar that is 85% as great as that produced after eating an equivalent amount of glucose.

Appendix 1 ('The glycaemic index and glycaemic load) gives the GI content of many popular foods. Most values lie somewhere between 20 and 100. Sports nutritionists find it useful to classify foods as *high GI* (71–100), *medium GI* (56–70) and *low GI* (0–55). This simply makes it easier to select the appropriate food before, during and after exercise. In a nutshell, the higher the GI, the higher the blood sugar levels after eating that food. In general, refined starchy foods, including potatoes, white rice and white bread, as well as sugary foods, such as soft drinks and biscuits, are high on the glycaemic index. For example, baked potatoes (GI 85) and white rice (GI 87) produce a rise in blood sugar almost the same as eating pure glucose (yes, you read correctly!). Less refined starchy foods – porridge, beans, lentils, muesli – as well as fruit and dairy products are lower on the glycaemic index. They produce a much smaller rise in blood sugar compared with glucose.

Only a few centres around the world provide a legitimate GI testing service. The Human Nutrition Unit at the University of Sydney in Australia has been at the forefront of GI research for over two decades, and has measured the GI of hundreds of foods. International Tables of Glycaemic Index have been published by the American Journal of Clinical Nutrition (Foster-

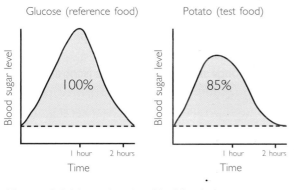

Figure 3.2 Measuring the GI of food

Powell and Brand-Miller, 1995; Foster-Powell *et al.*, 2002). But new and revised data are constantly being added to the list as commercial foods are reformulated and these are available on the website www.glycemicindex.com (note the US spelling of this website – not to be confused with www.glycaemicindex.com).

Table 3.2	FACTORS THAT INFLUENCE THE GI OF A FOOD	
Factor	**How it works**	**Examples of foods**
Particle size	Processing reduces particle size and makes it easier for digestive enzymes to access the starch. The smaller the particle size (i.e. the more processed the food), the higher the GI.	Most breakfast cereals, e.g. cornflakes and rice crispies, have a higher GI than muesli or porridge.
Degree of starch gelatinisation	The more gelatinised (swollen with water) the starch, the greater the surface area for enzymes to attack, the faster the digestion and rise in blood sugar, i.e. higher GI.	Cooked potatoes (high GI); biscuits (lower GI).
Amylose to amylopectin ratio	There are two types of starch: amylose (long straight molecule, difficult access by enzymes) and amylopectin (branched molecule, easier access by enzymes). The more amylose a food contains the slower it is digested, i.e. lower GI.	Beans, lentils, peas and basmati rice have high amylose content, i.e. low GI; wheat flour and products containing it have high amylopectin content, i.e. high GI.
Fat	Fat slows down rate of stomach emptying, slowing down digestion and lowering GI.	Potato crisps have a lower GI than plain boiled potatoes; adding butter or cheese to bread lowers GI.
Sugar (sucrose)	Sucrose is broken down into one molecule of fructose and one molecule of glucose. Fructose is converted into glucose in the liver slowly, giving a smaller rise in blood sugar.	Sweet biscuits, cakes, sweet breakfast cereals, honey.
Soluble fibre	Soluble fibre increases viscosity of food in the digestive tract and slows digestion, producing a lower blood sugar rise, i.e. lowers GI.	Beans, lentils, peas, oats, porridge, barley, fruit.
Protein	Protein slows stomach emptying and therefore carbohydrate digestion, producing a smaller blood sugar rise, i.e. lowers GI.	Beans, lentils, peas, pasta (all contain protein as well as carbohydrate). Eating chicken with rice lowers the GI of the rice.

WHAT MAKES ONE FOOD HAVE A HIGH GI AND ANOTHER FOOD A LOW GI?

Factors that influence the GI of a food include the size of the food particle, the biochemical make-up of the carbohydrate (the ratio of amylose to amylopectin), the degree of cooking (which affects starch gelatinisation), and the presence of fat, sugar, protein and fibre. How these factors influence the GI of a food is summarised in Table 3.2.

HOW CAN YOU CALCULATE THE GI OF A MEAL?

To date, only the GIs of single foods have been directly measured. In reality, it is more useful to know the GI of a meal, as we are more likely to eat combinations of foods. It is possible to *estimate* the GI of a meal by working out its total carbohydrate content, and then the contribution of each food to the total carbohydrate content. Table 3.3 shows how to calculate the overall GI of a typical breakfast.

Why does pasta have a low GI?

Pasta has a low GI because of the physical entrapment of ungelatinised starch granules in a sponge-like network of protein (gluten) molecules in the pasta dough. Pasta cooked al dente has a slighter lower GI than pasta that has been cooked longer until it is very soft. Pasta is unique in this regard and, as a result, pastas of any shape and size have a fairly low GI (30 to 60).

For a quick estimate of a simple meal, such as beans on toast, you may assume that half the carbohydrate is coming from the bread and half from the beans. So you can add the GI values of the two foods together and divide by 2: (70 + 48) ÷ 2 = 59.

If you have uneven proportions of two foods – for example 75% milk : 25% muesli – then 75% of the GI of milk can be added to 25% of the GI of muesli.

Table 3.3	HOW TO CALCULATE THE GI OF A MEAL			
Food	**Carbohydrate (g)**	**% total carbohydrate**	**GI**	**Contribution to meal GI**
Orange juice (150 ml)	13	21	46	21% × 46 = 10
Weetabix (30 g)	29	47	69	43% × 69 = 32
Milk (150 ml)	7	11	27	15% × 27 = 3
1 slice toast	13	21	70	27% × 70 = 15
Total	**62**	**100**		**Meal GI = 60**

Source: Adapted from Leeds et al., 2000.

However, this will give you only a rough guide, not an accurate prediction. Scientists at the University of Otago in New Zealand found that GI values significantly overestimate an individual's blood glucose response to a meal (Dodd *et al.*, 2011).

WHAT ARE THE DRAWBACKS OF THE GI?

The key to efficient glycogen refuelling – and minimal fat storage – is to maintain steady levels of blood glucose and insulin. When glucose levels are high (for example, after consuming high GI

Low GI diet at a glance

In essence, a low GI diet comprises carbohydrate foods with a low GI as well as lean protein foods and healthy fats:

- **Fresh fruit** – the more acidic the fruit, the lower the GI. Apples, pears, oranges, grapefruit, peaches, nectarines, plums and apricots have the lowest GI values, while tropical fruits such as pineapple, papaya and watermelon have higher values. However, as average portion size is small, the GL would be low.
- **Fresh vegetables** – most vegetables have a very low carbohydrate content and don't have a GI value (you would need to eat enormous amounts to get a significant rise in blood glucose). The exception is potatoes, which have a high GI. Eat them with protein/healthy fat or replace with low GI starchy vegetables (*see* below).
- **Low GI starchy vegetables** – these include sweetcorn (GI 46–48), sweet potato (GI 46) and yam (GI 37).
- **Low GI breads** – these include stoneground wholemeal bread (not ordinary wholemeal bread), fruit or malt loaf, wholegrain bread with lots of grainy bits, breads containing barley, rye, oats, soy and cracked wheat or those containing sunflower seeds or linseeds; chapatti and pitta breads (unleavened), pumpernickel (rye kernel) bread, sourdough bread.
- **Low GI breakfast cereals** – these include porridge, muesli and other oat or rye based cereals, and high bran cereals (e.g. All Bran).
- **Low GI grains** – these include bulgar wheat, noodles, oats, pasta, basmati (not ordinary brown or white) rice.
- **Beans and lentils** – chickpeas, red kidney beans, baked beans, cannellini beans, mung beans, black-eyed beans, butter beans, split peas and lentils.
- **Nuts and seeds** – almonds, brazils, cashews, hazelnuts, pine nuts, pistachios, peanuts; sunflower, sesame, flax and pumpkin seeds.
- **Fish, lean meat, poultry and eggs** – these contain no carbohydrate so have no GI value.
- **Low fat dairy products** – milk, cheese and yoghurt are important for their calcium and protein content. Opt for lower fat versions where possible.

foods), large amounts of insulin are produced, which shunts the excess glucose into fat cells. However, it is the combined effect of a large amount of carbohydrate as well as a food's GI value that really matters.

The biggest drawback of the GI is that it doesn't take account of the portion size you are eating. For example, watermelon has a GI of 72 – and is therefore classified as a high GI food – which puts it off the menu on a low GI diet. However, an average slice (120g) gives you only 6 g carbohydrate, not enough to raise your blood glucose level significantly. You would need to eat at least 6 slices (720 g) to obtain 50 g carbohydrate – the amount used in the GI test.

Similarly, many vegetables appear to have a high GI, which means they may be excluded on a low GI diet. However, their carbohydrate content is low and therefore their effect on blood glucose levels would be small. So despite having a high GI, the glycaemic load (GI × g carbohydrate per portion divided by 100) is low.

Another drawback is that some high fat foods have a low GI, which gives a falsely favourable impression of the food. For example, the GI of crisps or chips is lower than that of baked potatoes. Fat reduces the rate at which food is digested but high intakes of saturated and trans fats (*see* pp. 178 and 182) can increase blood cholesterol. It's important you don't select foods only by their GI – check the type of fat (i.e. saturated or unsaturated) and avoid those that contain large amounts of saturated or trans fats.

WHAT IS THE GLYCAEMIC LOAD?

You can gain a more accurate measure of the rise in your blood glucose (and insulin level) by using the glycaemic load (GL). This concept is derived from a mathematical equation developed by Professor Walter Willett from the Harvard Medical School in the US. It is calculated simply by multiplying the GI of a food by the amount of carbohydrate per portion and dividing by 100. One unit of GL is roughly equivalent to the glycaemic effect of 1 g of glucose. It gives you a good estimate of both the quality (GI) and quantity of carbohydrate:

- GL = (GI × carbohydrate per portion) ÷ 100

So, for watermelon:

- GL = (72 × 6) ÷ 100 = 4.3

	GI value	GL value	Daily GL total
Low	0–55	0–10	0–80
Medium	56–70	11–19	80–120
High	71–100	> 20	> 120

A high glycaemic load can result from eating a small quantity of a high carbohydrate, high GI food (e.g. white bread) or a larger quantity of a low GI food (e.g. pasta). This results in a large surge in blood glucose and insulin.

Conversely, eating smaller amounts of a low carbohydrate, high GI food (e.g. watermelon) or a larger quantity of a low GI food (e.g. beans) produces a low glycaemic 'load'. This results in a smaller and more sustained rise in blood glucose.

To optimise glycogen storage and minimise fat storage, aim to achieve a small or moderate glycaemic load – eat little and often, avoid overloading on carbohydrates, and stick to balanced combinations of carbohydrate, protein and healthy fat.

There's no need to cut out high glycaemic foods. The key is to eat them either in small amounts or combined with protein and/or a little healthy fat. This will evoke lower insulin levels and less potential fat storage. For example, have a baked potato (high GI food) with cheese, baked beans or tuna (low GI foods). Both protein and fat put a brake on the digestive process, slowing down the release of glucose.

Glycaemic response in athletes

Scientists have discovered that high GI foods have a smaller effect on blood glucose and insulin in regular exercisers compared with non-exercisers. That's because regular exercise increases insulin sensitivity and improves glucose uptake by body cells (Hawley & Lessard, 2008). In other words, your body learns to handle glucose more efficiently. Studies at the University of Sydney in Australia have found that when athletes are fed high GI foods, they produce much less insulin than would be predicted from GI tables. In other words, they don't show the same peaks and troughs in blood glucose and insulin as sedentary people do. This is thought to be related to increased activity of key proteins involved in the regulation of glucose uptake and insulin signalling in the muscles. Use the GI index only as a rough guide to how various foods are likely to behave in your body.

How much fibre?

Dietary fibre is the term used to describe the complex carbohydrates found in plants that are resistant to digestion. It includes cellulose, pectins, glucans, inulin and guar. The UK Scientific Advisory Committee recommends 30 g of fibre a day. The average intake in the UK is around 18 g/day, which is considerably less than the recommended level. Fibre helps your digestive system work properly and modifies the glycaemic effect of a meal. The soluble kind slows the digestion of carbohydrate, producing a slower blood glucose rise, and also helps reduce LDL cholesterol. The richest sources are beans, lentils, oats, rye, fruit and vegetables. Insoluble fibre – found mainly in wholegrain bread, whole grains and wholegrain breakfast cereals, wholewheat pasta, brown rice and vegetables – helps speed the passage of food through the gut, and prevents constipation and bowel problems.

SHOULD I USE GI OR GL?

GI remains the best researched and one of the most reliable indicators of health risk. In studies at Harvard University a low GI diet has been correlated with a low risk of chronic diseases like heart disease, type 2 diabetes and cancer of the bowel, upper gastrointestinal tract and pancreas. In particular, low GI is linked to high levels of HDL ('good') cholesterol (*see* p. 178). So if you have a low GI diet, the chances are you have a high 'good cholesterol' level and a lower risk of heart disease. In 1999 the World Health Organization (WHO) and Food and Agriculture

Organization (FAO) recommended that people base their diets on low GI foods in order to prevent chronic diseases.

However, the risk of disease is also predicted by the GL of the overall diet. In other words, GL simply strengthens the relationship, which suggests that the more frequently people eat high GI foods, the greater their health risk.

The downside to GL is that you could end up eating a low carbohydrate diet with a lot of fat and/or protein. Use the GI table (Appendix 1) to compare foods within the same category (e.g. different types of bread) and don't worry about the GI of those foods with a very low carbohydrate content (e.g. watermelon).

Carbohydrate timing

BEFORE EXERCISE

What, when and how much you eat before exercise will affect your performance, strength and endurance. Paradoxically, consuming carbohydrate increases carbohydrate burning in the muscle cells yet still delays the onset of fatigue. Numerous studies have concluded that consuming carbohydrate before exercise results in improved performance when compared with exercising on an empty stomach (Chryssanthopoulos *et al.*, 2002; Neufer *et al.*, 1987; Sherman *et al.*, 1991; Wright *et al.*, 1991).

DOES EXERCISE ON AN EMPTY STOMACH BURN MORE BODY FAT?

Exercising in a fasted state – such as first thing in the morning – may encourage your body to burn a slightly higher percentage of calories from fat and a lower percentage from carbohydrate. That's because blood glucose levels and insulin levels are at their lowest and glucagon levels are at their highest after an overnight fast. This increases the amount of fat that leaves your fat cells and travels to your muscles, where the fat is burned. However, it does not necessarily mean that you will burn more calories or lose more body fat. What matters most when it comes to fat loss is consuming fewer calories than you burn over 24 hours. On the downside, you may fatigue sooner or drop your exercise intensity and therefore end up burning fewer calories – and less body fat! If performance is your main goal, exercising in a fasted state will almost certainly reduce your endurance. And if strength and muscle mass are important goals, you will be better off exercising after a light meal. After an overnight fast, when muscle glycogen and blood glucose levels are low, your muscles will burn more protein for fuel. So you could end up losing hard-earned muscle!

WHEN IS THE BEST TIME TO EAT BEFORE EXERCISE?

Ideally, you should eat between 2 and 4 hours before training, leaving enough time for your stomach to settle so that you feel comfortable – not too full and not too hungry. This helps increase liver and muscle glycogen levels and enhances your subsequent performance (Hargreaves *et al.*, 2004). Clearly, the exact timing of your pre-exercise meal will depend on your daily schedule and the time of day you plan to train.

Researchers at the University of North Carolina found that performance during moderate to high intensity exercise lasting 35–40 minutes was improved after eating a moderately high carbohydrate, low fat meal 3 hours before exercise (Maffucci & McMurray, 2000). In this study, the volunteers were able to run significantly longer. Researchers asked the athletes to run on treadmills at a moderate intensity for 30 minutes, with high intensity 30 second intervals, and then until they couldn't run any longer, after eating a meal either 6 hours or 3 hours beforehand. The athletes ran significantly longer if they had eaten the meal 3 hours before training compared with 6 hours.

If you leave too long an interval between eating and training, you will be at risk of hypoglycaemia – low blood glucose – and this will certainly compromise your performance. You will fatigue earlier and, if you feel light-headed, risk injury too. On the other hand, training with steady blood glucose levels will allow you to train longer and harder.

HOW MUCH CARBOHYDRATE?

The size and timing of your pre-training meal are inter-related. The closer you are to the start of your training session, the smaller your meal should be (to allow for gastric emptying), whereas larger meals can be consumed when more time is available before training or competition. Intakes between 1–4 g/kg BW consumed 1–4 hours before exercise have been recommended (Burke, 2007). Most studies suggest 200–300 g carbohydrate or 2.5 g carbohydrate/kg of body weight about 3 hours before exercise (Rodriguez *et al.*, 2009). Researchers at Loughborough University found that this pre-exercise meal improved endurance running capacity by 9% compared with a no-meal trial (Chryssanthopoulos *et al.*, 2002). So, for example, if you weigh 70 kg, that translates to 175 g carbohydrate. You may need to experiment to find the exact quantity of food or drink and the timing that works best

for you. Some athletes can consume a substantial meal in the 2–4 hours before exercise with no ill effects, while others may experience discomfort and prefer to eat a snack or liquid meal.

WHAT ARE THE BEST FOODS TO EAT BEFORE EXERCISE?

Whether to eat high GI or low GI foods pre-exercise has long been a controversial area. Many experts recommend a low GI meal based on the idea that such a meal would supply sustained energy during exercise. Indeed, a number of well-designed studies carried out at the University of Sydney have supported this recommendation. For example, the researchers found that when a group of cyclists ate a low GI pre-exercise meal of lentils (GI = 29) 1 hour before exercise, they managed to keep going 20 minutes longer than when they consumed high GI foods (glucose drink, GI = 100; or baked potatoes, GI = 85) (Thomas *et al.*, 1991). Lentils were used in this study because they have one of the lowest GI values, but there are, of course, plenty of other low GI foods or food combinations that you can choose. For example, most fresh fruit, milk or yoghurt would be suitable, or a combination of carbohydrate, protein and healthy fat – for example, cereal with milk, a chicken sandwich or a baked potato with cheese. The box on p. 60 gives further suggestions for pre-exercise snacks and meals.

In other studies (Thomas *et al.*, 1994; DeMarco *et al.*, 1999), the researchers took blood samples at regular intervals from cyclists and found that low GI meals produce higher blood sugar and fatty acid levels during the latter stages of exercise, which is clearly advantageous for endurance sports. In other words, the low GI

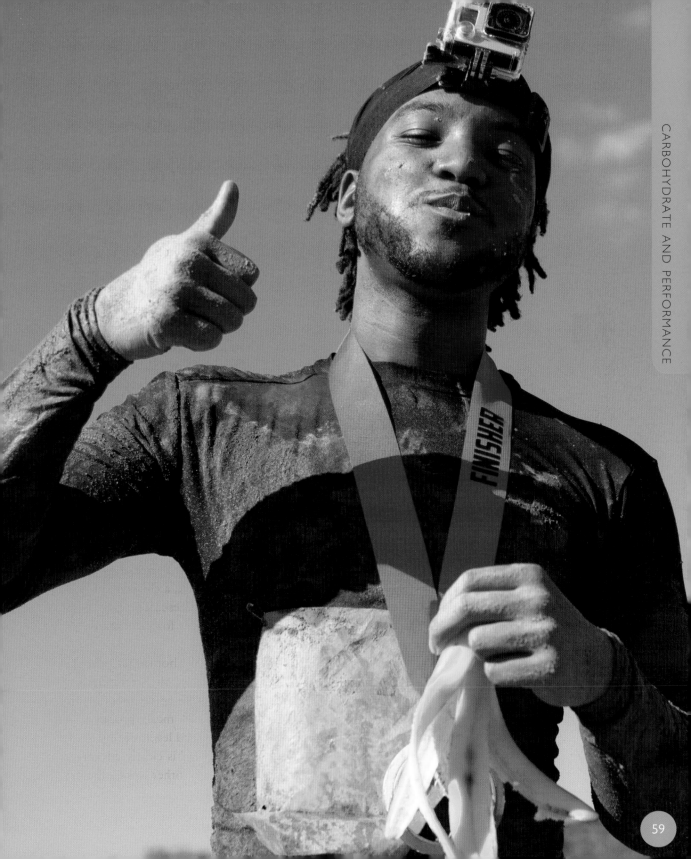

meals produce a sustained source of carbohydrate throughout exercise and recovery.

A UK study confirmed that athletes burn more fat during exercise following a low GI meal of bran cereal, fruit and milk compared with a high GI meal of cornflakes, white bread, jam and sports drink (Wu *et al.*, 2003). The benefits kick in early during exercise – the difference in fat oxidation is apparent even after 15 minutes.

A 2006 study at the University of Loughborough, UK, found that runners who consumed a low GI meal 3 hours before exercise were able to run longer (around 8 minutes) than after a high GI pre-exercise meal (Wu & Williams, 2006). The researchers suggest that the improvements in performance were due to increased fat oxidation following consumption of the low GI meal, which helped compensate for the lower rates of glycogen oxidation during the latter stages of the exercise trial. In other words, the low GI meal allowed the volunteers to burn more fat and less glycogen during exercise, which resulted in increased endurance.

This isn't necessarily a rule of thumb, as other studies have found that the GI of the pre-exercise meal has little effect on performance, with cyclists managing to keep going for the same duration whether they ate lentils (low GI) or potatoes (high GI) (Febbraio & Stewart, 1996). A Greek study also found that ingestion of high GI or low GI foods (containing the same quantity of carbohydrate) 30 minutes before exercise did not result in any differences in exercise performance in a group of 8 cyclists (Jamurtas *et al.*, 2011). It's certainly not a clear-cut case but what you have to consider is the timing of your pre-exercise meal. High GI foods are more 'risky' to your performance, particularly if you are sensitive to blood sugar

Pre-workout meals
2–4 hours before exercise:
- Sandwich/roll/bagel/wrap filled with chicken, fish, cheese, egg or peanut butter and salad
- Jacket potato with beans, cheese, tuna, coleslaw or chicken
- Pasta with tomato-based pasta sauce and cheese and vegetables
- Chicken with rice and salad
- Vegetable and prawn or tofu stir fry with noodles or rice
- Pilaf or rice/fish/vegetable dish
- Mixed bean hot pot with potatoes
- Chicken and vegetable casserole with potatoes
- Porridge made with milk
- Wholegrain cereal (e.g. bran or wheat flakes, muesli or Weetabix) with milk or yoghurt
- Fish and potato pie

Pre-workout snacks
1–2 hours before exercise:
- Fresh fruit
- Dried apricots, dates or raisins
- Smoothie (home-made or ready-bought)
- Yoghurt
- Shake (home-made or a meal replacement shake)
- Energy or nutrition bar
- Cereal bar or flapjack
- Toast with honey or jam
- Porridge or wholegrain cereal with milk

fluctuations (Burke *et al.*, 1998). Get the timing wrong, and you may be starting exercise with mild hypoglycaemia – remember, they produce a rapid rise in blood sugar and, in some people, a short-lived dip afterwards. The safest strategy may be to stick with low GI pre-exercise and then top up with high GI carbohydrate during exercise if you are training for more than 60 minutes.

DURING EXERCISE

For endurance activities lasting less than 45 minutes to 1 hour, consuming anything other than water is unnecessary provided your pre-exercise muscle glycogen levels are high, i.e. you have consumed sufficient carbohydrate during the previous few days and eaten a meal containing carbohydrate 2–4 hours before exercise (Burke *et al.*, 2011; IOC, 2011; Desbrow *et al.*, 2004). Muscle glycogen is generally not a limiting factor to performance during exercise lasting less than 1 hour.

It is well established that consuming carbohydrate during prolonged exercise (more than 1–2 hours) can enhance performance but research since the late 1990s has suggested that very small amounts of carbohydrate ('mouth-rinsing') may be beneficial for high intensity exercise (> 75% VO_2max) lasting 45–75 minutes (Carter *et al.*, 2004; Below, 1995; Jeukendrup *et al.*, 1997). The reasons are quite different.

Exercise lasting 45–75 minutes

With carbohydrate mouth-rinsing, the performance enhancing effect is mediated by the central nervous system (the brain), and not by any increase in carbohydrate uptake. Researchers have found that simply rinsing the mouth with a carbohydrate drink for 5–10 seconds improves performance even when you do not swallow the drink (Carter, 2004; Burke *et al.*, 2011).

A study at Loughborough University, found that mouth-rinsing enabled runners to run faster and cover more distance during a 30-minute treadmill run compared with a placebo (Rollo *et al.*, 2008). In a study at Ghent University, Belgium, cyclists were able to complete a 1-hour high intensity time trial 2.4 minutes faster after mouth-rinsing compared with a placebo (Pottier *et al.*, 2010). However, ingesting the carbohydrate drink did not improve performance compared with the placebo. A systematic review of 11 studies by Brazilian and Australian researchers found that 9 out of 11 (i.e. not all studies) showed a significant increase in performance during moderate to high intensity exercise lasting approximately 1 hour, ranging from 1.5% to 11.6% (de Ataide e Silva *et al.*, 2013).

The benefits of mouth-rinsing may be greater when exercising in a glycogen depleted state or when fasted rather than after a meal, i.e. when 'training low' (*see* p. 39). 'Training low' is a strategy used by some athletes to induce greater training-induced adaptations and promote a greater use of fat for fuel during endurance training (*see* pp. 36–43). The main drawback is that high intensity exercise feels harder and athletes often cannot train as hard. However, this may be counteracted to some extent by using a carbohydrate mouth rinse.

Researchers at RMIT University, Australia, found that glycogen depleted cyclists performed better in a 1-hour simulated time trial following an overnight fast compared with after a meal (Lane *et al.*, 2013). The performance benefits appear to be even greater when mouth-rinsing is combined with caffeine during high intensity exercise. In a randomised double-blind study at Liverpool John Moores University, glycogen depleted athletes were given carbohydrate mouth rinse with or without caffeine during a morning 45-minute steady run followed by a high intensity interval set until they reached the point of exhaustion (i.e. they 'trained low') (Kasper *et al.*, 2015). Those who used a carbohydrate rinse were able to exercise 16 minutes longer than the control (placebo) group but those who *also* took caffeine were able to keep going 29 minutes longer (52 min, 36 min and 65 minutes respectively). This strategy would therefore be advantageous for athletes training in a glycogen depleted state ('training low').

The ergogenic effects of mouth-rinsing are thought to be due to carbohydrate receptors in the mouth signalling to the brain that food is on its way. These sensors activate the brain's pleasure and reward centres and override the perception of effort and fatigue so you are able to continue exercising despite not actually consuming any carbohydrate. In other words, you get the performance enhancing effects of carbohydrate without consuming it.

In practice, then, for exercise lasting 45–75 minutes, you don't have to consume any carbohydrate – simply swilling or rinsing a carbohydrate drink, or sucking a sweet, will be enough to give you a performance boost. This strategy may be beneficial for those athletes who find it difficult to consume anything during exercise without experiencing gastrointestinal problems. Unfortunately, gastrointestinal problems are especially common among runners and endurance athletes due to a variety of mechanical, physiological and nutritional causes, but there are ways of alleviating them (*see* box, p. 285).

Exercise lasting 1–2½ hours

For moderate–high intensity exercise lasting longer than 60–90 minutes, consuming carbohydrate can help maintain blood glucose levels, delay fatigue and enable you to perform longer at a higher intensity (Pöchmüller et al, 2016; Coggan & Coyle, 1991; Coyle, 2004; Jeukendrup, 2004). It may also help you to continue exercising when your muscle glycogen stores are depleted.

During that first hour of exercise, most of your carbohydrate energy comes from muscle glycogen. After that, muscle glycogen stores deplete significantly, so the exercising muscles must use carbohydrate from some other source. That's where blood sugar (glucose) comes into its own. As you continue exercising hard, the muscles take up more and more glucose from the bloodstream. Eventually, after 2–3 hours, your muscles will be fuelled entirely by blood glucose and fat.

Sounds handy, but, alas, you cannot keep going indefinitely because blood glucose supplies eventually dwindle. Some of this blood glucose is derived from certain amino acids and some comes from liver glycogen. When liver glycogen stores run low, your blood glucose levels will fall, and you will be unable to carry on exercising at the same intensity. That's why temporary hypoglycaemia is common after 2–3 hours of exercise without consuming carbohydrate. In this state, you would feel very fatigued and light-headed, your muscles would feel very heavy and the exercise would feel very hard indeed. In other words, the depletion of muscle and liver glycogen together with low blood sugar levels would cause you to reduce exercise intensity or stop completely. This is sometimes called 'hitting the wall' in marathon running.

Clearly, then, consuming additional carbohydrate would maintain your blood sugar levels and allow you to exercise longer. An analysis of 73 previous studies by researchers at Auckland University of Technology, New Zealand, found that carbohydrate consumption during exercise led to an improvement in performance of up to 6% (Vandenbogaerde & Hopkins, 2011).

The consensus recommendation is an intake of 30–60 g carbohydrate/hour (IOC, 2011; Burke *et al.*, 2011; Rodriguez *et al.*, 2009; Coggan & Coyle, 1991). This matches the maximum amount of a single type of carbohydrate (e.g. glucose) that can be oxidised by the muscles during aerobic exercise because the transporter responsible for carbohydrate absorption in the intestine becomes saturated. Consuming more than 60 g glucose per hour would not improve your energy output or reduce fatigue.

Exercise lasting longer than 2½ hours

For intense exercise lasting more than 2½ hours, it would be beneficial to consume greater amounts of carbohydrate, up to 90 g/hour. Research at the University of Birmingham has found that this can be achieved by consuming a mixture of carbohydrates ('multiple transportable carbohydrates') – glucose + fructose, or maltodextrin + fructose in a 2:1 ratio – which overcomes the problems of glucose transporter saturation and therefore increases the uptake of carbohydrates from the intestines and also the oxidation rate in the muscles (IOC, 2011; Jeukendrup, 2008). It may also increase fluid uptake.

Glucose and fructose are absorbed via different transporter molecules in the small intestine. The transport capacity of these molecules is limited. For example, glucose is transported by sodium-dependent glucose transporter 1 (SGLT1) at a maximum rate of 60 g/hour. This means that you will gain no further performance benefit by consuming more than 60 g glucose/hour since the glucose transporters will be fully saturated. The excess glucose will simply stay in the intestine longer. However, by consuming fructose along with glucose, you can make use of the fructose transporters (GLUT5) and thus enhance the amount of carbohydrate absorbed and delivered to the muscles. This is advantageous during intense prolonged endurance activities such as triathlon, long distance cycling and ultra-distance running. One study found that performance in a cycling time trial improved by 8% when drinking a glucose/fructose drink compared with a glucose-only drink and 19% when compared with water (Currell & Jeukendrup, 2008).

WHICH FOODS OR DRINKS SHOULD I CONSUME DURING EXERCISE?

It makes sense that the carbohydrate you consume during exercise should be easily digested and absorbed. You need it to raise your blood sugar level and reach your exercising muscles rapidly. Thus, high or moderate GI carbohydrates are generally the best choices (*see* Table 3.5 on p. 64). Whether you choose solid or liquid carbohydrate makes little difference to your performance, provided you drink water with solid carbohydrate (Pfeiffer *et al.*, 2010a; Kennerly *et al.*, 2011; Mason *et al.*, 1993). Most athletes find liquid forms of carbohydrate (i.e. sports drinks) more convenient. Carbohydrate-containing drinks have a dual benefit because they provide fluid as well as fuel, reducing dehydration and fatigue. Obviously, you do not have to consume a commercial drink; you can make your own from fruit juice, or sugar, or squash, and water (*see* Chapter 7). A study at the University of Birmingham, UK, found that there was no difference in the rates of carbohydrate oxidation (91 g/hour) during 3 hours of cycling after consuming a bar or a drink containing a 2:1 glucose plus fructose mixture (Pfeiffer *et*

Table 3.4	SUMMARY OF RECOMMENDATIONS FOR CARBOHYDRATE INTAKE DURING EXERCISE	
Exercise duration	**Recommended amount of carbohydrate**	**Type of carbohydrate**
< 45 minutes	None	None
45–75 minutes	Very small amounts (mouth rinse)	Any
1–2 hours	Up to 30 g/h	Any
2–3 hours	Up to 60 g/h	Glucose, maltodextrin
> 2.5 hours	Up to 90 g/h	Multiple transportable carbohydrates (glucose + fructose, or maltodextrin + fructose in 2:1 ratio)

Source: Jeukendrup, 2014.

Table 3.5	SUITABLE FOODS AND DRINKS TO CONSUME DURING EXERCISE	
Food or drink	**Portion size providing 30 g carbohydrate**	**Portion size providing 60 g carbohydrate**
Isotonic sports drink (6 g/100 ml)	500 ml	1000 ml
Glucose polymer drink (12 g/100 ml)	250 ml	500 ml
Energy bar	½–1 bar	1–2 bars
Diluted fruit juice (1:1)	500 ml	1000 ml
Raisins or sultanas	1 handful (40 g)	2 handfuls (80 g)
Cereal or breakfast bar	1 bar	2 bars
Energy gel	1 sachet	2 sachets
Bananas	1–2 bananas	2–3 bananas

al., 2010a). Another study by the same researchers showed there was no difference in carbohydrate oxidation rate when they compared a gel and a drink (Pfeiffer *et al.*, 2010b). The choice, therefore, boils down to individual preference.

A range of commercial sports drinks, gels and bars containing a mixture of carbohydrates is widely available. If you prefer to consume food as well as drinks during exercise, energy or 'sports nutrition' bars, sports gels, ripe bananas, raisins or dried fruit bars are all suitable. Have a drink of water at the same time. In one study at Appalachian State University, there was no difference in exercise performance when cyclists were given equal amounts of carbohydrate either in the form of a banana or a 6% carbohydrate sports drink (Kennerly *et al.*, 2011). You should experiment with different drinks and foods during training to develop your own fuelling strategy.

It is important to begin consuming carbohydrate *before* fatigue sets in. It takes 30–40 minutes for the carbohydrate to be absorbed into the bloodstream (Coggan & Coyle, 1991). For workouts longer than 60–90 minutes, the best strategy is to begin consuming carbohydrate after about 30–40 minutes.

While consuming carbohydrate during exercise can delay fatigue, perhaps by up to 45 minutes, it will not allow you to keep exercising hard indefinitely. Eventually, factors other than carbohydrate supply will cause fatigue.

AFTER EXERCISE

The length of time that it takes to refuel depends on four main factors:

- how depleted your glycogen stores are after exercise;

- the extent of muscle damage;
- the amount and the timing of carbohydrate you eat;
- your training experience and fitness level.

Depletion

The more depleted your glycogen stores, the longer it will take you to refuel, just as it takes longer to refill an empty fuel tank than one that is half full. This, in turn, depends on the intensity and duration of your workout.

The higher the *intensity*, the more glycogen you use. For example, if you concentrate on fast, explosive activities (e.g. sprints, jumps or lifts) or high intensity aerobic activities (e.g. running), you will deplete your glycogen stores far more than for low intensity activities (e.g. walking or slow swimming) of equal duration. The minimum time it would take to refill muscle glycogen stores is 20 hours (Coyle, 1991). After prolonged and exhaustive exercise (e.g. marathon), it may take up to 7 days.

The *duration* of your workout also has a bearing on the amount of glycogen you use. For example, if you run for 1 hour, you will use up more glycogen than if you run at the same speed for half an hour. If you complete 10 sets of shoulder exercises in the gym, you will use more glycogen from your shoulder muscles than if you had completed only 5 sets using the same weight. Therefore, you need to allow more time to refuel after high intensity or long workouts.

Muscle damage

Certain activities that involve eccentric exercise (e.g. heavy-weight training, plyometric training or hard running) can cause muscle fibre damage. Eccentric exercise is defined as the forced lengthening of active muscle. Muscle damage, in turn, delays glycogen storage and complete glycogen replenishment could take as long as 7–10 days.

Carbohydrate intake

The higher your carbohydrate intake, the faster you can refuel your glycogen stores. Figure 3.3(a) shows how glycogen storage increases with carbohydrate intake.

This is particularly important if you train on a daily basis. For example, cyclists who consumed a low carbohydrate diet (250–350 g/day) failed to replenish fully their muscle glycogen stores (Costill *et al.*, 1971). Over successive days of training, their glycogen stores became progressively lower. However, in a further study, cyclists who consumed a high carbohydrate diet (550–600 g/day) fully replaced their glycogen stores in the 22 hours between training sessions (Costill, 1985) (*see* Fig. 3.3(b)).

More recently, a study from the University of Bath highlighted the importance of carbohydrate for short-term recovery when performing two workouts a day (Alghannam *et al.*, 2016). They found that runners who consumed a high carbohydrate drink (1.2 g/kg body weight) after the first workout were able to run significantly longer (80 min versus 48 minutes) before reaching the point of exhaustion in the second workout than those who drank a low carbohydrate drink (0.3 g/kg body weight). Muscle biopsies showed that in both cases, exhaustion corresponded to when their muscles reached a critically low level of glycogen. A high carbohydrate intake is essential for glycogen recovery and subsequent performance for those training twice a day.

Therefore, if you wish to train daily or twice a day, make sure that you consume enough carbohydrate. If not, you will be unable to train as hard or as long, you will suffer fatigue sooner and achieve smaller training gains.

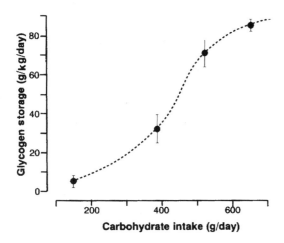

Figure 3.3(a) Glycogen storage depends on carbohydrate intake

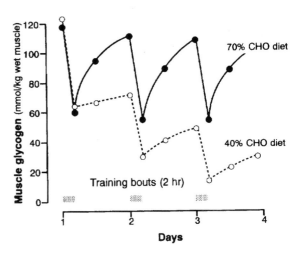

Figure 3.3(b) A low carbohydrate intake results in poor refuelling

Training experience

Efficiency in refuelling improves automatically with training experience and raised fitness levels. Thus, it takes a beginner longer to replace his glycogen stores than an experienced athlete eating the same amount of carbohydrate. That's why elite sportspeople are able to train almost every day while beginners cannot and should not!

Another adaptation to training is an increase in your glycogen storing capacity, perhaps by as much as 20%. This is an obvious advantage for training and competition. It is like upgrading from a 1-litre saloon car to a 3-litre sports car.

HOW SOON SHOULD I EAT AFTER EXERCISE?

When the recovery period between training sessions is less than 8 hours, you should eat as soon as practical after the first workout to maximise recovery as glycogen storage is faster during this post-exercise 'window' than at any other time. It may be more effective to consume several smaller high carbohydrate snacks than larger meals during the early recovery phase, according to researchers at the Australian Institute of Sport (Burke *et al.*, 2004). It makes no difference to the glycogen storage rate whether you consume liquid or solid forms of carbohydrate (Keizer *et al.*, 1986).

Research has shown that glycogen storage following exercise takes place in three distinct stages. During the first 2 hours, replenishment is most rapid – at approximately 150% (or one-and-a-half times) the normal rate (Ivy *et al.*, 1988). During the subsequent 4 hours the rate slows but remains higher than normal; after this period, glycogen manufacture returns to the normal rate. Therefore, eating carbohydrate

Post-exercise snacks

Each of the following provides 60–90 g carbohydrate and 15–25 g protein:

- 500 ml flavoured milk, one cereal bar, one banana
- Two bananas, 500 ml of semi-skimmed milk
- A wholemeal tuna sandwich (two slices of bread, 50 g tuna), one pot (150 g) yoghurt
- Recovery milkshake – mix 300 ml low fat milk, one pot (150 g) fruit yoghurt, one banana, 100 g strawberries and two heaped tsp (30 g) honey in a blender
- A wholemeal cheese sandwich (two slices bread, 40 g cheese), 100 g dried apricots
- 200 g baked beans on two slices wholemeal toast
- Two cereal bars plus 500 ml skimmed milk
- 60 g raisins and 50 g nuts
- Two Weetabix, 300 ml low fat milk, one pot (150 g) fruit yoghurt, 30 g sultanas
- A jacket potato (200 g) with 200 g baked beans and 40 g cheese
- Cooked pasta (85 g uncooked weight) with 130 g chicken breast
- Three oatcakes, 60 g hummus, 500 ml low fat milk

during this time speeds glycogen recovery. This is most important for those athletes who train twice a day.

There are two reasons why glycogen replenishment is faster during the post-exercise period. Firstly, eating carbohydrate stimulates insulin release, which, in turn, increases the amount of glucose taken up by your muscle cells from the bloodstream, and stimulates the action of the glycogen-manufacturing enzymes. Secondly, post-exercise, the muscle cell membranes are more permeable to glucose, so they can take up more glucose than normal.

However, for recovery periods of 24 hours or longer, the type and timing of carbohydrate intake is less critical, provided you consume enough energy (calories) and carbohydrate over a 24-hour period.

HOW MUCH CARBOHYDRATE?

For rapid recovery, most researchers recommend consuming 1–1.2 g/kg body weight early in the post-exercise period and, ideally, within 4 hours (Burke *et al.*, 2004; Burke *et al.*, 2011; ACSM/AND/DC, 2016). So, for example, if you weigh 70 kg you need to consume 70–84 g carbohydrate within 4 hours of exercise. Even if you finish training late in the evening, you still need to start the refuelling process, so do not go to bed on an empty stomach! For efficient glycogen refuelling, you should continue to eat carbohydrate at regular intervals. If you leave long gaps without eating, glycogen storage and recovery will be slower.

ARE HIGH GI OR LOW GI CARBOHYDRATES BEST FOR RECOVERY?

Since high GI foods cause a rapid increase in blood glucose levels, it seems logical that foods with a high GI would increase glycogen replenishment during the initial post-exercise period. Indeed, a number of studies have shown that you get faster glycogen replenishment during

the first 6 hours after exercise (and, in particular, the first 2 hours) with moderate and high GI carbohydrates compared with low GI (Burke *et al.*, 2004; Burke *et al.*, 1993).

However, Danish researchers discovered that, after 24 hours, muscle glycogen storage is about the same on a high GI as on a low GI diet (Kiens *et al.*, 1990). In other words, high GI foods post-exercise get your glycogen recovery off to a quick start, but low GI foods will result in the same level of recovery 24 hours after exercise.

But there are other performance benefits of a low GI recovery diet – it may improve your endurance the next day. Researchers at Loughborough University found that when athletes consumed low GI meals during the 24-hour period following exercise, they were able to exercise longer before exhaustion compared with those who had consumed high GI meals (Stevenson *et al.*, 2005). Further tests showed that they used a greater amount of fat to fuel their muscles during exercise. In other words, a low GI diet encourages greater fat burning, which not only benefits your performance but may also help you achieve faster weight (body fat) loss.

The bottom line is that if you are training intensely every day or twice a day, make sure you consume high GI foods during the first 2 hours after exercise. However, if you train once a day (or less frequently), low GI meals increase your endurance and performance during your subsequent workout.

DOES PROTEIN COMBINED WITH CARBOHYDRATE IMPROVE RECOVERY?

It is not always practical to consume large amounts of carbohydrate after exercise. But combining a small amount of protein (0.2–0.4 g

/kg BW/h) with less carbohydrate (0.8 g/kg BW/h) has been shown to be equally or more effective in promoting glycogen recovery than carbohydrate alone (Beelen *et al.*, 2010). This is because protein-carbohydrate mixtures stimulate a greater output of insulin, which, in turn, speeds the uptake of glucose and amino acids from the bloodstream into the muscle cells – thereby promoting glycogen and protein synthesis – and blunts the rise in cortisol that would otherwise follow exercise. Cortisol suppresses the rate of protein synthesis and stimulates protein catabolism.

Consuming protein stimulates muscle synthesis, inhibits protein breakdown and promotes positive protein balance in the muscle after both resistance and endurance exercise (Howarth *et al.*, 2009).

Endurance exercise

One of the first studies to demonstrate the advantages of consuming a carbohydrate-protein drink after exercise was carried out at the University of Texas at Austin in 1992 (Zawadski *et al.*, 1992). Researchers found that a carbohydrate-protein drink (112 g carbohydrate, 40 g protein) increased glycogen storage by 38% compared with a carbohydrate-only drink. Other studies subsequently have noted similar results (Ready *et al.*, 1999; Tarnopolsky *et al.*, 1997; Beelen *et al.*, 2010).

Researchers at the University of Texas at Austin measured significantly greater muscle glycogen levels 4 hours after 2.5 hours intense cycling when cyclists consumed a protein-carbohydrate drink (80 g carbohydrate, 28 g protein, 6 g fat) compared with a carbohydrate-only drink (80 g carbohydrate, 6 g fat) (Ivy *et al.*, 2002).

A joint study by researchers at the University of Bath and Loughborough University found that subsequent exercise performance after a carbohydrate-protein recovery drink was greater compared with consumption of a carbohydrate-only drink (Betts *et al.*, 2007). The runners in the study were able to run longer following a 4-hour recovery period during which they consumed a drink containing 0.8 g carbohydrate and 0.3 g protein/kg body weight/hour. More recently, Scandinavian researchers found that consuming a mix of carbohydrate and protein in the 2-hour post-exercise window after exhaustive cycling improved endurance performance the following day compared with consuming carbohydrate-only (Rustad et al, 2016). Cyclists were able to keep going for 63.5 minutes compared with 49.8 minutes.

Researchers at James Madison University have shown that a carbohydrate-protein drink also reduces post-exercise muscle damage and muscle soreness (Luden *et al.*, 2007).

Resistance exercise

Consuming a protein-carbohydrate drink also appears to enhance recovery and muscle protein synthesis (MPS) following resistance exercise compared with carbohydrate alone. Researchers at the University of Texas Medical Branch measured higher levels of protein retention in athletes after consuming a recovery drink containing a mixture of carbohydrate, protein and amino acids, compared with a carbohydrate-only drink that provided the same number of calories (Borsheim *et al.*, 2004). According to researchers at Ithaca College, New York, consuming a protein-carbohydrate drink immediately after resistance exercise promotes more efficient muscle tissue growth as well as faster glycogen refuelling, compared with a carbohydrate-only drink or a placebo (Bloomer *et al.*, 2000). In this study, the researchers measured higher levels of anabolic hormones such as testosterone and lower levels of catabolic hormones such as cortisol for 24 hours after a weights workout when the volunteers consumed a protein-carbohydrate drink. Canadian researchers measured an increased protein uptake in the muscles after volunteers drank a protein-carbohydrate drink following resistance exercise (Gibala, 2000). A review of studies from Maastricht University in the Netherlands concluded that consuming a protein-carbohydrate drink following resistance exercise helps increase glycogen storage, stimulate protein synthesis and inhibit protein breakdown (Van Loon, 2007). For more information about protein intake after exercise, *see* p. 81.

WHICH FOODS ARE BEST BETWEEN WORKOUTS?

After you have taken advantage of the 6-hour post-exercise recovery window, when and which carbohydrates you eat for the rest of the day are still important for glycogen recovery. To optimise glycogen replenishment following intense endurance exercise, you should ensure a relatively regular supply of carbohydrates into the bloodstream. In practice, this means eating carbohydrates in several small meals regularly spaced throughout the day. Researchers at the Human Performance Laboratory of Ball State University have shown that slowly digested carbohydrate – that is, meals with a low GI – cause much smaller rises and falls in blood sugar and insulin and create the ideal environment for the optimal replenishment of glycogen stores (Costill, 1988). Avoid consuming large, infrequent meals or lots of high GI meals, as they will produce large fluctuations in blood sugar and insulin. This means there will be periods of time when blood sugar levels are low, so glycogen storage will be reduced. Surges of blood sugar and insulin are more likely to result in fat gain.

ARE THERE ANY OTHER BENEFITS OF A LOW GI DAILY DIET?

While a low GI diet is important for regular exercisers for promoting glycogen recovery, it also has numerous health benefits and is widely promoted to the general population for weight loss. Reducing the GI of the diet increases satiety (feelings of satisfaction after eating), improves appetite control and makes it easier to achieve a healthy body weight (Brand-Miller *et al.*, 2005; Warren *et al.*, 2003). Studies have shown that the lower the GI of a meal, the more satisfied and less hungry you are likely to be during the following 3 hours (Holt, 1992). A low GI diet has also been shown to increase the resting metabolic rate, which increases daily energy expenditure and increases the rate of weight loss (Pereira *et al.*, 2004). What's more, low GI diets can help reduce the risk of cardiovascular disease by lowering total and LDL ('bad') cholesterol levels (Sloth *et al.*, 2004). This is due to the lower insulin levels associated with low GI eating – high insulin levels stimulate cholesterol manufacture in the liver (Rizkalla *et al.*, 2004). Total cholesterol may drop by as much as 15% on a low GI diet (Jenkins *et al.*, 1987).

A low GI diet is also promoted for the management of type 2 diabetes. Studies have found that it can improve blood glucose control as well as lower levels of total and LDL ('bad') cholesterol, typically associated with type 2 diabetes (Rizkalla, 2004; Brand-Miller *et al.*, 2003). There is mounting evidence, too, that a low GI diet can help prevent and manage the metabolic syndrome – the concurrent existence of raised blood glucose, high blood pressure, obesity and insulin resistance – and also polycystic ovary syndrome.

Carbohydrate loading

Carbohydrate loading is a technique originally devised in the 1960s to increase the muscles' glycogen stores above normal levels. With more glycogen available, you may be able to exercise longer before fatigue sets in. This is potentially advantageous in endurance events lasting longer than 90 minutes (e.g. long distance running or cycling) or for events that involve several heats or matches over a short period (e.g. tennis tournaments or swimming galas). It is unlikely to benefit you if your event lasts less than 90 minutes because muscle glycogen depletion would not be a limiting factor to your performance. Carbohydrate loading increases time to exhaustion by about 20% and improves performance by about 2–3% (Hawley *et al.*, 1997). The classical 6-day regimen involved 2 bouts of glycogen depleting exercise separated by 3 days of low carbohydrate intake and followed by 3 days of high carbohydrate intake and minimal exercise (Ahlborg *et al.*, 1967; Karlsson & Saltin, 1971) (Table 3.6). The theory behind this 2-phase regimen is that glycogen depletion stimulates the activity of glycogen synthetase, the key enzyme involved in glycogen storage, resulting in above-normal levels of muscle glycogen.

But this regimen had a number of drawbacks. Not only did it interfere with exercise tapering, but the low carbohydrate diet left athletes weak, irritable and tired. Worse, many failed to achieve high glycogen levels even after 3 days of high carbohydrate intake.

Researchers at Ohio State University, Ohio, US developed a 6-day carbohydrate loading regimen that resulted in similar increases in glycogen levels but without the disadvantages described above (Sherman *et al.*, 1981). This required tapering training on 6 consecutive days while following a normal diet during the first 3 days followed by a carbohydrate-rich diet during the next 3 days (Table 3.7 on p. 72).

More recently, researchers at the University of Western Australia have found that equally high levels of glycogen can be achieved by taking in 10–12 g of carbohydrate per kilogram of body

Table 3.6	CARBOHYDRATE LOADING (CLASSICAL REGIMEN)						
Exhaustive prolonged exercise	Taper training	Taper training	Exhaustive prolonged exercise	Taper training	Taper training	Taper training	
Day 1	**Day 2**	**Day 3**	**Day 4**	**Day 5**	**Day 6**	**Day 7**	**Competition**
Normal diet	Low carbohydrate diet	Low carbohydrate diet	Low carbohydrate diet	High carbohydrate diet	High carbohydrate diet	High carbohydrate diet	

weight over the course of 36–48 hours following a 3-minute bout of high intensity exercise (Fairchild *et al.*, 2002; Bussau *et al.*, 2002). It appears that the rate of glycogen storage is greatly increased following such a workout. The advantage of this new regimen is that only 1 instead of 6 days is needed to achieve high glycogen levels, and very little change to your usual training programme needs to be made.

Table 3.8 shows a recommended programme for carbohydrate loading. On Day 1, carry out endurance training for about 1 hour to reduce the amount of glycogen in your liver and muscles. For the following 3 days, taper your training and eat a moderate carbohydrate diet (5–7 g carbo-

hydrate/kg body weight). For the final 36–48 hours, continue your exercise taper, or rest, and increase your carbohydrate intake to 10–12 g/kg body weight.

Since glycogen storage is associated with approximately 3 g water for each 1 g of glycogen, carbohydrate loading can produce a weight increase of 1–2 kg. This may or may not affect your performance.

If you decide to try carbohydrate loading, rehearse it during training to find out what works best for you. Never try anything new before an important competition. You may need to try the technique more than once, adjusting the types and amounts of foods you eat.

Table 3.7	CARBOHYDRATE LOADING (MODIFIED REGIMEN)						
Endurance training	Taper training	Taper training	Taper training	Taper training	Taper training	Taper training	
Day 1	**Day 2**	**Day 3**	**Day 4**	**Day 5**	**Day 6**	**Day 7**	**Competition**
Normal diet	Normal diet	Normal diet	Normal diet	High carbohydrate diet	High carbohydrate diet	High carbohydrate diet	

Table 3.8	CARBOHYDRATE LOADING (1 DAY REGIMEN)						
Endurance training	Taper training	Taper training	Taper training	Taper training	Taper training	Warm-up & 3 min training exercise (sustained sprint)	
Day 1	**Day 2**	**Day 3**	**Day 4**	**Day 5**	**Day 6**	**Day 7**	**Competition**
Normal diet	Low carbohydrate diet	Low carbohydrate diet	Low carbohydrate diet	High carbohydrate diet	High carbohydrate diet	High carbohydrate diet 10–12 g carbohydrate/kg BW/day	

Table 3.9	RECOMMENDATIONS FOR PRE- AND POST-EXERCISE CARBOHYDRATE INTAKE	
Dietary strategy	**When**	**Recommended carbohydrate intake**
Pre-exercise fuelling	Before exercise > 60 min	1–4 g/kg BW consumed 1–4 h before exercise
Post-exercise rapid refuelling	< 8 h recovery between two sessions	$1.0–1.2 \text{ g} \cdot \text{kg}-1 \cdot \text{h}-1$ for first 4 h then resume daily fuel needs
Carbohydrate loading	For events > 90 min of sustained/intermittent exercise	36–48 h of 10–12 g/kg BW/24 h

Source: Burke et al., 2011.

Putting it together: what, when and how much

Table 3.9 summarises the recommendations on carbohydrate intake covered in this chapter. The simplest way to plan your daily food intake is to divide the day into four 'windows': before, during and after exercise, and between training sessions. You can then work out how much and what type of carbohydrate to consume during each 'window' to optimise your performance and recovery.

Summary of key points

- A carbohydrate intake of 5–7 g/kg body weight/day is recommended for most regular exercisers, and 7–10 g/kg body weight/day is recommended during periods of intense training.
- LCHF diets might be beneficial for certain physiological adaptations but will reduce high intensity performance.
- Periodising carbohydrate around selected training sessions (i.e. doing your low intensity

sessions with low carbohydrate availability) may improve your muscles' ability to utilise both fat and carbohydrate as fuel during exercise of different intensities.

- The glycaemic index (GI) is a more useful way of categorising carbohydrates for athletes than the traditional 'complex' versus 'simple' classification.
- The GI is a ranking of carbohydrates based on their immediate effect on blood glucose (blood sugar) levels. Carbohydrates with a high GI produce a rapid rise in blood sugar; those with a low GI produce a slow rise in blood sugar.
- The glycaemic load (GL) takes into account the GI as well as the amount of carbohydrate (serving size) consumed and thus provides a measure of the total glycaemic response to a food or meal. GL = GI (%) × grams of carbohydrate per serving.
- Low GI foods consumed 2–4 hours before exercise may help improve endurance and delay fatigue. High GI foods consumed pre-exercise benefit some athletes but may produce temporary hypoglycaemia at the

start of exercise in those athletes sensitive to blood sugar fluctuations.

- The pre-exercise meal should contain approx. 1–4 g carbohydrate/kg body weight.

- For moderate to high intensity exercise lasting more than 60 minutes, consuming 30–60 g moderate or high GI carbohydrate (in solid or liquid form) during exercise can help maintain exercise intensity for longer and delay fatigue.

- Glycogen recovery takes, on average, 20 hours but depends on the severity of glycogen depletion, extent of muscle damage and the amount, type and timing of carbohydrate intake.

- Glycogen replenishment is faster than normal during the 2-hour post-exercise period. To kick-start recovery, it is recommended to consume 1 g moderate–high GI carbohydrate/kg body weight during this period.

- High or moderate GI carbohydrates produce faster glycogen replenishment for the first 6 hours post-exercise, which is most important for athletes who train twice a day.

- A low GI recovery diet may improve endurance the next day, and increase fat utilisation during subsequent exercise.

- Combining carbohydrate with protein has been shown to be more effective in promoting muscle glycogen recovery and muscle tissue growth compared with carbohydrate alone.

- A low GI daily diet comprising 4–6 small meals and supplying 5–10 g/kg body weight (depending on training hours and intensity) will promote efficient muscle glycogen recovery as well as improve satiety and appetite control, reduce cardiovascular risk factors and improve the management of type 2 diabetes.

- A modified form of carbohydrate loading may improve endurance capacity by 20% and performance by 2–3%.

Protein requirements for sport

4

The importance of protein – and the question of whether extra protein is necessary – for sports performance is one of the most hotly debated topics among sports scientists, coaches and athletes and has been contended ever since the time of the Ancient Greeks. Protein has long been associated with power and strength, and as the major constituent of muscle, it would seem logical that an increased protein intake would increase muscle size and strength.

Traditionally, scientists have held the view that athletes do not need to consume more than the reference nutrient intake (RNI) for protein and that consuming anything greater than this amount would produce no further benefit. However, research since the 1980s has cast doubt on this view. There is considerable evidence that the protein needs of active individuals are consistently higher than those of the general population.

This chapter will help to give you a fuller understanding of the role of protein during exercise, and enable you to work out how much you need. It will show how individual requirements depend on the sport concerned and the training programme, and also how they are related to carbohydrate intake. An example of a daily menu is given to show how to meet your own protein requirements, and to provide a basis for developing your own menu. As more athletes are giving up meat and choosing a vegetarian diet, this chapter explains how you can obtain sufficient protein and other nutrients for peak performance on a meat-free diet.

Protein supplementation is discussed in detail in Chapter 6.

Why do I need protein?

Protein makes up part of the structure of every cell and tissue in your body, including your muscle tissue, internal organs, tendons, skin, hair and nails. On average, it comprises about 20% of your total body weight. Protein is needed for the growth and formation of new tissue, for tissue repair and for regulating many metabolic pathways, and can also be used as a fuel for energy production. It is also needed to make almost all of the body enzymes as well as various hormones (such as adrenaline and insulin) and neurotransmitters. Protein has a role in maintaining optimal fluid balance in tissues, transporting nutrients in and out of cells, carrying oxygen and regulating blood clotting.

WHAT ARE AMINO ACIDS?

The 20 amino acids are the building blocks of proteins. They can be combined in various ways to form hundreds of different proteins in the body. When you eat protein, it is broken down in your digestive tract into smaller molecular units – single amino acids and dipeptides (two amino acids linked together).

Twelve of the amino acids can be made in the body from other amino acids, carbohydrate and nitrogen. These are called dispensable, or non-essential, amino acids (NEAAs). The other eight are termed indispensable, or essential, amino acids (EAAs) meaning they must be supplied in the diet. All 20 amino acids are listed in Table 4.1. Branched-chain amino acids (BCAAs) include the three EAAs with a branched molecular configuration: valine, leucine and isoleucine. They make up one-third of muscle protein and are a vital substrate for two other amino acids, glutamine and alanine, which are released in large quantities during intense aerobic exercise. Also they can be used directly as fuel by the muscles, particularly when muscle glycogen is depleted. Strictly speaking, the body's requirement is for amino acids rather than protein.

Protein and exercise

HOW DOES EXERCISE AFFECT MY PROTEIN REQUIREMENT?

Numerous studies involving both endurance and strength exercise have shown that the current recommended protein intake of 0.75 g/kg BW/day is inadequate for people who participate in regular exercise or sport (ACSM/AND/DC, 2016; IOC, 2011; Phillips & Van Loon, 2011). Additional protein is needed to compensate for

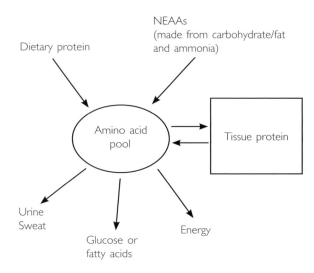

Figure 4.1 Protein metabolism

Protein metabolism

Tissue proteins are continually broken down (catabolised), releasing their constituent amino acids into the 'free pool', which is located in body tissues and the blood. For example, half of your total body protein is broken down and replaced every 150 days. Amino acids absorbed from food and non-essential amino acids made in the body from nitrogen and carbohydrate can also enter the free pool. Once in the pool, amino acids have four fates. They can be used to build new proteins, they can be oxidised to produce energy and they can be converted in glucose via gluconeogenesis or they can be converted into fatty acids. During energy production, the nitrogen part of the protein molecule is excreted in urine, or possibly in sweat.

Table 4.1	ESSENTIAL AND NON-ESSENTIAL AMINO ACIDS	
Essential amino acids (EAAs)	**Non-essential amino acids (NEAAs)**
Isoleucine	Alanine
Leucine	Arginine
Lysine	Asparagine
Methionine	Aspartic acid
Phenylalanine	Cysteine
Threonine	Glutamic acid
Tryptophan	Glutamine
Valine	Glycine
	Histidine*
	Proline
	Serine
	Tyrosine

* Histidine is essential for babies (not for adults)

the increased breakdown of protein during and immediately after exercise, and to facilitate repair and growth. Exercise triggers the activation of an enzyme that oxidises key amino acids in the muscle, which are then used as a fuel source. The greater the exercise intensity and the longer the duration of exercise, the more protein is broken down for fuel.

Your exact protein needs depend on the type, intensity and duration of your training. How these needs differ for endurance athletes

What is bioavailability?

Bioavailability is the 'usefulness' of the protein food or supplement. Foods that contain all eight EAAs are traditionally called 'complete' proteins. These include dairy products, eggs, meat, fish, poultry and soya. Plant foods, such as cereals and pulses, contain high amounts of several EAAs, but only very small amounts (or none) of the others. The EAA that is missing or in short supply is the limiting amino acid.

The ratio of EAAs to NEAAs and the amounts of specific amino acids is what determines the bioavailability of the protein food or supplement. E.g. the content of glutamine and the BCAAs (leucine, isoleucine and valine) determine the extent to which the protein is absorbed and utilised for tissue growth.

The bioavailability of a particular protein (BV) can be measured by its biological value, which indicates how close the proportions of amino acids are in relation to the body's requirements. It is a measure of the percentage of protein that is retained by the body for use in growth and tissue maintenance; in other words, how much of what is consumed is used for its intended purpose.

An egg has a BV of 100, which means, out of all foods, it contains the most closely matched ratio of EAAs and NEAAs to the body's needs. Therefore a high percentage of the egg protein can be used for making new body proteins. Dairy products, meat, fish, poultry, Quorn and soya have a higher BV (70–100); nuts, seeds, pulses and grains have a lower BV (less than 70).

and strength and power athletes is discussed in detail below.

Endurance training

Prolonged and intense endurance training increases your protein requirements for two reasons. Firstly, you will need more protein to compensate for the increased breakdown of protein during training. When your muscle glycogen stores are low – which typically occurs after 60–90 minutes of endurance exercise – certain amino acids, namely glutamate and the BCAAs valine, leucine and isoleucine (see p. 76), can be used for energy. One of the BCAAs, leucine, is converted into another amino acid, alanine, which is converted in the liver into glucose. This glucose is released back into the bloodstream and transported to the exercising muscles, where it is used for energy. In fact, protein may contribute up to 15% of your energy production when glycogen stores are low. This is quite a substantial increase, as protein contributes less than 5% of energy needs when muscle glycogen stores are high. Secondly, additional protein is needed for the repair and recovery of muscle tissue after intense endurance training. Prolonged endurance training causes substantial damage to muscle and body proteins. So, for endurance athletes, consuming protein together with carbohydrate in the post-training recovery period is important for muscle repair and remodelling (Moore et al., 2014).

Strength and power training

Strength and power athletes have additional protein needs compared with endurance athletes. After resistance training, the rate of protein breakdown and synthesis (building) increases, although for the first few hours the rate of break-down exceeds the rate of synthesis (Phillips et al., 1997; Phillips et al., 1999).

In addition, dietary protein provides an enhanced stimulus for muscle growth (Phillips et al., 2011; Phillips, 2012). To build muscle, you must be in 'positive nitrogen balance'. This means the body is retaining more dietary protein than is excreted or used as fuel. A suboptimal intake of protein will result in slower gains in strength, size and mass, or even muscle loss, despite hard training. In practice, the body is capable of adapting to slight variations in protein intake. It becomes more efficient in recycling amino acids during protein metabolism if your intake falls over a period of time. The body can also adapt to a consistently high protein intake by oxidising surplus amino acids for energy.

It is important to understand that a high protein diet alone will not result in increased strength or muscle size. These goals can be achieved only when an optimal protein intake is combined with heavy resistance (strength) training.

CAN I MINIMISE PROTEIN BREAKDOWN DURING EXERCISE?

Protein is broken down in increased quantities when muscle glycogen stores are low. Thus, during high intensity exercise lasting longer than 1 hour, protein can make a substantial contribution to your energy needs (up to 15%). Clearly, it is advantageous to start your training session with high muscle-glycogen stores. This will reduce the contribution protein makes to your energy needs at any given point during training.

If you are on a weight/fat loss programme, make sure you do not reduce your carbohydrate too drastically, otherwise protein will be used as an energy source, making it unavailable for tissue growth. To minimise muscle loss, reduce your calorie intake from carbohydrate in proportion to your calorie reduction (*see* Chapter 9 on weight loss).

HOW MUCH PROTEIN DO I NEED FOR MAXIMUM PERFORMANCE?

At low–moderate exercise intensities (< 50% VO_2max), it appears there is no significant increase in protein requirements (Hargreaves & Snow, 2001). Thus, for both sedentary people and recreational exercisers, the daily protein requirement is 0.75 g protein/kg BW daily.

For higher training intensities, the protein requirements are greater. Current guidelines recommend an intake in the range 1.2–2.0 g/kg BW/day (ACSM/AND/DC, 2016). That's equivalent to 84–140 g/day for an athlete weighing 70 kg, or 96–160 g/day for an 80 kg athlete. These recommendations encompass a range of training programmes and allow for adjustment according to individual needs and experience. Previously, separate recommendations were made for endurance and strength athletes but these are no longer considered accurate (ACSM/AND/DC, 2016). Instead, scientists recommend adjusting your protein intake in line with the specific goals of your training sessions and body composition goals (Phillips *et al.*, 2007; Tipton & Witard, 2007). For example, a higher protein intake would be appropriate following a resistance workout, and an intake at the higher end of the range (between 1.4 and 2.0 g/kg BW/day) is generally recommended (Phillips *et al.*, 2007; Tipton *et al.*, 2007; Williams, 1998; Tarnopolsky *et al.*, 1992; Lemon *et al.*, 1992).

A lower protein intake, around 1.2–1.4 g/kg body weight/day is generally recommended for

> ### Do beginners need more or less protein than experienced athletes?
>
> Contrary to popular belief, studies have shown that beginners have slightly higher requirements for protein per kg body weight compared with more experienced athletes (Phillips & Van Loon, 2011). When you begin a training programme, your protein needs rise due to increases in protein turnover (Gontzea *et al.*, 1975). After about 3 weeks of training, the body adapts to the exercise and becomes more efficient at recycling protein. Broken down protein can be built up again from amino acids released into the amino acid pool. The body also becomes more efficient in conserving protein. One study has shown that the requirements per kg body weight of novice bodybuilders can be up to 40% higher than those of experienced bodybuilders (Tarnopolsky, 1988).

endurance training (Rodrigues, 2009; Phillips *et al.*, 2007; Tipton *et al.*, 2007; Lemon, 1998; Williams & Devlin, 1992; Williams, 1998; ACSM, 2000) but a higher protein intake would also be appropriate when doing more frequent, prolonged or high intensity endurance sessions, or when training with low glycogen availability (pp. 36–43). Similarly, during a period of reduced energy availability (weight loss), increasing your dietary protein helps preserve muscle mass and prevent excessive protein breakdown (*see* 'Should I consume more protein if I want to lose weight?, p. 80). Also, experienced athletes generally require less protein than novices (*see* 'Do beginners need more or less protein than experienced athletes?', p 79).

University of Stirling researchers found that consuming extra protein can improve immune function (Witard *et al.*, 2014), mood and time trial performance during a period of high intensity training that mimicked a training camp situation (Witard *et al.*, 2011). In a trial involving 10 cyclists, those who consumed a post-training whey shake experienced fewer upper respiratory infections compared with those who consumed a carbohydrate drink (Witard *et al.*, 2014).

SHOULD I CONSUME MORE PROTEIN IF I WANT TO LOSE WEIGHT?

When cutting calories to lose body fat, you risk losing muscle mass as well. A higher protein intake can offset some of the muscle wasting effects associated with any weight reducing programme. Researchers recommend increasing your protein intake to 1.8–2.7 g/kg BW/day (or 2.3–3.1 g/kg fat-free mass), while cutting your daily energy intake by a modest amount (approximately 500 kcal) and including some form of resistance training in order to prevent lean mass losses (Murphy *et al.*, 2015; Helms *et al.*, 2014; Phillips & Van Loon, 2011). For example, a 70 kg athlete would need to consume 126–189 g protein/day. Protein timing is important and it is recommended that protein intake should be evenly spaced throughout the day. Ideally, your post-exercise meal should contain 0.25–0.3 g/kg BW protein, ideally from foods that are rapidly digested and absorbed and have a high leucine content, such as milk.

What's more, it may even be possible to lose fat while gaining muscle – something that most

Protein and satiety

Protein plays an important role in appetite regulation. It has been shown to promote satiety (the feeling of fullness and reduction in hunger after eating) more than carbohydrate, which is why it is particularly useful when you're trying to lose weight or prevent weight regain (Westerterp-Plantenga et al., 2012). It slows stomach emptying, thus helping you feel full longer. It also triggers the release of appetite-regulating hormones in the gut, such as glucagon-like peptide-1 (GLP-1), peptide YY (PYY) and glucagon; and reduces levels of 'hunger' hormones such as ghrelin. These hormones signal to the appetite control centre in the brain that you are satiated, so you stop eating. Researchers at the University of Copenhagen gave 25 volunteers different amounts of protein and found that there was a dose-dependent effect on levels of appetite hormones and satiety (Belza et al., 2013). Increasing doses of protein stimulated corresponding increases in responses of these hormones after eating, as well as increases in subjective feelings of satiety. The greater the protein intake, the higher the levels of GLP-1, PYY and glucagon and the greater the satiety experienced by the volunteers.

scientists previously believed to be impossible. A study at McMaster University, Ontario, US found that volunteers who consumed 2.4 g protein/kg BW in combination with a 40% calorie deficit and an intense resistance training programme lost significantly more body fat (4.8 kg vs. 3.5 kg) and gained significantly more muscle (1.2 kg vs. 0.1 kg) over 4 weeks than a control group who consumed 1.2 g protein/kg BW (Longland *et al.*, 2016). However, the training programme was very hard and may, therefore, not be sustainable for most.

TIMING OF PROTEIN INTAKE

The timing of your protein intake around exercise is just as important as your total daily protein requirement when it comes to metabolic adaptation, muscle repair and muscle protein synthesis (MPS). The amount of protein consumed during and post exercise, as well as the type and distribution of protein intake throughout the day, all affect the rate of muscle recovery and MPS. As a result, guidelines for protein intake have moved towards the expression of recommendations on a 'per meal' basis rather than a total daily basis.

PROTEIN BEFORE AND DURING EXERCISE

A number of studies suggest that consuming protein plus carbohydrate before and during prolonged, high intensity exercise stimulates MPS during exercise, minimises protein breakdown, improves recovery from exercise and results in less muscle damage (Beradi *et al.*, 2008; Saunders, 2007; Luden *et al.*, 2007; Romano-Ely *et al.*, 2006). This would be likely to help improve your subsequent performance.

Researchers at the University of Texas Medical Branch, US, found that consuming a drink containing protein and carbohydrate before exercise was more effective in stimulating post-exercise MPS than consuming the same drink immediately after exercise (Tipton *et al.*, 2001). Another study by researchers at Maastricht University found that consuming a drink containing equal amounts of protein plus carbohydrate at regular intervals during a 2-hour resistance workout resulted in significantly increased MPS rates and reduced protein breakdown during exercise compared with a carbohydrate-only drink (Beelen *et al.*, 2008).

Consuming protein plus carbohydrate may also increase performance during endurance exercise. A study at the University of Texas found that cyclists were able to exercise 36% longer when they consumed a carbohydrate-protein drink immediately before, and then every 20 minutes, during exercise, compared with a carbohydrate-only drink (Ivy *et al.*, 2003). Researchers at James Madison University, Vancouver, measured a 29% increase in endurance when cyclists consumed a carbohydrate-protein drink every 15 minutes compared with a carbohydrate-only drink (Saunders *et al.*, 2004). The exact amount of each ingredient is not clear, but most of the trials used drinks containing a carbohydrate to protein ratio of approximately 2:1 or 1:1 (e.g. 0.8 g carbohydrate/kg BW plus 0.4 g protein/kg BW) (Beelen *et al.*, 2010).

PROTEIN AFTER EXERCISE

Consuming protein in the post-exercise period increases training adaptation and enhances performance for both strength and endurance athletes. Following resistance training, protein in your diet is used to rebuild contractile proteins in the muscle fibres (actin and myosin), which, over time, results in bigger, stronger muscles. Following endurance training, instead of rebuilding contractile proteins, dietary protein is used to rebuild mitochondrial proteins, which is where energy production occurs (ATP). Therefore, consuming protein immediately after exercise would be advantageous for both resistance and endurance performance.

A review of studies concluded that protein consumed early in the post-exercise recovery phase increases the rate of MPS, promotes muscle repair and increases muscle adaptation to prolonged exercise (Van Loon, 2014). However, it is not necessary to consume protein immediately after exercise as the post-exercise anabolic window is thought to be as wide as several hours or perhaps more. One study found no difference in muscle mass, size or strength after pre-workout or post-workout protein consumption (Schoenfeld et al, 2017).

Several studies suggest that the optimal post-exercise protein intake is 0.25 g/kg BW, which translates to 20 g for an athlete weighing 80 kg (ACSM/AND/DC, 2016; Phillips & Van Loon, 2011; Moore et al., 2009; IOC, 2011; Rodriguez et al., 2009). In a study at McMaster University, volunteers consumed either 5, 10, 20 or 40 g egg protein immediately after resistance training (Moore et al., 2009). Scientists then measured the rate of MPS in the following 4 hours and found there was a dose-response relationship between protein intake and MPS up to a maximum, which occurred with 20 g protein. Higher doses (40 g) produced no further increase in MPS. Any excess is simply used as an energy source (oxidised) and the amino nitrogen converted into urea and excreted in the urine.

More recently, researchers at the University of Stirling measured the increase in the MPS in the 4-hour post-exercise period after consuming different quantities of whey protein (0, 10, 20 or 40 g) (Witard et al., 2014). They, too, found that 20 g of whey protein was the optimal dose for stimulating maximum MPS after resistance training. But these studies involved leg-only workouts and more recent research suggests that when a larger amount of muscle mass is involved, then larger amounts of protein may be optimal. The same research group found that consuming 40g protein after a whole-body resistance workout resulted in greater MPS than 20g protein (Macnaughton et al, 2016). In other words, when larger muscle groups are trained then a higher protein intake may be required. Although the studies used protein supplements, this was to eliminate confounding dietary factors and isolate the benefits of protein; it is quite feasible that consuming protein in food form, such as milk, eggs, yoghurt or meat, will have the same benefits. Supplements are not essential!

Furthermore, most of the athletes in the studies weighed approximately 80 kg, so it is likely that heavier athletes would require more (20–25 g) and lighter athletes would need less (15–20 g) to stimulate maximum MPS (Phillips et al., 2011).

Older athletes over 65 years old, on the other hand, may need more than 25g to stimulate maximum MPS. An analysis by Canadian and UK researchers found that healthy older men are less sensitive to low protein intakes and required a higher protein intake (0.4 g/kg BW per meal) than younger men (0.24 g/kg BW per meal) (p. 268) to stimulate maximum MPS (Moore et al., 2015). This equates to 32 g for an older athlete weighing 80 kg.

DISTRIBUTION OF PROTEIN INTAKE THROUGHOUT THE DAY

The window of opportunity to allow MPS to be elevated is not limited to the few hours immediately after exercise. Scientists have shown that this 'anabolic window' extends at least 24 hours

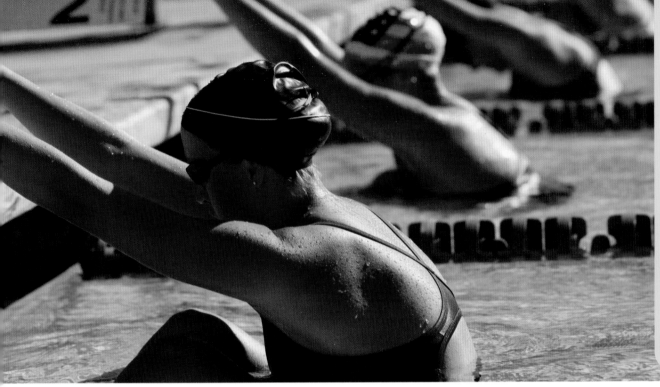

(particularly following resistance training), which means it would be beneficial to consume protein throughout the day, not only immediately after exercise (Schoenfeld *et al.*, 2013; Burd *et al.*, 2011). Consuming an optimal amount of protein at regular intervals throughout the day results in a more sustained delivery of amino acids to the muscles and promotes increased MPS.

A study at RMIT University, Australia, measured the rate of MPS during a 12-hour recovery period following a resistance workout when volunteers consumed 80 g protein either as 2 × 40 g every 6 hours; 4 × 20 g every 3 hours or 8 × 10 g every 1.5 hours (Areta *et al.*, 2013). They found that MPS was 31–48% higher when 20 g protein was consumed every 3 hours compared with the other protocols.

Similarly, researchers at the University of Texas Medical Branch, US, found that evenly distributing 90 g protein at breakfast (30 g), lunch (30 g) and dinner (30 g) resulted in 25% higher rate of MPS compared with a meal pattern that skewed most of the protein towards dinner (63 g) with small amounts at breakfast (10 g) and lunch (16 g) (Mamerow *et al.*, 2014).

In other words, for maximum MPS, it is advantageous to distribute your protein intake evenly throughout the day. You should also aim to consume 0.25 g/kg BW or 15–25 g protein at each meal or snack. This may mean rethinking your breakfast options, as most people focus on carbohydrates (e.g. cereal, toast) at this meal. Try including extra milk, a milk-based drink, eggs or yoghurt.

PROTEIN BEFORE SLEEP

The 'anabolic window' probably also extends to overnight recovery during sleep. Scientists have recently evaluated the benefits of consuming protein after an evening resistance training session and before sleep. One study at Maastricht University in the Netherlands found that protein synthesis was 22% higher in volunteers who consumed 40 g of protein (in the form of a casein drink) after a resistance workout and before sleep, compared with those who consumed a placebo (Res *et al.*, 2012). Casein was chosen as it is digested and absorbed relatively slowly so produced a sustained rise in amino acids in the bloodstream.

A further study found that consuming 28 g protein (in the form of a drink containing 28 g protein and 15 g carbohydrate) after a resistance workout and before sleep for 12 weeks resulted in significantly greater gains in muscle strength and size compared to a placebo (Snijders *et al.*, 2015). However, the athletes consuming the pre-bed protein drink consumed 1.9 g protein/kg BW/day while the placebo group consumed 1.3 g/kg BW/day. So it is not clear whether consuming protein before sleep is more effective than consuming protein at other times of the day, or whether there is an optimal dose or whether there is any advantage of liquid over solid forms of protein.

WHAT TYPE OF PROTEIN IS BEST AFTER EXERCISE?

Most studies suggest that 'high quality' proteins (i.e. proteins that contains all eight essential amino acids (EAAs) and are rapidly digested and absorbed) such as milk and egg are the best type of protein to consume after exercise (Phillips *et al.*, 2011; Tipton *et al.*, 2007). EAAs act as a stimulus for MPS in a dose-dependent manner: the greater the concentration of EAAs in the bloodstream, the greater the rate of MPS. Therefore, foods that contain high levels of EAAs would be most beneficial.

Milk-based proteins (such as whey and casein) have been shown to promote greater protein uptake in the muscle as well as greater muscle protein synthesis compared with soy protein (Wilkinson *et al.*, 2007; Tipton *et al.*, 2004; Tipton *et al.*, 2007). A study at McMaster University found that those who consumed milk after resistance training gained more muscle mass than those who consumed soy drinks (Phillips *et al.*, 2005).

In a study at the University of Connecticut, volunteers gained significantly more muscle when they consumed a daily whey supplement over a 9-month period while following a resistance training programme, compared with soy protein or carbohydrate supplements containing the same calories (Volek *et al.*, 2013). This is thought to be partly because whey is a 'fast' protein, which means it is digested and absorbed relatively fast, producing a rapid rise in EAAs in the bloodstream, and partly due to its higher content of leucine (Tang *et al.*, 2009; Boirie *et al.*, 1997; Dangin *et al.*, 2001). This amino acid is an important trigger and substrate for protein synthesis (Phillips & Van Loon, 2011; Burd *et al.*, 2009; Tang *et al.*, 2009). Although the exact mechanism isn't clear, whey seems to be the most effective protein in stimulating muscle growth because it produces the most rapid rise in blood leucine levels (Phillips *et al.*, 2011) (*see* 'Leucine and muscle protein synthesis', opposite).

Newer research suggests that consuming a mixture of 'fast' and 'slow' proteins may have additional benefits compared with whey protein since different proteins are digested at different rates. A study at the University of Texas Medical Branch has shown that a supplement containing a 19 g blend of whey, casein and soy protein produced a more sustained rise in blood

Leucine and muscle protein synthesis

Studies have shown that the amino acid leucine is responsible for the stimulatory effect of MPS (Anthony et al., 2001; Norton & Laymen, 2006). Without it, protein synthesis cannot take place. Much of the MPS-enhancing property of dairy protein is thought to be due to its high content of leucine. Leucine is a branched-chain amino acid (see p. 76), and acts as both a substrate (building block) and a trigger for MPS. It initiates the process of regenerating and building muscles so it is particularly important for those wanting to build strength and muscle mass. Leucine increases MPS by stimulating the mTOR (mammalian target of rapamycin) signalling pathway, which results in the formation of new muscle proteins.

It has been hypothesised that to maximise MPS, a 'leucine threshold' must be surpassed. This is the intake required to achieve maximum MPS and is thought be 2–3 g leucine per meal, perhaps as high as 3.5 g in older athletes (Drummond & Rasmussen, 2008; Katsanos et al., 2006). If leucine concentration is too low, mTOR deactivates and no MPS occurs.

In a study at the University of Maastricht, athletes who consumed a leucine/carbohydrate/protein supplement after resistance training had less muscle protein breakdown and greater MPS than those who consumed a supplement without leucine (Koopman et al., 2005).

Leucine is found widely in animal proteins, including eggs, milk and dairy products, meat, fish and poultry. It is found in particularly high concentrations in whey protein, which explains why whey supplements have been shown to increase MPS more than other sources. Table 4.2 shows the amounts of various foods that you would need to consume to get 2 g leucine and 20 g protein.

levels of amino acids and therefore a longer period of increased MPS following resistance exercise compared with the same amount of whey protein (Reidy et al., 2013). Whether this is more effective than consuming protein-rich foods (such as milk) is unclear but given that foods naturally contain a mixture of proteins (milk is a blend of casein and whey), plus they are sources of many other nutrients, natural food sources may be better options than supplements for most people.

It is not clear whether it is advantageous to consume liquid forms of protein, such as milk or whey protein shakes, rather than solid forms of protein (such as meat or eggs). A study at the

Table 4.2	FOODS SUPPLYING 2 G LEUCINE AND 20 G PROTEIN
600 ml milk	
85 g Cheddar cheese	
450 g plain yoghurt	
3 eggs	
85 g meat or poultry	
100 g fish	
17 g whey powder	

Australian Institute of Sport found that consuming liquid protein produced a more rapid rise in amino acid levels in the bloodstream following exercise (Burke *et al.*, 2012) . While this may increase MPS in the immediate post-exercise period, it does not necessarily mean that MPS is any different over 24 hours or that it results in bigger strength or muscle mass gains.

MILK AS A RECOVERY DRINK

Milk is a near-perfect recovery drink, in terms of glycogen replenishment, muscle protein synthesis and rehydration. Researchers at the University of Connecticut were among the first to demonstrate that skimmed milk produces a more favourable hormonal environment immediately following exercise compared with a carbohydrate sports drink (Miller *et al.*, 2002). This, they suggest, may spare body protein and encourage protein anabolism during recovery. Since then, milk as a recovery drink has been extensively investigated. University of Texas researchers found that drinking milk (any type: whole, semi-skimmed and skimmed) after resistance training resulted in muscle synthesis (Elliot, 2006). Several studies have shown that dairy milk promotes muscle manufacture and muscle gains more effectively than soy milk (Wilkinson, 2007; Phillips, 2005).

Milk appears to have a favourable effect on body composition. Canadian researchers found that when novice male weight trainers consumed skimmed milk as part of a 12-week resistance training programme, it promoted greater hypertrophy than isoenergetic soy or carbohydrate drinks (Hartman *et al.*, 2007). A similar study with women found that drinking skimmed milk after resistance exercise for 12 weeks reduced body fat levels and increased lean mass and strength (Josse *et al.*, 2010). Milk's beneficial effect on MPS is thought to be due to its whey content, which is rich in leucine and other branched-chain amino acids.

What's more, milk has been proven to be an effective rehydration drink. In 2007, researchers at Loughborough University showed that skimmed milk resulted in better post-exercise rehydration than either sports drinks or water (Shireffs *et al.*, 2007). Studies have also shown that consuming milk after training can help alleviate symptoms of exercise induced muscle damage, including delayed onset muscle soreness and reductions in muscle performance. The original benefits were demonstrated based on drinking quite a large volume of milk (1 litre) but recently, a smaller volume (500 ml) of milk was found to have similar effects on muscle performance, blood measures and muscle soreness in comparison to the larger volume (Cockburn *et al.*, 2012). In this study, 24 men consumed either 500 ml semi-skimmed milk, 1 litre semi-skimmed milk or 1 litre water after performing leg exercises. Those drinking either 500 ml or 1 litre milk experienced less muscle damage than those drinking water, with no difference between the two milk-drinking groups.

Many studies have highlighted the benefits of chocolate milk as a recovery drink, particularly after endurance exercise. Flavoured milk contains a 3 to 1 ratio of carbohydrate to protein and is therefore a good option for a recovery drink. In the first of these studies, researchers at Indiana University, US, showed that cyclists who consumed chocolate milk after an interval workout were able to recover faster and perform better than those consuming carbohydrate drink in an endurance workout performed 4 hours later (Karp *et al.*, 2006).

A 2008 study by researchers at Northumbria University found that athletes who drank 500 ml of semi-skimmed milk or chocolate milk immediately after training had less muscle soreness and more rapid muscle recovery compared with commercial sports drinks or water (Cockburn *et al.*, 2008).

A 2009 study from James Madison University, US, found that chocolate milk promoted better muscle recovery compared with a commercial sports drink (Gilson *et al.*, 2009). Football players who drank chocolate milk after training had less muscle damage and faster muscle recovery compared with those who consumed a sports drink with the same amount of calories.

University of Texas researchers found that chocolate milk not only promotes muscle glycogen recovery but also results in greater aerobic capacity, lean body mass and reduced body fat compared with carbohydrate (sports) drinks (Ferguson-Stegall *et al.*, 2011). The exact mechanism is not clear, but it is thought that the peptides released during the digestion of milk protein are responsible for alterations in protein metabolism and increasing training adaptations.

For longer, harder training sessions, extra carbohydrate may be needed to refuel energy stores. Researchers at the University of Texas at Austin found that consuming a bowl of wholegrain cereal plus milk was as effective at refuelling glycogen stores as sports drinks after 2 hours of moderate exercise (Kammer *et al.*,

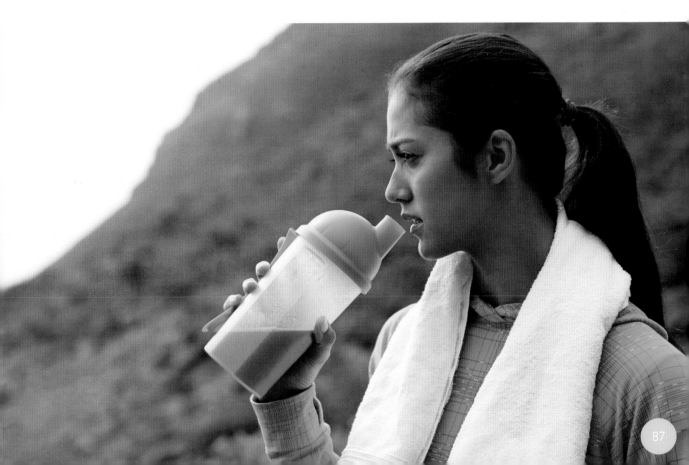

2009). It also promoted greater MPS compared with the sports drink.

ARE PROTEIN SUPPLEMENTS BETTER THAN FOOD SOURCES?

While many studies have used supplements, this was to isolate the effects of protein, it does not necessarily mean that supplements are better than good sources of protein.

Indeed, food sources of protein, such as milk, have been found to be just as effective as supplements (Wilkinson, 2007; Phillips, 2005). A US study found that consuming 237 ml of either whole milk or skimmed milk within an hour following resistance training resulted in greater protein synthesis (Elliot *et al.*, 2006). A Canadian study found that adding whey protein to a sports drink did not make any difference to the performance of cyclists in a 80 km time trial (Van Essen & Gibala, 2006). There is no evidence that protein supplements improve prformance or promote recovery better than food sources.

How can I meet my protein needs?

In practice, protein intakes generally reflect total calorie intake, so provided you are meeting your calorie needs from a wide variety of foods, you are likely to be getting enough protein. Dietary surveys show that most athletes already consume diets providing protein intakes above the maximum recommended level without the use of protein supplements.

But if you reduce your calorie intake or cut out entire food groups (for example, if you eat a vegan diet or you have a dairy allergy), you may find it more difficult to meet your protein needs.

Table 4.3 lists a wide range of foods containing protein. Animal sources generally provide higher levels of essential amino acids, but plant sources can also make a significant contribution to your daily protein intake. The key is to eat a wide variety of foods containing protein. This will not only ensure that you get a better balance of amino acids but also increases your intake of other nutrients such as fibre, vitamins, minerals and carbohydrate. For example, combining rice with pulses gives a better complement of amino acids needed to make new body proteins than eating either of these foods on their own. However, it is not necessary to always combine proteins within a single meal. Our bodies pool the amino acids we need as we eat them over a 24-hour period, and we use them as needed.

IS MORE PROTEIN BETTER?

Although some strength athletes and bodybuilders consume as much as 2–3 g/kg BW/day, there is no evidence that these high daily intakes result in further muscle mass and strength gains (Tipton & Wolfe, 2007.

Consuming more protein than you need certainly offers no advantage in terms of health or physical performance. Once your requirements have been met, additional protein will not be converted into muscle, nor will it further increase muscle size, strength or stamina.

The nitrogen-containing amino group of the protein is converted into a substance called urea in the liver. This is then passed to the kidneys and excreted in the urine. The remainder of the protein is converted into glucose and used as an energy substrate. It may either be used as fuel immediately or stored, usually as glycogen. If you are already eating enough carbohydrate to

Table 4.3	GOOD SOURCES OF PROTEIN		
Food		**Portion size**	**Protein (g)**
Meat and fish	Beef, fillet steak, grilled, lean	2 slices 105 g	31
	Chicken breast, grilled meat only	1 breast 130 g	39
	Turkey, light meat, roasted	2 slices 140 g	47
	Cod, poached	1 fillet 120 g	25
	Mackerel, grilled	1 fillet 150 g	31
	Tuna, canned in brine	1 small tin (100 g)	24
Dairy products and eggs	Cheese, cheddar	1 slice (25 g)	6
	Cottage cheese	2 tbsp (100 g)	12
	Milk (all types)	1 glass (250 ml)	8
	Low fat yoghurt, plain	1 carton (125 g)	6
	Low fat strained Greek yoghurt	3 tbsp (150 g)	15
	Eggs	2	12
Nuts and seeds	Peanuts, roasted and salted	1 handful (25 g)	7
	Cashew nuts, roasted and salted	1 handful (25 g)	5
	Walnuts	1 handful (25 g)	4
	Sunflower seeds	2 tbsp (32 g)	6
	Sesame seeds	2 tbsp (24 g)	4
Pulses	Baked beans	1 small tin (205 g)	10
	Red lentils, boiled	4 tbsp (200 g)	18
	Beans, boiled	4 tbsp (200 g)	18
	Chickpeas, boiled	4 tbsp (200 g)	18
Soya products	Soya 'milk', plain	1 glass (250 ml)	8
	Soya 'yoghurt', plain	1 carton (125 g)	5
	Tofu	Half a pack (100 g)	13
Quorn products	Quorn mince	4 tbsp (100 g)	15
	Quorn sausages	3 (100 g)	14
Grains and 'pseudograins'	Wholemeal bread	5 heaped tbsp (80 g)	8
	Wholemeal pasta, boiled	5 heaped tbsp (250 g)	10
	Brown rice, boiled	5 heaped tbsp (180 g)	7
	Quinoa, cooked	5 heaped tbsp (250 g)	11
	Oats	4 tbsp (50 g)	7

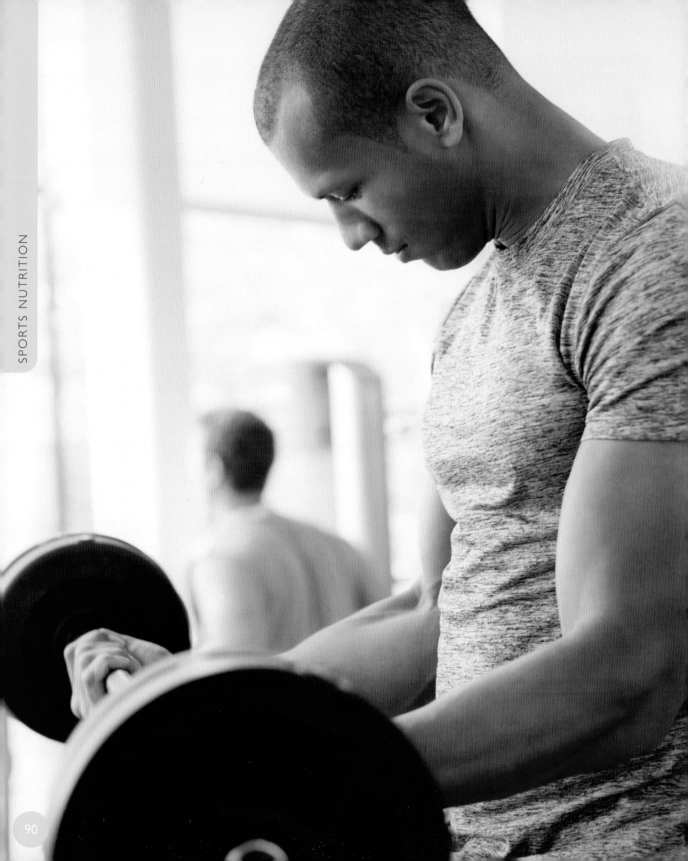

refill your glycogen stores, excess glucose may be converted into fat. However, in practice this does not occur to a great extent. Fat gain is usually the result of excessive calorie consumption. Recent studies have shown that eating protein increases the metabolic rate, so a significant proportion of the protein calories are oxidised and given off as heat (*see* Chapter 9). Thus, a slight excess of protein is unlikely to be converted into fat.

In a study carried out at McMaster University, Ontario, strength athletes were given either a low protein diet (0.86 g/kg body weight/day – similar to the RNI), a medium protein diet (1.4 g/kg body weight/day) or a high protein diet (2.3 g/kg body weight/day) for 13 days (Tarnopolsky *et al.*, 1992). The low protein diet, which was close to the RNI for sedentary people, caused the athletes to lose muscle mass. Both the medium and high protein diets resulted in an increased muscle mass, but the amount of the increase was the same for the two groups. In other words, no further benefits were gained by increasing the protein intake from 1.4 g to 2.4 g/kg body weight/day.

Similar findings were reported at Kent State University, Ohio. Researchers gave 12 young volunteers either a protein supplement (total daily protein was 2.62 g/kg body weight) or a carbohydrate supplement (total daily protein was 1.35 g/kg body weight) for 1 month, during which time they performed intense weight training 6 days a week (Lemon *et al.*, 1992). Nitrogen balance measurements were carried out after each diet and the researchers found that an intake of 1.4–1.5 g/kg body weight/day was needed to maintain nitrogen balance, although strength, muscle mass and size were the same with either level of protein intake.

The researchers concluded two main points. First, strength training approximately doubles your protein needs (compared with sedentary people). Secondly, increasing your protein intake does not enhance your strength, mass or size in a linear fashion. Once your optimal intake has been reached, additional protein is not converted into muscle.

IS TOO MUCH PROTEIN HARMFUL?

It was once thought that excess protein might cause liver or kidney damage and place excessive stress on these organs. However, this has never been demonstrated in healthy people, so it remains only a theoretical possibility (Tipton & Wolfe, 2007). Those with liver or kidney problems, however, are advised to consume a low protein diet.

It has also been claimed that eating too much protein leads to dehydration because extra water is drawn from the body's fluids to dilute and excrete the increased quantities of urea. The only evidence for this comes from a study reported at the 2002 Experimental Biology meeting in New Orleans, which found that a high protein diet (246 g daily) consumed for 4 weeks caused dehydration in trained athletes. Their blood urea nitrogen – a clinical test for proper kidney function – reached abnormal levels and they produced more concentrated urine. According to the researchers at the University of Connecticut, this could have been avoided by increasing their fluid intake. This is unlikely to be a problem if you drink enough fluids.

Fears that high protein diets cause an excessive excretion of calcium, increasing the risk of osteoporosis, are largely unfounded too. A study at the University of Maastricht, The Netherlands, found that a 21% protein diet produced no negative effect on calcium status compared with a 12% protein diet (Pannemans *et al.*, 1997).

In conclusion, while eating too much protein is unlikely to be harmful in the short term, it also offers no advantages.

Summary of key points

- Protein is needed for the maintenance, replacement and growth of body tissue. It is used to make the enzymes and hormones that regulate the metabolism, maintain fluid balance, and transport nutrients in and out of cells.
- Athletes require more than the current RNI for protein of 0.75 g/kg body weight/day for the general population.
- Additional protein is needed to compensate for the increased breakdown of protein during intense training and for the repair and recovery of muscle tissue after training.
- Strength and power athletes have additional needs to facilitate muscle protein synthesis.
- Current guidelines recommend an intake in the range 1.2–2.0 g/kg BW/day.
- During weight loss, a higher protein intake of 1.8–2.7 g/kg BW/day (or 2.3–3.1 g/kg fat-free mass), in conjunction with an energy deficit plus resistance training, may help prevent lean mass losses.
- Consuming protein plus carbohydrate before and during prolonged, high intensity exercise increases MPS during exercise and minimises protein breakdown.
- Consuming 0.25 g protein/kg BW in the post-exercise period increases training adaptation and enhances performance for both strength and endurance athletes. Older athletes may need as much as 0.4 g/kg BW per meal to stimulate maximum MPS.
- For maximum MPS, consume 0.25 g protein/kg BW in each meal and distribute your protein intake evenly throughout the day.
- 'High quality' proteins, such as milk and egg, are the best type of protein to consume after exercise.
- Leucine acts as both a substrate (building block) and a trigger for MPS.
- Protein intake above your optimal requirement will not result in further muscle mass or strength gains and is used as an energy substrate. However, there is no evidence that excess protein is harmful.
- Milk is a particularly valuable recovery food and has been shown to increase MPS, promote muscle repair, reduce post-exercise muscle soreness, promote rehydration, improve body composition and increase muscle mass and strength.
- Athletes should be able to meet their protein needs from a well-planned diet that matches their calorie needs.

Vitamins //and Minerals 5

Vitamins and minerals are often equated with vitality, energy and strength. Many people think of them as health enhancers, a plentiful supply being the secret to a long and healthy life.

In fact, vitamins and minerals do not in themselves provide energy. They are nutrients that, though required in tiny amounts, are essential for health as well as for physical performance. It is tempting to think that extra vitamins and minerals lead to better performance but consuming too much can sometimes be just as harmful as consuming too little.

This chapter explains what vitamins and minerals do, where they come from, and how exercise affects requirements. It considers whether athletes need more than the recommended daily amount and whether they need to take supplements.

The functions, sources, requirements and Safe Upper Limits (SULs) of vitamins and minerals are given in the Glossary of Vitamins and Minerals (Appendix 2). The table also examines the claims made for supplementation of vitamins and minerals and whether they could benefit athletic performance.

WHAT ARE VITAMINS?

Vitamins are required in tiny amounts for growth, health and physical well-being. There are 13 vitamins that your body cannot make (or which are only made in small amounts), so they must be supplied in your diet. Many form the essential parts of enzyme systems that are involved in energy production and exercise performance. Others are involved in the functioning of the immune system, the hormonal system and the nervous system.

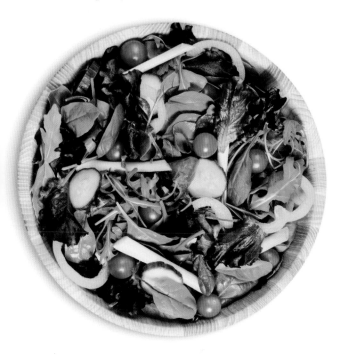

WHAT ARE MINERALS?

Minerals are inorganic elements that have many regulatory and structural roles in the body. There are about 20 minerals and trace elements that are essential for health. Some (such as calcium and phosphorus) form part of the structure of bones and teeth. Others are involved in controlling the fluid balance in tissues, muscle contraction, nerve function, enzyme secretion and the formation of red blood cells. Like vitamins, they cannot be made in the body and must be obtained in the diet.

HOW MUCH DO I NEED?

Everyone has different nutritional requirements. These vary according to age, size, level of physical activity and individual body chemistry. It is, therefore, impossible to state an intake that would be right for everyone. To find out your exact requirements, you would have to undergo a series of biochemical and physiological tests.

However, scientists have studied groups of people with similar characteristics, such as age and level of physical activity, and have come up with some estimates of requirements. The Reference Nutrient Intake (RNI) is the measure used in the UK, but the RNI value for a nutrient can vary from country to country. European Union (EU) regulations require Nutrient Reference Values (NRVs) to be shown on food and supplement labels. In the US, labels show the Daily Value (DV). RNIs are said to apply to 'average adults' and are only very rough guides.

RNI values are derived from studies of the physiological requirements of healthy people. For example, the RNI for a vitamin may be the amount needed to maintain a certain blood concentration of that vitamin. The RNI is not the amount of a nutrient recommended for optimum health or for athletic performance.

WHAT ARE DIETARY REFERENCE VALUES (DRVS)?

In 1991 the Department of Health published *Dietary Reference Values for Food Energy and Nutrients for the United Kingdom* (Department of Health, 1991). A Dietary Reference Value (DRV) is a generic term for various daily dietary recommendations and covers three values that have been set for each nutrient:

1. The **Estimated Average Requirement** (**EAR**) is the amount of a nutrient needed by an average person, so 50% of the population will need more and 50% will need less.
2. The **Reference Nutrient Intake** (**RNI**) is the amount of a nutrient that should cover the needs of 97.5% of the population. It is more than most people require, and only a very few people (2.5%) will exceed it.
3. The **Lower Reference Nutrient Intake** (**LRNI**) is the amount of a nutrient that is enough for the small number of people who have low needs (about 2.5% of the population). Most people will need more than this amount.

Individual nutritional requirements vary widely and these values are based on population groups, not individuals. Athletes and sportspeople may exceed the upper limits because they have the highest requirements. EARs are used for energy, RNIs are often used as a reference amount for population groups.

The RNI is not a target intake to aim for – it is only a guideline. It should cover the needs of most people but, of course, it is possible that many athletes may need more than the RNI, due to their higher energy expenditure.

In practice, if you are eating consistently less than the RNI, you may be lacking in that particular nutrient.

How are DRVs set?

First of all, scientists have to work out what is the minimum amount of a particular nutrient that a person needs to be healthy. Once this has been established, scientists usually add on a safety margin, to take account of individual variations. No two people will have exactly the same requirement. Next, a storage requirement is assessed. This allows for a small reserve of the nutrient to be kept in the body.

Unfortunately, scientific evidence of human vitamin and mineral requirements is fairly scanty and contradictory. A lot of scientific guesswork is inevitably involved, and results are often extrapolated from animal studies.

In practice, DRVs are arrived at through a compromise between selected scientific data and good judgement. They vary from country to country and are always open to debate.

CAN A BALANCED DIET PROVIDE ALL THE VITAMINS AND MINERALS I NEED?

Most athletes eat more food than the average sedentary person. With the right food choices, this means you should automatically achieve a higher vitamin and mineral intake. However, in practice many athletes do not plan their diets well enough, or they may restrict their calorie intake so it can be difficult to obtain sufficient amounts of vitamins and minerals from food. Vitamin losses also occur during food processing,

preparation and cooking, thus further reducing your actual intake. Intensive farming practices have resulted in crops with a lower nutrient content. For example, the use of agro-chemicals has depleted the mineral content of the soil so plants have a smaller mineral content. EU pricing policy, which keeps prices artificially high, has resulted in mountains of cauliflowers, cabbages and other produce, which remain in storage for up to a year before being sold in supermarkets. Obviously, considerable vitamin losses may have occurred during that time.

Eating a balanced diet may not always be easy in practice, particularly if you travel a lot, work shifts or long hours, train and eat at irregular times, eat on the move or are unable to purchase and prepare your own meals. Planning and eating a well-balanced diet requires considerably more effort under these circumstances, so you may not be getting all the vitamins and minerals you need. A deficient intake is also likely if you are on a restricted diet (e.g. eating less than 1500 calories a day for a period of time or excluding a food group from your regular diet).

A number of surveys have shown that many sportspeople do not achieve an adequate intake of vitamins and minerals from their diet (Short & Short, 1983; Steen & McKinney, 1986; Bazzare et al., 1986). Low intakes of certain minerals and vitamins are more common among female athletes compared with males. A study of 60 female athletes found that calcium, iron and zinc intakes were less than 100% of the RNI (Cupisti et al., 2002). US researchers also measured low intakes of vitamin E, calcium, iron, magnesium, zinc and phosphorus in US national figure skaters (Ziegler, 1999). This was correlated with lower than recommended intakes of fruit, vegetables, dairy and high protein foods. Study of US elite female heptathletes by researchers at the University of Arizona found that while average nutrient intakes were greater than 67% of the RNI, vitamin E intakes fell below this minimum level (Mullins, 2001). However, more than half of the athletes were taking vitamin and mineral supplements, which would boost their overall intake. A study of 58 swimmers found that 71% of males and 93% of females did not meet the recommended intakes for at least one of the antioxidant vitamins (Farajian *et al.*, 2004).

All these results suggest that athletes do not consume a well-balanced diet, with not enough fruit and vegetables in particular.

HOW DOES EXERCISE INCREASE MY REQUIREMENTS OF VITAMINS AND MINERALS?

Regular intense exercise places additional demands on your body, which means the requirement for many micronutrients is likely to be higher than the RDAs for the general population. Micronutrients play an important role in energy production, haemoglobin synthesis, bone health, immune function, and protection of the body against oxidative damage. They help with synthesis and repair of muscle tissue during recovery. As a result, greater intakes of micronutrients may be required to cover increased needs for building, repair and maintenance of lean body mass in athletes. Failure to get enough micronutrients could leave you lacking in energy and susceptible to minor infections and illnesses.

Vitamin E

Vitamin E is a fat-soluble vitamin found in nuts, seeds, plant oils, oily fish, avocados and egg yolk, as well as a powerful antioxidant, which helps prevent the oxidation of fatty acids in cell membranes and protects the cell from damage. Early studies suggested that vitamin E supplementation reduced the amount of free radical damage following prolonged intense cycling to exhaustion, compared with a placebo (Rokitzki *et al.*, 1994).

However, more recent studies have shown that supplementation may reduce training adaptations and result in decreased performance (*see also* 'Antioxidants', p. 109). For example, triathletes who took vitamin E supplements (800 IU) daily for 2 months performed no better than those who took a placebo (Nieman *et al.*, 2004). Although blood levels of vitamin E were higher, this did not reduce markers of oxidative stress or translate into any improvement in performance. Similarly, another study found that 8 weeks of vitamin E supplementation did not reduce markers of oxidative stress or improve exercise performance (Gaeini *et al.*, 2006). And more recently, Norwegian researchers showed that supplementation with vitamins E and C did not improve endurance performance compared with a placebo (Paulsen *et al.*, 2013). This is because the vitamin supplements interfered with exercise-induced cell-signalling in cell muscle fibres.

Taking high doses of vitamin E supplements will not confer any performance advantage and may blunt training adaptations. Aim to get your vitamin E from food rather than supplements.

Vitamin C

Vitamin C has several exercise-related functions. It is required for the formation of connective tissue and certain hormones (e.g. adrenaline), which are produced during exercise; it is involved in the formation of red blood cells, which enhances iron absorption; it is a powerful anti-oxidant, which, like vitamin E, can also protect against exercise-related cell damage.

However, there is little evidence that vitamin C supplementation improves performance in athletes who are not deficient in the vitamin. In fact, rather than improving exercise performance, high doses (more than 1000 mg) of vitamin C may have detrimental effects. In a double blind randomised study, athletes who took vitamin C supplements (1000 mg/day) experienced a reduction in endurance capacity after 8 weeks (Gomez-Cabrera *et al.*, 2008). That's because supplements prevented muscle cell adaptations (e.g. an increase in enzyme production) to exercise, resulting in no improvement in aerobic capacity.

Norwegian researchers found that people who took high dose supplements of vitamins C (1000 mg) and E (235 mg) for 11 weeks gained no performance benefit compared with those taking a placebo (Paulsen *et al.*, 2013). Those taking the supplements produced fewer extra mitochondria, which are needed to improve endurance. The researchers concluded that vitamins C and E should be used with caution as they may 'blunt' the way muscles respond to exercise.

A review of studies concluded that vitamin C supplementation reduced the benefits of training and resulted in slower recovery and strength gains (Adams *et al.*, 2014).

Lower doses of vitamin C (< 1000 mg/day) may be useful if you are involved in prolonged high intensity training because it may stabilise

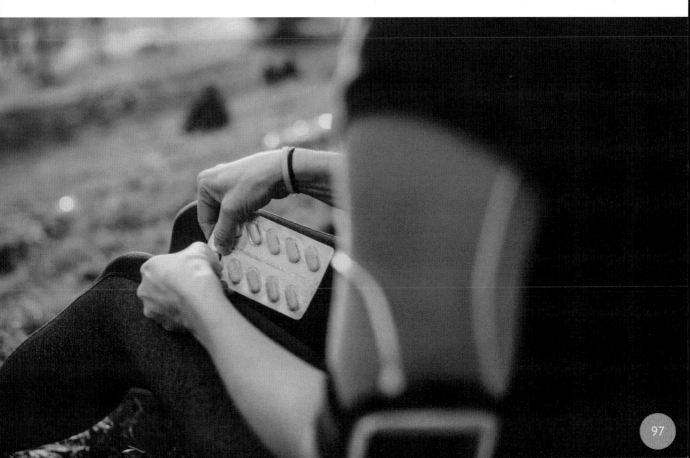

cell membranes and protect against viral attack. One study (Peters *et al.*, 1993) found a reduced incidence in upper respiratory tract infections in ultra-marathon runners after taking 600 mg vitamin C for 21 days prior to the race. Another study at the University of North Carolina, US, found that vitamin C supplementation before and after resistance exercise reduced post-exercise muscle soreness and muscle damage and promoted recovery (Bryer & Goldfarb, 2006). However, you should aim to get your vitamin C from food before considering supplements.

Vitamin D

The role of this vitamin in maintaining bone health is well recognised, but following the discovery of the vitamin D receptor in muscle tissue, recent research has focused on its role in muscle structure and function. Several studies suggest that vitamin D deficiency is widespread among athletes, particularly those in northern latitudes who train mainly indoors or get little sun exposure, or who do not consume vitamin D-rich foods (Larson-Meyer & Willis, 2010; Lovell, 2008; Meier *et al.*, 2004). One study measured low serum vitamin D levels (less than 50 ng/ml) in 38 out of 61, (62%) UK athletes (Close *et al.*, 2013). This is an area of concern because there is increasing evidence that a deficiency reduces muscle function, strength and performance (Hamilton, 2011). Potentially, vitamin D deficiency may also increase the risk of injury and illness risk, and have a detrimental effect on your training and performance (Halliday, 2011).

Several studies have observed a correlation between vitamin D status and athletic performance (Larson-Meyer & Willis, 2010). Low levels are associated with reduced performance while high levels may enhance performance. A review of studies has highlighted a seasonal variation in performance (Cannell, 2009). The latter found that performance peaks in the summer months (when vitamin D levels peak), declines in winter months (when vitamin D levels decline), and reaches its lowest point when vitamin D levels are at their lowest. Peak athletic performance seems to occur when vitamin D levels approach those obtained by natural, full body, summer sun exposure, which is above 50 ng/ml. An adequate vitamin D status may also help protect against acute and chronic medical conditions, such as stress fractures, muscle weakness, impaired muscle function and reduced performance. Getting adequate levels of vitamin D, whether from sun exposure or diet, is therefore important for optimal performance.

Supplementation is a controversial area and scientific opinion is divided. Some believe that it would be beneficial for those who get little sun exposure or perhaps during the winter months when levels of vitamin D are low (IOC, 2011; Halliday, 2011). Others say that vitamin D supplements may not benefit athletic performance (Powers *et al.*, 2011). If you think you may be at risk of vitamin D deficiency, you should consult your doctor and/or sports nutritionist, who may recommend a simple blood test to determine whether you would benefit from vitamin D supplements. The US Institute of Medicine classifies blood serum vitamin D3 below 50 nmol/l as inadequate (Heaney, 2011). The optimal level of vitamin D is not established but researchers recommend a blood concentration above 75 ng/ml (Heaney, 2013).

Because Vitamin D is found only in a small number of foods (oily fish, egg yolk, liver and some fortified breakfast cereals, yogurts and spreads), it may be difficult to get enough from food alone. From April to September most of us can get all the vitamin D we need from sunlight exposure but in winter months Public Health England recommends taking a 10 mcg supplement. People at high risk of deficiency (with dark skin or with little outdoor access) should take a supplement all year round.

B vitamins

The B vitamins thiamin (B_1), riboflavin (B_2) and niacin (B_3) are involved in releasing energy from food. Since requirements for these are based on the amount of carbohydrate and calories consumed, athletes do need more than sedentary people. In general, it is easy to obtain these vitamins from wholegrain bread, breakfast cereals, oatmeal and brown rice. If you are restricting your calorie intake (e.g. on a fat-loss programme) or you eat lots of refined rather than wholegrain carbohydrates, you may be missing out on B vitamins. To compensate for any shortfall, you may benefit from a multivitamin supplement that contains at least 100% of the RNI of the B vitamins.

Vitamin B6 is involved in protein and amino acid metabolism. It is needed for making red blood cells and new proteins, so getting the right amount of vitamin B6 is very important to athletes.

Pantothenic acid (vitamin B_5) is necessary for making glucose and fatty acids from other metabolites in the body. It is also used in the manufacture of steroid hormones and brain chemicals. Obviously, a deficiency would be detrimental to health and athletic performance.

Folic acid and vitamin B12

These are both involved with red blood cell production in the bone marrow. They are also needed for cell division, and protein and DNA manufacture. Clearly, exercise increases all of these processes and therefore your requirements for folic acid and vitamin B_{12}. Vegans, who eat no animal products, must obtain vitamin B_{12} from fortified foods such as Marmite and breakfast cereals or fermented foods such as tempeh and miso. Taking a multivitamin supplement is a good insurance.

Beta-carotene

Beta-carotene is one of 600 carotenoid pigments that give fruit and vegetables their yellow, orange and red colours. They are not vitamins but act as antioxidants by protecting cells from free radical damage. Beta-carotene enhances the antioxidant function of vitamin E, helping to regenerate it after it has disarmed free radicals. However, carotenoids function most effectively together, so it is best to take these nutrients packaged together, in a supplement or in food.

Calcium

Calcium is an important mineral in bone formation, but it also plays an important role in muscle growth, muscle contraction and nerve transmission. While the body is able to increase or decrease the absorption of this mineral according to its needs, extra calcium is recommended for female athletes with low oestrogen levels (*see* p. 222). Weight-bearing exercise, such as running and weight training, increases bone mass and calcium absorption so it is important to get enough calcium in your diet.

Iron

Iron is important for athletes. Its major function is in the formation of haemoglobin (which transports oxygen in the blood) and myoglobin (which transports oxygen in the muscle cells).

Many muscle enzymes involved in energy metabolism require iron. Clearly, athletes have higher requirements for iron compared with sedentary people. Furthermore, iron losses may occur during exercise that involves pounding of the feet, such as running, aerobics and step aerobics. Also at risk of iron deficiency are women who have been pregnant in the last year (lower iron stores) and athletes who eat less than about 2000 kcal a day. Athletes who tend to avoid red meat, a rich source of iron, need to ensure they get iron from other sources or supplements. Iron deficiency and sports anaemia are discussed in detail in Chapter 11 (*see* p. 223). Rich food sources of iron include meat and offal, wholegrain cereals, egg yolks, beans, lentils, green leafy vegetables, dried apricots, nuts, seeds, sardines and tuna.

CAN VITAMIN AND MINERAL SUPPLEMENTS IMPROVE YOUR PERFORMANCE?

Many studies have been carried out over the years using varying doses of supplements. In the vast majority of cases, scientists have been unable to measure significant improvements in the performance of healthy athletes. Where a beneficial effect has been observed – for example, increased endurance – this has tended to be in athletes who started with a suboptimal vitamin or mineral status. Taking supplements simply restored the athletes' nutrient stores to 'normal' levels.

In other words, low body stores or deficient intakes can adversely affect your performance, but vitamin and mineral supplements taken in excess of your requirements will not necessarily produce a further improvement in performance. More does not mean better!

The scientific consensus is that vitamin and mineral supplements are unnecessary for those consuming a varied diet that provides enough energy to maintain your body weight (Rodrigues *et al.*, 2009).

To find out if your diet is deficient in any nutrient, you should consult a registered nutritionist or registered dietitian (look for the initials RNutr or RD, *see* online resources on pp. 377–78) who will be able to analyse your diet and give you advice about whether supplements will have health benefits for you in your particular circumstances.

WHO MAY BENEFIT FROM TAKING SUPPLEMENTS?

Research shows that one in three people take some form of vitamin or mineral supplement –

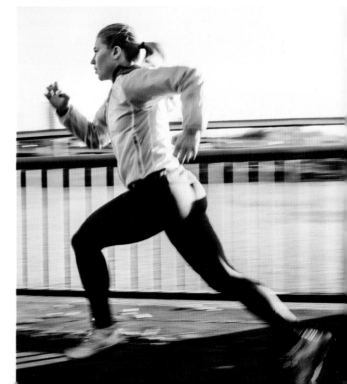

the most popular being multivitamins. A study of male triathletes found that over 60% routinely took vitamin supplements (Knez & Peake, 2010). All athletes consumed less vitamin D than the recommended daily intake but everyone consumed adequate amounts of all other nutrients. Obviously, supplements are not a substitute for poor or lazy eating habits. If you think you may be lacking in vitamins and minerals, try to adjust your diet to include more vitamin- and mineral-rich foods.

As a temporary measure, you may benefit from taking supplements if:

• you have erratic eating habits
• you eat less than 1500 kcal a day
• you are pregnant (folic acid)
• you eat out a lot/rely on fast foods
• you are a vegan (vitamin B$_{12}$ and possibly other nutrients)
• you are anaemic (iron)
• you have a major food allergy or intolerance (e.g. milk)
• you are a heavy smoker or drinker
• you are ill or convalescing.

CAN HIGH DOSES OF SUPPLEMENTS BE HARMFUL?

Except perhaps in the case of vitamin A from liver (owing to modern animal feeding practices), it is almost impossible to overdose on vitamins and minerals from food. Problems are more likely to arise from the indiscriminate use of supplements, so always follow the guidelines on the label or the advice of a registered nutritionist or dietitian. As a rule of thumb, never take more than 10 times the RNI of the fat-soluble vitamins A and D, and no more than the RNI for any mineral.

Certain vitamins and minerals taken in high doses can be harmful. The Expert Group on Vitamins and Minerals in the UK have published safe upper levels for vitamins and minerals (Food Standards Agency, 2003). In particular, it warns against high doses of:

• Chromium in the form of chromium picolinate – may cause cancer, although up to 10 mg/day of other forms of chromium is unlikely to be harmful.
• Vitamin C – although excess vitamin C is excreted in the urine, levels above 1000 mg/day may result in stomach cramps, diarrhoea and nausea.
• Iron – levels above 17 mg/day may result in constipation and discomfort through an upset or bloated stomach.
• Vitamin D – large doses can cause weakness, thirst, increased urination and, if taken for a long period, result in high blood pressure and kidney stones.
• Vitamin A – large doses over a prolonged period can cause nausea, skin changes such as flakiness, liver damage and birth defects in unborn babies. Pregnant women are advised to avoid vitamin A supplements, fish liver oils and concentrated food sources of vitamin A such as liver and liver paté.
• Vitamin B$_6$ – doses over 10 mg/day taken for a long period may lead to numbness, persistent pins and needles and unsteadiness (a type of neuropathy).

HOW ARE SUPPLEMENTS REGULATED?

Vitamin and mineral supplements are regulated under the EU Food Supplements Directive

(2002, amended August 2005). Manufacturers can only use nutrients and ingredients from a 'permitted' list, and then within maximum limits. Each ingredient must undergo extensive safety tests before it is allowed on the permitted list and, therefore, into a supplement. Manufacturers must also provide scientific proof to support a product's claims and ensure that it is clearly labelled.

CAN SUPPLEMENTS CAUSE IMBALANCES?

Taking single vitamins or minerals can easily lead to imbalances and deficiencies. Many interact with each other, competing for absorption, or enhancing or impairing each other's functions. For example, iron, zinc and calcium share the same absorption and transport system, so taking large doses of iron can reduce the uptake of zinc and calcium. For healthy bones, a finely tuned balance of vitamin D, calcium, phosphorus, magnesium, zinc, manganese, fluoride, chloride, copper and boron is required. Vitamin C enhances the absorption of iron, converting it from its inactive ferric form to the active ferrous form. Most of the B vitamins are involved in energy metabolism, so a short-term shortage of one may be compensated for by a larger than normal use of another.

If in doubt about supplements, it is safest to choose a multivitamin and mineral formulation rather than individual supplements. Single supplements should be taken only upon the advice of your doctor or nutritionist.

ARE 'NATURAL' VITAMIN SUPPLEMENTS BETTER THAN SYNTHETIC?

There is no proof that so-called 'natural' or 'food state' vitamin supplements are better absorbed than synthetic vitamins. The majority have an identical chemical structure. In other words, they are the same thing and such terms on supplement labels are meaningless. Tests have shown that a relatively new type of supplement called 'food form' vitamins and minerals are more readily absorbed than synthetic vitamins. 'Food form' vitamins and minerals are micronutrients that are grown from food-based (yeast) cultures in the lab and are therefore intricately bound to protein, in a similar way as naturally occurring vitamins in food. That means you need to take lower doses for maximum effect.

ARE TIME-RELEASE SUPPLEMENTS BETTER THAN NORMAL SYNTHETIC SUPPLEMENTS?

Time-release vitamins are coated with protein and embedded in micropellets within the supplement. In theory, the supplement should take longer to dissolve, with the protein coating slowing down vitamin absorption. However, there is little evidence that this is the case or that they are better for you. Some may not even dissolve fully and end up passing straight through the digestive tract. If you take any supplement with a meal, the absorption of the vitamins and minerals is retarded anyway by the carbohydrate/fat/protein in the food. So, it is not worth paying extra money for time-release supplements.

HOW SHOULD I CHOOSE A MULTIVITAMIN/MINERAL SUPPLEMENT?

If you are consuming a healthy diet that meets your calorie and macronutrient requirements, you probably won't benefit from multivitamin supplements. High doses will not enhance exercise performance or health. While diet should always come first, a well-formulated multivitamin and mineral supplement acts as a nutritional safety net to ensure you obtain all the nutrients you need from your diet. Here are some basic guidelines.

- Check it contains at least 23 vitamins and minerals.
- Check the percentages. In general, the amounts of each vitamin should be approximately 100% of the NRV stated on the label, but below the safe upper limit (*see* Appendix 2).
- Avoid supplements containing more than 100% of the NRV of any mineral as these nutrients compete for absorption and can be harmful in doses higher than the NRV.
- Choose beta-carotene rather than vitamin A – it is a more powerful antioxidant and has no harmful side effects in high doses.
- Avoid supplements with unnecessary ingredients such as sweeteners, colours, artificial flavours and talc (a bulking agent).
- Check the supplement contains at least 5 mcg (200 IU) vitamin D, the EU NRV (10 mcg or 400 IU in US).
- For women, check the supplement contains 14 mg iron, the EU NRV (18 mg in US).
- Take with food and water.

Antioxidants

WHAT ARE ANTIOXIDANTS?

Antioxidants are enzymes and nutrients in the blood that 'disarm' free radicals (*see* right) and render them harmless. They work as free radical scavengers by donating one of their own electrons to 'neutralise' the free radicals. Fortunately, your body has a number of natural defences against free radicals. They include various enzymes (e.g.

superoxide dismutase, glutathione, peroxidase) which have minerals such as manganese, selenium and zinc incorporated in their structure; vitamins C and E, as well as hundreds of other natural substances in plants, called phytochemicals. These include carotenoids (such as beta-carotene), plant pigments, bioflavonoids and tannins.

WHAT ARE FREE RADICALS?

Free radicals are atoms or molecules with an unpaired electron and are produced all the time in our bodies as a result of normal metabolism and energy production. They can easily generate other free radicals by snatching an electron from any nearby molecule, and exposure to cigarette smoke, pollution, exhaust fumes, UV light and stress can increase their formation.

In large numbers, free radicals have the potential to wreak havoc in the body. Free radical damage is thought to be responsible for heart disease, many cancers, aging and post-exercise muscle soreness, as unchecked free radicals can damage cell membranes and genetic material (DNA), destroy enzymes, disrupt red blood cell membranes, and oxidise LDL cholesterol in the bloodstream, thus also increasing the risk of atherosclerosis or the furring of arteries – the first stage of heart disease. Studies have demonstrated increased levels of free radicals following exercise and these have been held partly responsible for muscle soreness, pain, discomfort, oedema (fluid retention) and tenderness post-exercise (Halliwell & Gutteridge, 1985).

Not all free radicals are damaging. Some help to kill germs, fight bacteria and heal cuts. The problem arises when too many are formed and they cannot be controlled by the body's defence system.

Table 5.1	FOOD SOURCES OF ANTIOXIDANTS	
	Antioxidant	**Source**
Vitamins	Vitamin C	Most fruit and vegetables, especially blackcurrants, strawberries, oranges, tomatoes, broccoli, green peppers, baked potatoes
	Folate	Spinach, broccoli, curly kale, green cabbage and other green leafy vegetables
	Vitamin E	Sunflower/safflower/corn oil, sunflower seeds, sesame seeds, almonds, peanuts, peanut butter, avocado, oily fish, egg yolk
Minerals	Selenium	Whole grains, vegetables, meat
	Copper	Whole grains, nuts, liver
	Manganese	Wheatgerm, bread, cereals, nuts
	Zinc	Bread, wholegrain pasta, grains, nuts, seeds, eggs
Carotenoids	Beta-carotene	Carrots, red peppers, spinach, spring greens, sweet potatoes, mango, cantaloupe melon, dried apricots
	Alpha- and gamma-carotene	Red coloured fruit, red and green coloured vegetables Tomatoes, watermelon
Flavonoids	Flavanols and polyphenols	Fruit, vegetables, tea, coffee, red wine, garlic, onions
Phytochemicals	Canthaxanthin	Tomatoes, watermelon
	Coumaric acid	Green peppers, tomatoes, carrots
	Allicin saponins	Onions, garlic, leeks
	Glucosinolates	Broccoli, cabbage, cauliflower, Brussels sprouts
	Sulforaphane	Broccoli
	Lycopene	Tomatoes
	Lutein	Green vegetables
	D-limonene	Pith of citrus fruits
	Quercetin	Onions, garlic, apples, grapes
	Phenols	Grapes
	Resveratrol	Grape skins, red wine
	Ellagic acid	Grapes, strawberries, cherries

HOW DOES EXERCISE AFFECT FREE RADICAL LEVELS?

Because exercise increases oxygen consumption, there is an increased generation of free radicals. No one knows exactly how or why exercise does this, but it is thought to be connected to energy metabolism. During the final steps of ATP production (from carbohydrates or fats), electrons (the negative particles of atoms) sometimes get off course and collide with other molecules, creating free radicals.

Another source is the damage done to muscle cell membranes during high intensity eccentric exercise, such as heavy-weight training or plyometrics exercise, causing minor tears and injury to the muscles that results in the production of free radicals.

Other factors such as increased lactic acid production, increased haemoglobin breakdown and heat generation may be involved too. In essence, the more you exercise, the more free radicals you generate.

WHAT ARE THE BEST SOURCES OF ANTIOXIDANTS?

The best source of antioxidants is the natural one: food! There are hundreds of natural substances in food called phytochemicals. These substances, which are found in plant foods, have antioxidant properties that are not present in supplements. Each appears to have a slightly different effect and to protect against different types of cancer and other degenerative diseases. For example, the phytochemicals in soya beans may prevent the development of hormone dependent cancers, such as breast, ovarian and prostate cancer, while those in garlic can slow down tumour development. It is therefore wise to obtain as wide a range of phytochemicals from food as possible.

Table 5.1 lists the food sources for the various antioxidants.

Summary of key points

- Vitamin and mineral requirements depend on age, body size, activity level and individual metabolism.
- DVRs should be used as a guide for the general population; they are not targets and do not take account of the needs of athletes.
- Regular and intense exercise increases the requirements for a number of vitamins and minerals. However, there are no official recommendations for athletes.
- Low intakes can adversely affect health and performance. However, high intakes exceeding requirements will not necessarily improve performance.
- Vitamins A, D and B_6 and a number of minerals may be toxic in high doses (more than 10 × RNI). Indiscriminate supplementation may lead to nutritional imbalances and deficiencies.
- Due to an erratic lifestyle or restricted food intake, many athletes consume suboptimal amounts of vitamins and minerals. Therefore a supplement containing a broad spectrum of vitamins and minerals would benefit their long-term health and performance.
- A well-formulated supplement should contain 100% of the NRV for vitamins (but below the safe upper limit) and no more than 100% of the NRV for minerals.

Sports
// supplements

6

The most effective way to develop your natural sports ability and achieve your fitness goals is through consistent and efficient training combined with optimal nutrition. But there is a huge variety of sports supplements marketed to athletes, including pills, powders, drinks, gels and bars, promising greater stamina, improved strength, quicker recovery and less body fat.

Many athletes believe supplements are an essential component for sports success and it has been estimated that the majority of elite athletes are using some form of performance-enhancing agent. A study of 440 elite male and female athletes at the University of Calgary Sport Medicine Centre found that 87% used supplements regularly (Lun *et al.*, 2012). A study of Canadian varsity athletes found that 99% took supplements (Kristiansen *et al.*, 2005). A US study of collegiate varsity athletes found that 65% used some type of supplement regularly (Herbold *et al.*, 2004). The most commonly used supplements in the studies were vitamin/minerals, carbohydrate supplements, creatine and protein supplements. Creatine and ephedra are more popular among bodybuilders than other athletes, according to a study at Long Island University, New York, US (Morrison *et al.*, 2004). Most athletes in the studies said they took supplements to improve their health and athletic performance, reduce body fat or increase muscle mass.

Sifting through the multitude of products on offer can be an overwhelming task for athletes. It can be hard to pinpoint which ones work,

Definition of sports supplements and ergogenic aids

Sports supplements are a category of nutritional supplements whose purpose is to supplement the normal diet to improve general health and well-being or enhance sporting performance. They may include tablets, capsules, powders, drinks and bars, which claim to help with building muscle, increasing endurance, weight gain or loss, improving suppleness, rehydrating, aiding recovery or overcoming a mineral deficiency.

Ergogenic aids are defined as any external influence created to enhance sport performance. They can include sports supplements as well as illegal drugs and methods.

especially when advertising claims sound so persuasive. Scientific research may be exaggerated or used selectively by manufacturers trying to sell a product. Testimonials from well-known athletes are also a common ploy that is used to hype products. In this chapter, guidelines are given for evaluating the claims of supplements. But you need to be wary of all ergogenic products because of the risk of contamination with prohibited substances not listed on the label. Some supplements, such as ephedrine, are sold

Legislation

There are no specific compositional or labelling rules for sports products and supplements in the European Union (EU). They are regulated by general EU food legislation. According to the European Food Safety Authority (EFSA), sports nutrition products should be considered as 'normal foods', not specialist products (EFSA, 2015).

Guidelines for evaluating the claims of sports supplements*

How valid is the claim?

- Does the claim made by the manufacturer of the product match the science of nutrition and exercise, as you know it? If it sounds too good to be true, then it probably isn't valid.
- Does the amount and form of the active ingredient claimed to be present in the supplement match that used in the scientific studies on this ergogenic aid?
- Does the claim make sense for the sport for which the claim is made?

How good is the supportive evidence?

- Is the evidence presented based on testimonials or scientific studies?
- What is the quality of the science? Check the credentials of the researchers (look for university-based or independent) and the journal in which the research was published (look for a peer-reviewed journal reference). Did the manufacturer sponsor the research?
- Read the study to find out whether it was properly designed and carried out. Check that it contains phrases such as 'double-blind placebo controlled', i.e. that a 'control group' was included in the study and that a realistic amount of the ergogenic substance/placebo was used.
- The results should be clearly presented in an unbiased manner with appropriate statistical procedures. Check that the results seem feasible and the conclusions follow from the data.

Is the supplement safe and legal?

- Are there any adverse effects?
- Does the supplement contain toxic or unknown substances?
- Is the substance contraindicated in people with a particular health problem?
- Is the product illegal or banned by any athletic organisations?

* Adapted from ACSM/ADA/DC (2000), Butterfield (1996), Clark (1995).

through the internet, but are banned in sport and could result in a positive doping test.

This chapter examines the evidence for some of the most popular supplements and provides an expert rating on their effectiveness and safety.

Are sports supplements safe?

There is currently no specific European or national legislation governing the safety of sports supplements. As they are classified as foods, supplements are not subject to the same strict manufacturing, safety testing or labelling requirements as licensed medicines. This means that there is no guarantee that a supplement lives up to its claims.

Moreover, as many supplements are sold through the internet, it is difficult to regulate the market and there remains the risk of purchasing contaminated products. Contaminants – anabolic androgenic steroids and other prohibited stimulants – have been found in many different supplements. In 2012, 44% of UK Anti-Doping's positive tested cases were caused by prohibited substances contained in supplements (LGC, 2015). Inadvertent contamination may be caused by cross-contamination during manufacturing or through poor raw ingredient sourcing.

The largest survey was from the International Olympic Committee-accredited laboratory in Cologne. They looked for steroids in 634 supplements and found 15% contained substances – including nandrolone – that would lead to a failed drugs test (Geyer, 2004); 19% of UK samples were contaminated. In another report, Swiss researchers found different substances than those declared on the labels, including testosterone, in seven out of 17 pro-hormone supplements, i.e. 41% of the supplements (Kamber, 2001).

Advice to UK athletes on the use of supplements

In light of concerns about contamination and poor labelling of supplements, UK Sport, the British Olympic Association, the British Paralympic Association, National Sports Medicine Institute and the Home Country Sports Councils have issued a position statement on supplements. They advise UK athletes to be 'extremely cautious' about the use of any supplement. No guarantee can be given that any particular supplement, including vitamins and minerals, ergogenic aids and herbal remedies, is free from prohibited substances as these products are not licensed and are not subject to the same strict manufacturing and labelling requirements as licensed medicines. Anti-doping rules are based on the principle of strict liability and therefore supplements are taken at an athlete's risk. Athletes sign a code of conduct agreeing that they are responsible for what they take. Athletes are advised to consult a medical practitioner, accredited sports dietitian or registered nutritionist before taking supplements. For more information about drugs in sports, see The Global Drug Information Database www.globaldro.com.

An analysis of 58 supplements purchased through standard retail outlets in the USA by HFL Sport in 2007 found that 25% contained steroids and 11% were contaminated with stimulants. In 2008, HFL undertook an analysis of 152 supplements purchased through standard retail outlets within the UK and found that over 10% were contaminated with steroids and/or stimulants (Judkins, 2008).

A 2012 investigation by the Medicines and Healthcare Products Regulatory Agency (MHRA) found 84 illegal products such as energy and muscle gain products containing dangerous ingredients such as steroids, stimulants and hormones (MHRA, 2012).

The most common supplements associated with inadvertent doping include pre-workout formulas, 'fat burners' and testosterone boosters. These may contain banned substances such as ephedrine, androstenedione, androstenediol, dehydroepiandrosterone (DHEA), 19-Norandrostenedione, 19-Norandrostenediol, amphetamines and ma huang.

How can I minimise the risk of inadvertent doping?

While the risk of using a contaminated supplement will never be eliminated, should you decide to take a supplement you can minimise the risk of inadvertent doping by looking for voluntary certifications by companies such as Informed Sport or NSF Certified for Sport (US) on the label. This indicates that the product has been independently tested for banned substances. You'll find all registered products listed on the companies' websites: www.informed-sport.com and www.nsfsport.com. However, it is important to realise that even when using certified products, you are still risking a positive drug test. Any product can be contaminated since there is no regulation in place to prevent this.

Antioxidant supplements

WHAT ARE THEY?

Antioxidant supplements may contain one or more of the following nutrients: beta-carotene, vitamin C, vitamin E, zinc, magnesium, copper, lycopene (a pigment found in tomatoes), selenium, co-enzyme Q10, catechins (found in green tea), methionine (an amino acid) and anthocyanidins (pigments found in purple or red fruit).

WHAT DO THEY DO?

The traditional theory, the so-called antioxidant-exercise hypothesis, suggests that intense exercise produces high levels of free radicals, or reactive oxygen species (ROS). These damage cell membranes and DNA and impair muscle function, hastening fatigue. The imbalance is sometimes called 'oxidative stress'. The idea behind antioxidant supplementation is to offset exercise-induced ROS damage and to speed recovery.

WHAT IS THE EVIDENCE?

Although previous studies have suggested supplementation may be beneficial, these are no longer considered valid due to small subject numbers and poor study design. Newer studies suggest that antioxidant supplements either have no effect on performance or can actually decrease training efficiency and prevent adaptation of muscles to training – the very opposite of what athletes want (Nikolaidis *et al.*, 2012). Although supplements reduce post-exercise oxidative stress, this isn't a good thing because oxidative stress is needed to stimulate muscle growth. In other words, oxidative stress and inflammation are desirable and are considered essential for training adaptations. Reactive oxygen species generated during intense exercise signal to the body that it needs to adapt to the stress of training by becoming stronger and more efficient. By prematurely quenching these ROS with high doses of antioxidant supplements, you could be preventing muscle adaptations.

Studies suggest that exercise itself increases the oxidative capacity of muscles by enhancing the action of antioxidant enzymes such as glutathione peroxidase and superoxide dismutase (Draeger *et al.*, 2014). Thus, taking supplements will provide no further benefit. A review of more than 150 studies by Australian researchers concluded that there is insufficient evidence that antioxidant supplements improve performance (Peternelj & Coombes, 2011).

A double-blind randomised controlled trial found that vitamin C (1000 mg) and E (235 mg) supplements blunted the endurance training induced increase of mitochondrial proteins, which is important for improving muscular endurance. (Paulsen *et al.*, 2013). There was no difference in aerobic capacity (VO$_2$max) or performance between those taking supplements or a placebo. The researchers concluded that vitamins C and E hampered cellular adaptations in the muscles and therefore provided no performance benefit.

In another study, cyclists taking antioxidant supplements experienced no performance benefit during 12 weeks of strenuous endurance training compared with those taking a placebo (Yfanti *et al.*, 2010). Similarly, another study found that vitamin C and vitamin E supplementation had no effect on muscle performance or recovery following 4 weeks of eccentric training (Theodorou *et al.*, 2011). In another, footballers who took an antioxidant supplement experienced no increase in aerobic capacity (VO$_2$max) after 6 weeks of training, while those taking a placebo did (Skaug *et al.*, 2014). In other words, supplementation with antioxidants appears to reduce rather than improve the benefits of training.

DO I NEED THEM?

There is no benefit to be gained from taking high dose antioxidant supplements. Instead of improving performance or promoting recovery, supplements may actually hamper it by disrupting the mechanisms designed to deal with exercise-derived oxidative stress. The consensus statement by the American College of Sports Medicine cautions against the use of antioxidant supplements (Rodrigues *et al.*, 2009).

Getting your vitamins and minerals through a varied and balanced diet remains the best approach to maintain an optimal antioxidant status. There's good evidence to suggest that a diet rich in foods that are naturally high in antioxidants is associated with better health outcomes.

ARE THERE ANY SIDE EFFECTS?

Antioxidant supplementation may delay recovery and even result in reduced performance.

Branched-chain amino acid supplements

WHAT ARE THEY?

Branched-chain amino acids (BCAAs) include valine, leucine and isoleucine. These three essential amino acids make up one-third of muscle proteins.

WHAT DO THEY DO?

The theory behind BCAA supplements is that they can help prevent the breakdown of muscle tissue during intense exercise. They are converted into two other amino acids – glutamine and alanine – which are released in large quantities during intense aerobic exercise. Also, they can be used directly as fuel by the muscles, particularly when muscle glycogen is depleted.

WHAT IS THE EVIDENCE?

Studies at the University of Guelph, Ontario, suggest that taking 4 g BCAA supplements during and after exercise can reduce muscle breakdown (MacLean *et al.*, 1994). They may help preserve muscle in athletes on a low carbohydrate diet (Williams, 1998) and, taken before resistance training, reduce delayed onset muscle soreness (Nosaka *et al.*, 2006; Shimomura *et al.*, 2006). A study by researchers at Florida State University found that BCAA supplementation before and during prolonged endurance exercise reduced muscle damage (Greer *et al.*, 2007). However, similar benefits were obtained following consumption of a carbohydrate drink and it is not clear whether chronic BCAA supplementation benefits performance. Studies with long distance cyclists at the University of Virginia found that supplements taken before and during a 100 km bike performance test did not improve performance compared with a carbohydrate drink (Madsen *et al.*, 1996). In other words, BCAAs may not offer any advantage over carbohydrate drinks taken during exercise.

DO I NEED THEM?

If sufficient calories, protein and carbohydrate are being consumed then there appears to be little benefit in taking BCAA supplements. But if you are in calorie deficit or consuming little

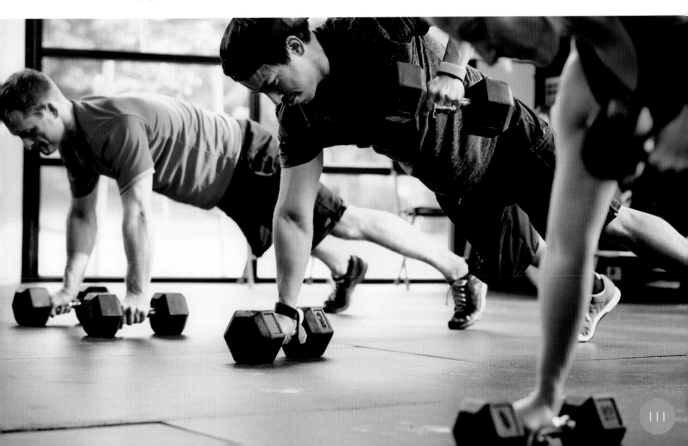

carbohydrate or protein then doses of 6–15 g may help improve your recovery during hard training periods by reducing muscle protein breakdown. Given that many recovery drinks contain a mixture of carbohydrate, protein and amino acids, there is little point taking a separate BCAA supplement.

ARE THERE ANY SIDE EFFECTS?

BCAAs are relatively safe because they are normally found in protein in the diet. Excessive intake may reduce the absorption of other amino acids.

Beta-alanine

WHAT IS IT?

Beta-alanine is an amino acid that is used to make carnosine (a dipeptide formed from beta-alanine and histidine). Carnosine is an important buffer in muscles – it buffers the acidity (hydrogen ions) produced during high intensity exercise.

WHAT DOES IT DO?

Taking beta-alanine supplements increases muscle carnosine levels. Taking 5–6 g/day increases muscle carnosine content by 60% after 4 weeks and 80% after 10 weeks (Harris *et al.*, 2006). This raises the buffering capacity of the muscles, increasing the ability of muscles to tolerate high intensity exercise for longer. Normally, a build-up of acidity results in fatigue. Supplementation may therefore increase power output and performance in anaerobic exercise, and decrease perceived exertion.

WHAT IS THE EVIDENCE?

A systematic review of 19 randomised controlled (i.e. high quality) studies concluded that beta-alanine supplementation leads to improved performance in short duration, high intensity activities (Quesnele *et al.*, 2014). According to an analysis of 15 studies, the average performance improvement is 2.85% (Hobson *et al.*, 2012).

In a study at Ghent University, Belgium, beta-alanine supplements reduced fatigue when performing a set of knee extensions (Derave *et al.*, 2007). Another study at the College of New Jersey found that beta-alanine supplements resulted in increased training volume and reduced subjective feelings of fatigue in football players (Hoffman *et al.*, 2008).

Australian researchers found that runners who took beta-alanine supplements for 28 days achieved significantly faster 800 m race times compared with those who took a placebo (Ducker *et al.*, 2013). Another study measured significant improvements in power output and time trial performance in cyclists after 4 weeks of beta-alanine supplementation (Howe *et al.*, 2013). Similarly, a study by Belgian researchers found that beta-alanine supplementation for 8 weeks significantly enhanced sprint performance at the end of a simulated endurance cycle race (Van Thienen *et al.*, 2009).

DO I NEED IT?

Beta-alanine supplements may be beneficial for sports involving high intensity efforts lasting between 1 and 4 minutes, or intermittent sports such as football and tennis that involve repeated sprints. They may also be advantageous for bodybuilders and those following a strength training programme. The optimum dose appears to be around 3 g (4 × 800 mg) per day for 6 weeks followed by a maintenance dose of 1.2 g/day (Stegen *et al.*, 2014). However, the research to date has involved relatively small numbers of athletes, so recommendations may change as further research is carried out.

ARE THERE ANY SIDE EFFECTS?

There have been reports of parathesia (skin tingling), although this appears to be harmless, and is associated mainly with higher doses. Smaller doses or sustained-release formulations are less likely to cause side effects. Importantly, the long-term effects of beta-alanine supplements are not known.

Beetroot juice (nitrate)

WHAT IS IT?

Beetroot juice (and beetroot) is a rich source of nitrate. Nitrate is also found in smaller amounts in other vegetables, such as spinach, rocket, celeriac, cabbage, endive, leeks and broccoli. Nitrate may also be taken in the form of sodium nitrate supplements.

WHAT DOES IT DO?

Beetroot juice increases the amount of nitrate in the blood. Nitrate is then converted into nitric oxide (NO) in the body. This gas plays an important role in vasodilation and regulating blood pressure. Increasing NO levels prior to exercise could be an advantage, as it means blood vessels become more dilated, aiding the delivery of oxygen and nutrients to muscles during exercise, and helping improve exercise efficiency, i.e. reducing the energy required to exercise at a given intensity.

WHAT IS THE EVIDENCE?

Nitrate appears to be a very potent ergogenic aid. A number of studies have shown that nitrate in the form of beetroot juice enhances stamina and performance. It also reduces resting blood pressure and the oxygen cost of exercise, meaning that athletes can tolerate higher intensity levels for longer. For example, researchers at the University of Exeter, UK, found that drinking 500 ml beetroot juice a day for a week enabled volunteers to run 15% longer before experiencing fatigue (Lansley *et al.*, 2011). This was due to the higher levels of nitrate measured in the blood, which reduced muscle uptake of oxygen and made them more fuel-efficient. A further study by the same researchers found that cyclists given 500 ml beetroot juice 2½ hours before a time trial race improved their performance by 2.8% in a 4 km race and 2.7% in a 16.1 km race (Lansley *et al.*, 2011). University of Maastricht researchers found that 170 ml beetroot juice concentrate over 6 days improved 10 km time trial performance and power output in cyclists (Cermak *et al.*, 2012). But whole beetroot works equally well. Athletes who consumed 200 g cooked beetroot an hour before exercise were able to run faster in the latter stages of a 5 km run (Murphy *et al.*, 2012). These results suggest that the nitrates in beetroot juice reduce maximal oxygen uptake, improve exercise economy and allow athletes to exercise longer. This may give you the edge in events lasting 4–30 minutes or during intense intermittent exercise and team sports.

A review of 17 studies by UK and Australian researchers concluded that nitrate either in the form of beetroot juice or sodium nitrate significantly improved endurance, as measured by time to exhaustion (Hoon *et al.*, 2013a). Although time to exhaustion isn't a direct measure of performance, this finding could translate into a 1–2% reduction in race times. More recently, studies have suggested that beetroot juice also has the potential to improve performance in high intensity sports that require a high recruitment of fast-twitch muscle fibres. Exeter University researchers found that consuming 70ml (1 shot) of concentrated beetroot juice for 5 days improved their 20m sprint and high-intensity intermittent running performance in competitive team sport players (Thompson *et al*, 2016).

However, the majority of studies showing a positive effect involved untrained or recreational athletes, not elite athletes. Whether beetroot juice also benefits performance in elite athletes is unclear. Australian researchers found that beetroot juice supplementation did not improve performance in competitive cyclists (Lane *et al*., 2013). Even when combined with caffeine, beetroot juice (2 × 70 ml shots) made no difference to their performance in a 60-minute simulated time trial. Another study with competitive cyclists found little difference in time trial performance following beetroot juice supplementation (Hoon *et al*., 2014). So, to date, beetroot juice appears to be a more effective ergogenic aid for non-elite than elite athletes.

DO I NEED IT?

Beetroot may help improve your performance time in endurance activities lasting between 4 and 30 minutes, as well as in high intensity activities involving single or multiple sprints. The optimal dose is likely to be 0.6 g nitrate, equivalent to 2 × 70 ml concentrated beetroot 'shots' (Wylie *et al*., 2013), although it has also proved to benefit performance in studies using 0.3–0.4 g (0.62 mg/kg body weight), equivalent to 500 ml beetroot juice or a single 70 ml concentrated 'shot' or 200 g cooked beetroot.

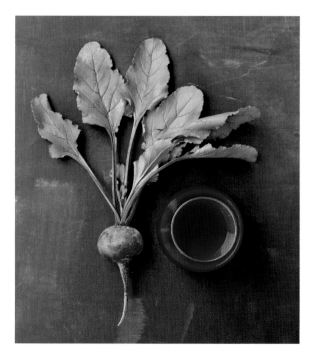

The optimal timing appears to be 2–3 hours pre-exercise as NO levels in the blood peak 2–3 hours after consumption and then gradually fall over 12 hours. Alternatively, you may prefer 'nitrate loading' for 3–7 days prior to a competition to ensure blood levels of NO remain high (Cermak *et al*., 2012).

Avoid using antibacterial mouthwash as this removes the beneficial bacteria in the mouth that convert some of the nitrate to nitrite and thus reduces the benefits of beetroot juice.

ARE THERE ANY SIDE EFFECTS?

No side effects of beetroot have been reported to date apart from a harmless, temporary pink coloration of urine and stools. There have been questions whether beetroot juice could theoretically increase cancer risk (dietary nitrates can be converted to nitrite in the body and then go on to react with amino acids to produce carcino-genic compounds called nitrosamines). However, research has shown that these harmful effects are associated with nitrates and nitrites from processed meat, not from vegetables (Gilchrist *et al.*, 2010; Hord *et al.*, 2009).

Bicarbonate

WHAT IS IT?
Sodium bicarbonate is a 'pH buffer', an extra-cellular anion that helps maintain pH gradients between the cells and blood. It is also a raising agent and a main ingredient of baking powder.

WHAT DOES IT DO?
Bicarbonate is already found in the blood, but consuming supplements ('bicarbonate load-ing') will increase the concentration further. Bicarbonate increases the pH of the blood, making it more alkaline. During high intensity (anaerobic) exercise, hydrogen ions are produced, which gradually accumulate and result in fatigue ('the burn'!). However, by raising the pH of the blood, hydrogen ions can pass more easily from the muscle cells to the blood, where they can be removed (buffered), which allows you to continue exercising at a high intensity a little longer. It also means lactate is removed faster so you can recover faster.

WHAT IS THE EVIDENCE?
Research has shown improvement in high inten-sity events lasting 1–7 minutes. One meta-anal-ysis found an improvement of 1.7% for events lasting about 1 minute with a bicarbonate dose of 0.3 g/kg BW (Carr *et al.*, 2011). A study with elite cyclists found that bicarbonate supplemen-tation significantly improved 4-minute cycling performance compared with a placebo (Driller *et al.*, 2012).

However, not all studies have shown beneficial effects of bicarbonate. For example, an Australian study with 8 swimmers found that bicarbonate loading did not result in faster times in 200 m freestyle (approximately 2 minutes duration) compared with taking a placebo (Joyce *et al.*, 2012). Another study with New Zealand rugby players found that bicarbonate loading produced no difference in performance in rugby-specific skills (Cameron *et al.*, 2010). The discrepancies in findings may be explained by the fact that elite athletes already have enhanced muscle buffering capacity so stand to benefit less than recreational athletes from bicarbonate loading.

DO I NEED IT?
You may benefit from bicarbonate if you are competing in high intensity events lasting 1–7 minutes – for example, sprint and middle distance swimming, running and rowing events – or in events that involve multiple sprints, e.g. tennis, football, rugby. However, the side effects may cancel out any potential improvement.

The most common dose for bicarbonate load-ing is 0.2–0.3 g/kg. This equates to 14–21 g for a 70 kg person. It should be consumed gradually with at least 500 ml water 60–90 minutes before the start of exercise to minimise GI symptoms.

ARE THERE ANY SIDE EFFECTS?
Typical side effects include gastrointestinal upset, nausea, stomach pain, diarrhoea and vomiting. Bicarbonate loading may also cause water retention, which may be a disadvantage in many events. These side effects could negate

any possible performance advantage. Symptoms may be reduced by taking the loading dose in divided doses over a 2–2½ hour period before the event, along with a small carbohydrate-rich meal and plenty of water. Alternatively, if you will be competing in several events over a few days, you could try taking 0.5 g/kg/day over the course of 1–3 days and then stop 12–24 hours before the event. Theoretically, the benefits will persist but with less risk of side effects.

Blackcurrant extract

WHAT IS IT?
Blackcurrant extract is a concentrated powdered form of blackcurrants, available as capsules.

WHAT DOES IT DO?
Blackcurrants contain a high concentration of anthocyanins, a sub-class of flavonoids (phytonutrients) that have powerful antioxidant properties and anti-inflammatory effects. They are thought to help enhance performance and reduce post-exercise inflammation, soreness and muscle damage. New Zealand-grown blackcurrants have 1.5 times more anthocyanins than those grown in Europe.

WHAT IS THE EVIDENCE?
Animal studies show that anthocyanins act as powerful vasodilators (Ziberna et al., 2013). It is thought that the anthocyanins in blackcurrant extract have the same effect in humans, increasing peripheral blood flow and oxygen delivery to the muscles during exercise and thus improving performance (Willems et al., 2014).

Researchers at The New Zealand Institute for Plant and Food Research found that 240 mg blackcurrant extract consumed immediately before and after 30 minutes of moderate intensity aerobic exercise reduced exercise-induced oxidative stress and muscle damage compared with a placebo (Lyall et al., 2009).

More recent research at the University of Chichester has found that 7 days of supplementation with 300 mg blackcurrant extract improved performance in a series of repeated treadmill sprints (6 × 19 s) and also improved lactate clearance (i.e. hastened muscle recovery) after exercise (Perkins et al., 2015).

A further study with 14 cyclists showed that blackcurrant supplementation increased fat oxidation by 27% during moderate intensity cycling (65% VO_2max) and also improved 16.1 km time trial cycling performance by an average of 2.4% (Cook et al., 2015). Researchers also found that supplements resulted in a higher lactate tolerance during the time trial, which suggests you would be able to exercise at higher intensities before reaching exhaustion.

Triathletes who consumed blackcurrant extract for 7 days had 14% lower levels of blood lactate when cycling at an intensity corresponding to their VO_2max and up to 27% at lower cycling intensities (Willems et al., 2015).

DO I NEED IT?
To date, only a few small studies have been carried out with athletes so it is not possible to make firm recommendations. However, the results are positive and suggest that blackcurrant extract may benefit performance by increasing oxygen delivery, increasing fat oxidation, reducing muscle soreness and improving recovery.

ARE THERE ANY SIDE EFFECTS?
No side effects have been reported to date.

Caffeine

WHAT IS IT?

Caffeine is a stimulant and has a pharmacological action on the body so is classed as a drug rather than a nutrient. It was once classed as a banned substance but was removed from the World Anti-Doping Agency (WADA) Prohibited List in 2004. This change was based on the recognition that caffeine enhances performance at doses that are indistinguishable from everyday caffeine use, and that the previous practice of monitoring caffeine use via urinary caffeine concentrations is not reliable.

It is found in everyday drinks and foods such as coffee, tea and cola, herbs such as guarana, and chocolate. It is also added to a number of energy drinks and sports drinks and gels. Table 6.1 (*see* p. 118) lists the caffeine content of popular drinks and foods. The amounts used in research range from 3–15 mg/kg BW, which is equivalent to 210–1050 mg for a 70 kg athlete. Studies normally used caffeine pills rather than drinks.

WHAT DOES IT DO?

Caffeine acts on the central and peripheral nervous system, blocking a sleep-inducing brain chemical called adenosine, thus increasing alertness and concentration, reducing the perception of effort and allowing exercise to be maintained at a higher intensity for a longer period.

It was once believed that caffeine enhances endurance performance because it promotes an increase in the utilisation of fat as an exercise fuel and 'spares' the use of glycogen. In fact, studies now show that the effect of caffeine on 'glycogen sparing' during sub-maximal exercise is short-lived and inconsistent – not all athletes respond in this way. Therefore, it is unlikely to explain the enhancement of exercise capacity and performance seen in many studies.

WHAT IS THE EVIDENCE?

Most studies of caffeine and performance have been carried out in laboratories rather than during real-life sports events. Nevertheless, there is sound evidence that caffeine may enhance the performance of a range of sports:

- Endurance sports (> 60 min)
- High intensity sports (1–60 min)
- Team and intermittent sports

There is a huge amount of research evidence suggesting that caffeine improves endurance as well as performance in anaerobic and high intensity activities (Goldstein *et al.* 2010; Dodd, 1993; Graham & Spriet, 1991; Spriet, 1995).

An analysis by UK researchers of 40 studies on caffeine and performance concluded that it significantly improves endurance, on average by 12% (Doherty & Smith, 2004). In a 2009 study at the University of Texas, cyclists who consumed caffeine in the form of an energy drink completed a 1-hour time trial 3 minutes 4 seconds faster than those who took a placebo (Ivy *et al.*, 2009).

A study at the University of Saskatchewan found that consuming caffeine in amounts equivalent to 2 mg caffeine/kg of body weight 1 hour before exercise significantly increased bench press muscle endurance (Forbes *et al.*, 2007). Another study with footballers found that consuming a caffeinated drink 1 hour before training and then at 15 minute intervals improved sprinting performance and reduced the perception of fatigue (Gant *et al.*, 2010).

One study with swimmers showed a 23 second improvement in a 21 minute swim (MacIntosh, 1995). Researchers at RMIT University, Victoria, Australia found that caffeine improved performance by 4–6 seconds in competitive rowers during a 2000 metre row (Anderson *et al.*, 2000). However, not all studies have shown positive results. Researchers at the University of Stirling, UK, and the University of Cape Town, South Africa, found that caffeine had no effect on performance during a 100 km cycling time trial (Hunter *et al.*, 2002).

Table 6.1	THE CAFFEINE CONTENT OF POPULAR DRINKS AND FOODS
Product	**Caffeine content, mg/cup**
Instant coffee	60 mg
Espresso	45–100 mg
Cafetière/filter	60–120 mg
Tea	40 mg
Green tea	40 mg
Energy drinks	100 mg
Cola	40 mg
Energy gel (1 sachet)	25 mg
Dark chocolate (50 g)	40 mg
Milk chocolate (50 g)	12 mg

DO I NEED IT?

A large number of studies now show that caffeine intake can enhance performance for most types of endurance, power and strength activities at doses of 1–3 mg/kg, which is considerably less than once believed (6 mg/kg). There appears to be little increase in performance above 3 mg/kg. For a 70 kg person, this would be 210 mg, equivalent to about 2 cups of coffee or 2 cans of caffeinated energy drink.

Performance benefits occur soon after consumption, so caffeine may be consumed just before exercise, spread throughout exercise, or taken late in exercise as fatigue is beginning to occur. As individual responses vary, you should experiment during training to find the dose and protocol that suits you.

Australian researchers have found that 1.5 mg/kg (105 mg for a 70 kg athlete) taken in divided doses (e.g. 4 caffeine-containing energy gels over 2 hours) throughout an intense workout benefits performance in elite athletes (Armstrong, 2002).

It makes little difference to performance whether you take your caffeine in the form of pills, gels, energy drinks or coffee, according to a 2015 review of studies by University of Georgia researchers (Higgins *et al.*, 2015). Bear in mind, though, that the caffeine content in coffee can vary greatly depending on the preparation method, brand and variety. As individual responses vary, you should experiment in training – not during competition – to find the dose and protocol that suits you.

It was once thought that cutting down on caffeine for several days before competition results in a more marked ergogenic effect. However, studies show that there is no difference in the

Does caffeine promote dehydration?

Although caffeine is a diuretic, a daily intake of less than 4 mg/ kg (equivalent to 4 cups of coffee) provides similar hydrating qualities to water (Killer *et al*, 2014). At this level, caffeine is considered safe and unlikely to have any detrimental effect on performance or health (Armstrong, 2002). Taking caffeine regularly (e.g. drinking coffee) builds up your caffeine tolerance so you experience smaller diuretic effects.

According to a study from Ohio State University, caffeine taken immediately before exercise does not promote dehydration (Wemple, 1997). Six cyclists consumed a sports drink with or without caffeine over a 3-hour cycle ride. Researchers found that there was no difference in performance or urine volume during exercise. Only at rest was there an increase in urine output.

In another study, when 18 healthy men consumed 1.75 litres of three different fluids at rest, the caffeine-containing drink did not change their hydration status (Grandjean, 2000).

Researchers at the University of Maastricht found that cyclists were able to rehydrate after a long cycle equally well with water or a caffeine-containing cola drink (Brouns, 1998). Urine output was the same after both drinks. However, large doses of caffeine – over 600 mg, enough to cause a marked ergogenic effect – may result in a larger fluid loss. A study at the University of Connecticut, US, found that both caffeine-containing cola and caffeine-free cola maintained hydration in athletes (during the non-exercise periods) over 3 successive days of training (Fiala *et al.*, 2004). The athletes drank water during training sessions but rehydrated with either caffeinated or caffeine-free drinks. A further study by the same researchers confirmed that moderate caffeine intakes (up to 452 mg caffeine/kg body weight/day) did not increase urine output compared with a placebo and concluded that caffeine does not cause a fluid electrolyte balance in the body (Armstrong *et al.*, 2005).

performance response to caffeine between non-users and users of caffeine, and that withdrawing from caffeine does not increase the improvement in performance.

ARE THERE ANY SIDE EFFECTS?

The effects of an acute intake of caffeine follow a U-shaped curve. Low–moderate doses produce positive effects and a sense of well-being, but higher doses of caffeine (6–9 mg/kg BW) can have negative effects. It may increase the heart rate, impair fine motor control and technique, and cause anxiety or over-arousal, trembling and sleeplessness. Some people are more susceptible to these than others. If you are sensitive to caffeine, it is best to avoid it.

Scientific research shows, on balance, no link between long-term caffeine use and health problems such as hypertension and bone mineral loss. The connection between raised cholesterol levels and heavy coffee consumption is now known to be caused by certain fats in coffee, which are more pronounced in boiled coffee than instant or filter coffee.

Cherry juice

WHAT IS IT?

Montmorency cherry juice is available as a concentrate, or in freeze-dried powdered form as capsules.

WHAT DOES IT DO?

Montmorency cherry juice is a rich source of flavonoids and anthocyanins, which have potent antioxidant and anti-inflammatory effects. It is thought that these compounds can help alleviate delayed onset muscle soreness (DOMS) and reduce inflammation that occurs after an intense workout or event and quicken the recovery process.

WHAT IS THE EVIDENCE?

It's a relatively new supplement but studies to date suggest that Montmorency cherry juice promotes muscle recovery following intense exercise. Researchers at London South Bank University gave 10 athletes 30 ml of tart cherry juice concentrate twice daily for 7 days prior to and 2 days after an intense strength training regimen (Bowtell *et al.*, 2011). The researchers found that the athletes' muscle recovery after the cherry juice concentrate was significantly faster compared to a placebo. It is thought that the antioxidant flavonoid compounds in the cherry juice may well have reduced the oxidative damage to muscles, which normally occurs when muscles are worked to their max – allowing the muscles to recover more quickly.

A study in runners carried out at Northumbria University, UK, found that consuming cherry juice for 5 days before and 2 days after a marathon improved muscle recovery and reduced inflam-mation (Howatson *et al.*, 2010). And another study by the same researcher group demonstrated that cyclists who consumed 30 ml cherry juice concentrate for 5 days had less muscle damage and exercise-induced inflammation following a 109 minute cycling trial (Bell *et al.*, 2015).

DO I NEED IT?

Consuming 30 ml cherry juice concentrate for 4–5 days prior to and 2 days after a strenuous event (or a workout involving eccentric exercise) may reduce exercise-induced inflammation, muscle soreness and pain and accelerate recovery. Although the supplement speeds functional recovery, unlike high-dose antioxidant supplements (such as vitamins C and E) it does not interfere with the inflammation that is necessary for chronic training adaptations (*see* Antioxidants, p. 109). It therefore appears to be a better option than antioxidant supplements, which can actually interfere with post-training recovery.

ARE THERE ANY SIDE EFFECTS?

No side effects have been found.

Conjugated linoleic acid (CLA)

WHAT IS IT?

CLA is an unsaturated fatty acid (in fact, it is a mixture of linoleic acid isomers) found naturally in small amounts in full fat milk, meat and cheese. Supplements are made from sunflower and safflower oils.

WHAT DOES IT DO?

It is marketed as a fat loss supplement. It is thought that CLA works by stimulating the enzyme hormone sensitive lipase (which releases fat from fat cells) and suppressing the hormone lipoprotein lipase (which transports fat into fat cells).

WHAT IS THE EVIDENCE?

Most of the research evidence for CLA is based on animal studies, which suggested that it promotes fat loss, increases muscle mass and reduces muscle breakdown. For this reason, CLA has been marketed as a supplement for weight loss. But there have been relatively few studies with humans and these have produced mixed results. Some have found that CLA supplements reduce fat levels and increase strength while others found no change in body composition. In studies that found positive results, CLA was used in conjunction with other supplements, making it difficult to assess its true effect (Falcone *et al.*, 2015). A randomised controlled study involving 28 overweight women found that CLA supplementation in conjunction with an 8 week aerobic exercise programme had no effect on body composition compared with a placebo (Ribeiro *et al.*, 2016). Similarly, researchers at the University of Memphis found no significant difference in body composition, fat loss or strength following 28 days of resistance training between volunteers taking CLA supplements and those taking a placebo (Kreider *et al.*, 2002). A review of studies by Brazilian researchers found that there is very little evidence that CLA reduces body fat in humans (Lehnen *et al.*, 2015).

DO I NEED IT?

It is unlikely that CLA supplements help reduce your body fat or increase muscle mass.

ARE THERE ANY SIDE EFFECTS?

No side effects have been reported to date.

Colostrum

WHAT IS IT?

Colostrum supplements are derived from bovine colostrum, the milk produced in the first few days after the birth of a calf. It has a high concentration of immune and growth compounds, such as immunoglobulins and antimicrobial proteins.

WHAT DOES IT DO?

It is claimed that bovine colostrum supplements enhance immunity and improve performance, recovery and body composition.

WHAT IS THE EVIDENCE?

It is unclear whether supplements help reduce the suppression of the immune system associated with prolonged intense exercise. Some studies found a reduction in self-reported upper respiratory tract infections (Brinkworth & Buckley, 2003), but others have found no effect (Crooks *et al.*, 2006). University of Queensland researchers measured an increase in immunoglobulins but no significant difference in incidence of upper respiratory tract infection (URTI) among a group of cyclists during high intensity training (Shing *et al.*, 2007). A review of studies concluded that daily supplementation with bovine colostrum helps maintain intestinal barrier integrity and immune function and reduces the chances of URTI or URTI symptoms in athletes undertaking heavy training (Davison, 2012). Another review of studies concluded that colostrum supplements may benefit performance and recovery during periods of high intensity training as a result of increased plasma IGF-1, improved intramuscular buffering capacity, increases in lean body mass and increases in salivary IgA (Shing *et al.*, 2009).

There is inconclusive evidence that colostrum supplements improve performance, strength and power. One study at the University of South Australia suggests that supplements improve anaerobic power after 8 weeks (Buckley *et al.*, 2003). But another study by the same researchers found that supplements had no effect on body composition after 8 weeks of weight training (Brinkworth, 2004).

DO I NEED IT?

While supplements may help boost your immunity during periods of strenuous training, it is not certain whether they will reduce your risk of upper respiratory tract infection. It is unlikely that supplements have any benefit on your athletic performance.

You should not take colostrum supplements if you participate in drug-tested sport. The World Anti-Doping Agency (WADA) recommends that athletes adopt a safe approach and avoid the supplement due to the naturally high quantities of insulin-like growth factor 1 contained in colostrum, a substance on WADA's prohibited list.

ARE THERE ANY SIDE EFFECTS?

There are no known side effects.

Creatine

WHAT IS IT?

Creatine is a protein that is made naturally in the body from three amino acids (arginine, glycine and methionine), but can also be found in meat and fish or taken in higher doses as a supplement. It is most commonly available as creatine monohydrate, but it is often an ingredient in 'all-in-one' meal replacement drinks and supplement 'stacks'.

WHAT DOES IT DO?

Creatine combines with phosphorus to form phosphocreatine (PC) in your muscle cells. This is an energy-rich compound that fuels your muscles during high intensity activities, such as lifting weights or sprinting (p. 22). Creatine supplementation raises PC levels typically around 2% (Hultman *et al.*, 1996). This enables you to sustain all-out effort longer than usual and recover faster between sets so it would be beneficial for training that involves repeated high intensity efforts. Creatine supplements also help promote protein manufacture and muscle hypertrophy (by drawing water into the cells), increasing lean body mass; reduce muscle acidity (it buffers excess hydrogen ions), thus allowing more lactic acid to be produced before fatigue sets in; and reduce muscle protein breakdown following intense exercise, resulting in greater strength and improved ability to do repeated sets.

WHAT IS THE EVIDENCE?

Hundreds of studies have measured the effects of creatine supplements on anaerobic performance and the majority have proven it to be an effective aid for increasing strength and muscle mass as well as enhancing performance in high intensity activities (Gualano *et al.*, 2012). The greatest improvements are found in high power output efforts repeated for a number of bouts.

The International Society of Sports Nutrition (ISSN) describes creatine as 'the most effective ergogenic nutritional supplement currently available to athletes in terms of increasing high intensity exercise capacity and lean body mass during training'. A review of 22 studies concluded that creatine supplementation increases maximum strength (i.e. 1 rep maximum) by an average

8% as well as endurance strength, i.e. maximum reps at a sub-maximal load, by 14% (Cooper *et al.*, 2012; Rawson and Volek, 2003). Another review found that 70% of creatine studies showed a positive effect on performance, and 30% showed no effect (Kreider, 2003).

Creatine supplementation results in lean mass and total mass gains of typically 1–3% lean body weight (approx. 0.8–3 kg) after a 5 day loading dose, compared with controls – although not all studies show positive results (Buford *et al.*, 2007). The observed gains in weight are due partly to an increase in cell fluid volume (i.e. water weight) and partly to muscle synthesis.

Creatine appears to enhance performance in both men and women. Researchers at McMaster University, Ontario, gave 12 male and 12 female volunteers either creatine supplements or a placebo before a high intensity sprint cycling test (Tarnopolsky & McLennan, 2000). Creatine improved performance equally in both sexes.

Researchers at the Australian Institute of Sport found that creatine improved sprint times and agility run times in football players (Cox *et al.*, 2002). A study in former Yugoslavia found that creatine supplementation improved sprint power, dribbling and vertical jump performance in young football players, but had no effect on endurance (Ostojic, 2004).

If creatine improves the quality of resistance training over time, this would lead to faster gains in mass, strength and power. The vast majority of studies indeed show that short-term creatine supplementation increases body mass.

There is less evidence for the use of creatine with aerobic-based sports – only a few laboratory studies have shown an improvement in performance. This is probably due to the fact that the

How does creatine work?

The observed gains in weight are due partly to an increase in cell volume and partly to muscle synthesis. Creatine causes water to move across cell membranes. When muscle cell creatine concentration goes up, water is drawn into the cell, an effect that boosts the thickness of muscle fibres by around 15%. The water content of muscle fibres stretches the cells' outer sheaths – a mechanical force that can trigger anabolic reactions. This may stimulate protein synthesis and result in increased lean tissue (Haussinger *et al.*, 1996).

Creatine may have a direct effect on protein synthesis. In studies at the University of Memphis, athletes taking creatine gained more body mass than those taking the placebo, yet both groups ended up with the same body water content (Kreider *et al.*, 1996; Clark, 1997).

PC energy system is less important during endurance activities. However, one study at Louisiana State University suggests creatine supplements may be able to boost athletes' lactate threshold and therefore prove beneficial for certain aerobic-based sports (Nelson *et al.*, 1997).

DO I NEED IT?

If you train with weights or do any sport that includes repeated high intensity movements, such as sprints, jumps or throws (as in, say, rugby and football), creatine supplements may help increase your performance, strength and muscle mass. In some people (approx. 2 out of every 10), muscle creatine concentrations increase only very slightly. It may be partly due to differences in muscle fibre types. Fast-twitch (FT) fibres tend to build up higher concentrations of creatine than slow-twitch (ST) fibres. This means that athletes with a naturally low FT fibre composition may experience smaller gains from creatine supplements. Taking creatine with carbohydrate may help solve the problem as carbohydrate raises insulin, which, in turn, helps creatine uptake by muscle cells.

HOW MUCH CREATINE?

The most common creatine-loading protocol is 4×5–7 g doses per day over a period of 5 days, i.e. 20–25 g daily. It works, but that doesn't mean it's the best way to load up. In fact, it's a rela-tively inefficient way of getting creatine into your muscles and is more likely to produce side effects such as water retention. Around two-thirds of this creatine ends up in your urine and only one-third ends up in your cells. The key to efficient creatine supplementation is to take small quantities at a time – and to slow down the speed of absorption from the gut. That gives the maximum chance of all the creatine consumed ending up in your muscle cells and not your urine.

According to a Canadian study, relatively low doses of creatine supplementation can significantly improve weight training performance to the same extent as higher doses (Burke *et al.*, 2000). Volunteers who took 7.7 g creatine daily for 21 days were able to perform more repetitions on the bench press and maintain maximum power longer than those who took a placebo. They also gained significantly more muscle mass (2.3% versus a 1.4% increase with placebo).

Some researchers recommend taking 6 daily doses of 0.5–1 g (i.e. 6×1 g doses) with food to increase the absorption rate (Harris, 1998). Over a 5 or 6 day period, that will produce results equivalent to taking 20 g a day. After that, a maintenance dose of 2 g a day will maintain muscle creatine levels. Alternatively, you can load up with 3 g a day over 30 days. This technique also results in saturation of your muscles with creatine, and should produce the least water retention (Hultman *et al.*, 1996).

Studies have shown that insulin helps shunt creatine faster into the muscle cells (Green *et al.*, 1996; Steenge *et al.*, 1998). Taking creatine along with carbohydrate – which stimulates insulin release – will increase the uptake of creatine by the muscle cells and raise levels of PC. The exact amount of carbohydrate needed to produce

What is the best form of creatine?

Creatine monohydrate is the most widely available form of creatine. It is a white powder that dissolves readily in water and is virtually tasteless. It is the most concentrated form available commercially and the least expensive. Creatine monohydrate comprises a molecule of creatine with a molecule of water attached to it so it is more stable.

Although other forms of creatine such as creatine serum, creatine citrate and creatine phosphate are available, there is no evidence that they are better absorbed, produce higher levels of phosphocreatine in the muscle cells or result in greater increases in performance or muscle mass (Jäger *et al.*, 2011).

Will I lose strength when I stop taking creatine supplements?

When you stop taking supplements, elevated muscle creatine stores will drop very slowly to normal levels over a period of 4 weeks (Greenhaff, 1997). During supplementation your body's own synthesis of creatine is depressed but this is reversible. In other words, you automatically step up creatine manufacture once you stop supplementation. Certainly, fears that your body permanently shuts down normal creatine manufacture are unfounded. You may experience weight loss and there are anecdotal reports about athletes experiencing small reductions in strength and power, although not back to pre-supplementation levels.

It has been proposed that creatine is best taken in cycles, such as 3–5 months followed by a 1-month break.

an insulin spike is debatable but estimates range from 35 g to around 100 g. Some scientists recommend taking creatine with or shortly after eating a meal. The idea is to take advantage of the post-meal rise in insulin to get more creatine into the muscle cells. Taking creatine monohydrate is the least expensive way to achieve this. Creatine drinks and supplements containing carbohydrate are expensive and may add a lot of unwanted calories to your diet.

Creatine uptake is also greater immediately after exercise so adding creatine to the post-exercise meal will help to boost muscle creatine levels.

Canadian researchers have suggested that muscle creatine levels may be enhanced when alpha-lipoic acid (an antioxidant) is given at the same time (Burke *et al.*, 2001a). And researchers at St Francis Xavier University, Nova Scotia, found that those who supplemented with whey protein and creatine achieved greater increases in strength (bench press) and muscle mass compared with those who took only whey protein or placebo (Burke *et al.*, 2001b).

ARE THERE ANY SIDE EFFECTS?

Creatine appears to be safe in both the short and long term. The only side effect is weight gain. This is due partly to extra water in the muscle cells and partly to increased muscle tissue. While this is desirable for bodybuilders and people who work out with weights, it could be disadvantageous in sports where there is a critical ratio of body weight and speed (e.g. running) or in weight-category sports. In swimmers, a heavier body weight may cause more drag and reduce swim efficiency. It's a matter of weighing up the potential advantage of increased maximal power and/or lean mass against the possible disadvantage of increased weight.

There have been anecdotal reports about muscle cramping, gastrointestinal discomfort, dehydration, muscle injury, and kidney and muscle damage. However, there is no clinical data to support these statements (Lugares *et al.*, 2013; Williams *et al.*, 1999; Robinson *et al.*, 2000; Mihic *et al.*, 2000; Kreider, 2000; Greenwood *et al.*, 2003; Mayhew *et al.*, 2002; Poortmans & Francaux, 1999).

Energy bars

WHAT ARE THEY?

Energy bars consist mainly of sugar and malto-dextrin, and provide around 250 calories and 25–35 g of carbohydrate/bar. Some may also have added vitamins and minerals, cereals or soy flour to boost the nutritional content.

WHAT DO THEY DO?

Energy bars provide a convenient way of consuming carbohydrate before, during or after intense exercise lasting more than 1 hour.

WHAT IS THE EVIDENCE?

An Australian study compared an energy bar (plus water) with a sports drink during exercise; it was found that both boosted blood sugar levels and endurance equally (Mason *et al.*, 1993).

In a study at the University of Texas, cyclists were given either a sports drink (containing 10% carbohydrate), an energy bar with water, or a placebo (Yaspelkis *et al.*, 1993). Those who consumed some form of carbohydrate managed to keep going 21 minutes 30 seconds longer before reaching exhaustion than those taking a placebo. The reason? The extra carbohydrate helped fuel the cyclists' muscles, reducing the dependency on glycogen. After 3 hours in the saddle, the cyclists sipping the sports drink or eating food had 35% more glycogen than those who had no carbohydrate.

DO I NEED THEM?

Any form of high GI carbohydrate will help improve your endurance during high intensity exercise lasting longer than 1 hour. Whether you consume carbohydrate in the form of an energy bar, drink or any other form during exercise is down to personal preference. The main benefit of energy bars is their convenience: they are easy to carry and eat! Make sure that you have your bar with enough water to replace fluids lost in sweat as well as to digest the bar. They are an acquired taste and texture, and you may need to experiment with different flavours and brands.

ARE THERE ANY SIDE EFFECTS?

If you don't consume enough water, they may cause gastrointestinal discomfort. Some products may adhere to your teeth so ensure you rinse with water.

Energy gels

WHAT ARE THEY?

Energy gels come in small squeezy sachets and have a jelly-like texture. They consist of simple sugars (such as fructose and glucose) and malto-dextrin (a carbohydrate derived from corn starch, consisting of 4–20 glucose units). They may also contain sodium, potassium and, sometimes, caffeine. Most contain between 18 and 25 g of carbohydrate per sachet.

WHAT DO THEY DO?

Gels provide a concentrated source of calories and carbohydrate and are designed to be consumed during endurance exercise.

WHAT IS THE EVIDENCE?

Studies show that consuming 30–60 g of carbohydrate per hour during prolonged exercise delays fatigue and improves endurance. This translates into 1–2 sachets per hour. A 2007 study from Napier University, Edinburgh, showed that gels have a similar effect on blood sugar levels and performance as sports drinks (Patterson & Gray, 2007). Soccer players who consumed an energy gel (with water) immediately before and during high intensity interval training increased their endurance by 45% compared with a placebo.

DO I NEED THEM?

Energy gels provide a convenient way of consuming carbohydrate during intense endurance exercise lasting longer than an hour. But you need to drink around 350 ml of water with each (25 g carbohydrate) gel to dilute it to a 7% carbohydrate solution in your stomach. Try half a gel with 175 ml (6 big gulps) every 15–30 minutes. On the downside, some people dislike their texture, sweetness and intensity of flavour – it's really down to personal preference – and they don't do away with the need for carrying a water bottle with you.

ARE THERE ANY SIDE EFFECTS?

Energy gels don't hydrate you so you must drink plenty of water with them. If you don't drink enough, they can cause stomach discomfort. They are very concentrated in sugar, which drags water from your bloodstream into your stomach, increasing the risk of dehydration.

Ephedrine/ma huang/ 'fat burners'/thermogenic supplements

WHAT IS IT?

The main ingredient in 'fat burners' or thermogenics is ephedrine, a synthetic version of the Chinese herb ephedra or ma huang. Ephedrine is, strictly, a drug rather than a nutritional supplement. It is also used at low concentrations in cold and flu remedies (pseudoephedrine).

WHAT DOES IT DO?

Ephedrine is chemically similar to amphetamines, which act on the brain and the central nervous system. Athletes use it because it increases arousal, physical activity and the potential for neuromuscular performance. It is often combined with caffeine, which enhances the effects of ephedrine.

WHAT IS THE EVIDENCE?

Ephedrine is a proven stimulant. However, research studies generally show it has little effect on strength and endurance. This is probably because relatively low doses were used. What is more likely is that these products have a 'speed-like' effect; they make you feel more awake and alert, more motivated to train hard and more confident.

There is some evidence that ephedrine helps fat loss: partly due to an increase in thermogenesis (heat production), partly because it suppresses your appetite and partly because it makes you more active.

When taken as a 'caffeine–ephedrine stack', or a 'caffeine–ephedrine–aspirin stack', it is thought that ephedrine has a greater effect in terms of thermogenesis and weight loss. In one study, volunteers who took a combination of caffeine and ephedrine before a cycle sprint (anaerobic exercise) achieved a better performance than those who took caffeine only, ephedrine only or a placebo (Bell, 2001). However, the fat-burning effect of ephedrine seems to decrease over time, i.e. weight loss slows or stops after 12 weeks.

DO I NEED IT?

It is an addictive drug and I would strongly recommend avoiding any fat-burner containing ephedrine or ma huang because of the significant health risks. It is banned by WADA, whether in cold remedies or in supplements. Exercise and good nutrition are the safest methods for burning fat.

ARE THERE ANY SIDE EFFECTS?

Ephedrine is judged to be safe in doses containing around 18–25 mg; that's the amount used in decongestants and cold remedies. Taking too much can have serious side effects. These include increased heart rate, increased blood pressure, palpitations, anxiety, nervousness, insomnia, nausea, vomiting and dizziness. Very high doses (around 3000 mg) cause heart attacks and can even be fatal. Caffeine–ephedrine stacks produce adverse effects at even lower doses. A case of a sportsman who suffered an extensive stroke after taking high doses of 'energy pills' (caffeine–ephedrine) has been reported in the *Journal of Neurology, Neurosurgery and Psychiatry* (Vahedi, 2000).

In 2002, the American Medical Association called for a ban on ephedrine due to concerns over its side effects. Since 1997 the FDA in the US has documented at least 70 deaths and more than 1400 'adverse effects' involving supplements containing ephedrine. These included heart attacks, strokes and seizures. Ephedrine's risks far outweigh its potential benefits. It is addictive and people can develop a tolerance to it (you need to keep taking more and more to get the same effects).

Fat burners (ephedrine-free)

WHAT ARE THEY?

Certain fat-burning and weight loss supplements claim to mimic the effects of ephedrine, boost the metabolism and enhance fat loss but without harmful side effects. The main ingredients in these products include *citrus aurantium* (synephrine or bitter orange extract); green tea extract and *Coleus forskohlii* extract (a herb, similar to mint).

WHAT DO THEY DO?

Citrus aurantium is a weak stimulant, chemically similar to ephedrine and caffeine. It contains a compound called synephrine which, according to manufacturers, reduces appetite, increases the metabolic rate and promotes fat burning. However, despite the hype, there is no sound scientific evidence to back up the weight loss claims.

The active constituents in green tea are a family of polyphenols called catechins (the main type is epigallocatechin gallate, EGCG) and flavanols, which possess potent antioxidant activity. The theory behind *Coleus forskohlii* as a dietary supplement is that its content of forskolin can be used to stimulate adenyl cyclase activity, which will increase cAMP (cyclic adenosine monophosphate) levels in the fat cell, which will in turn activate another enzyme (hormone sensitive lipase) to start breaking down fat stores.

WHAT IS THE EVIDENCE?

Despite the hype, there is no sound scientific evidence to back up the weight loss claims of fat burners. The only ingredient that may have some value is green tea extract. Research suggests that it may stimulate thermogenesis, increasing calorie expenditure, fat burning and weight loss (Dulloo *et al.*, 1999). There are no published trials showing that *Coleus forskohlii* extract promotes weight loss.

DO I NEED THEM?

The research on ephedrine-free fat burners is not robust and any fat-burning boost they provide would be relatively small or none. The doses used in some brands may be too small to provide a measurable effect. A reduced calorie intake and exercise are likely to produce better weight loss results in the long term. The only positive data is for green tea, but you would need to drink at least six cups daily (equivalent to 100–300 mg EGCG) to achieve a significant fat-burning effect.

ARE THERE ANY SIDE EFFECTS?

While the herbal alternatives to ephedrine are generally safer, you may get side effects with high doses. *Citrus aurantium* can increase blood pressure as much, if not more, than ephedrine. High doses of forskolin may cause heart disturbances.

Fish oil/omega-3 fatty acids

WHAT ARE THEY?

Fish oil contains the two unsaturated fatty acids eicosapentaenoic acid (EPA) and docosahexaenoic acid (DHA), derived from the tissues of oily, cold-water fish such as tuna, cod (liver) and salmon.

WHAT DO THEY DO?

Omega-3 fatty acids are involved in a number of processes in the body, including the activation of 'locally acting hormones' known as eicosanoids, which control inflammation and immunity. They're also vital for the structure and fluidity of cell membranes. In addition, omega 3s are essential for growth, development, vision and the correct functioning of the brain and nervous system, with depletion associated with learning deficits. More recently, omega-3s have been linked with protection against depression, high blood pressure, heart disease, cancer, obesity and inflammation.

Theoretically, supplements are a good way of boosting omega-3 intake for people who do not eat oily fish regularly. Manufacturers claim they help reduce the risk of heart disease, cancer, type 2 diabetes, depression and degenerative diseases such as Parkinson's. For athletes, supplementation may be a good way to help reduce inflammation in the body, including post-exercise muscle soreness, and improve muscle functioning, blood vessel elasticity and delivery of oxygen to muscles.

WHAT IS THE EVIDENCE?

Fish oil supplementation in conjunction with exercise appears to have beneficial effects. A study at the University of South Australia showed that overweight people who took fish oils while following an exercise programme lost more body fat, lowered their blood fats and increased HDL cholesterol levels compared with those taking a placebo (Hill *et al.*, 2007). In a 2010 study, scientists at Gettysburg College in Pennsylvania supplemented diets of healthy, active adults with either safflower oil or fish oil (Noreen *et al.*, 2010). After 6 weeks, those taking the fish oil benefited from a significant increase in lean body mass and reduction in fat mass. One study found that omega-3s increased blood flow by up to 36% during exercise (Walser *et al.*, 2006). However, a more recent study at the University of Stirling found that fish oil supplements (in conjunction with protein supplementation) made no significant difference to muscle protein synthesis following an 8-week resistance training programme (McGlory *et al.*, 2016).

Omega-3s also appear to play a key role in immune function. Researchers found 3 g fish oil supplementation for 60 days before a marathon prevented a drop in immune function induced by the race, although the researchers did not measure whether this led to a reduced incidence of colds or infection (Santos *et al.*, 2013). Another found that supplementation for 14 days reduced levels of inflammation after intense exercise (Phillips *et al.*, 2003).

However, not all studies have produced positive results. In one, supplementation with 3.6 g fish oil/day for 6 weeks had no effect on delayed-onset muscle soreness compared with a placebo (Lenn *et al.*, 2002).

DO I NEED THEM?

Fish oil and omega-3s appear to have a number of benefits for athletes, including improved blood flow and reduced inflammation, but it is unclear whether they can reduce post-exercise muscle soreness. If you don't eat oily fish regularly, 2 capsules of fish oil will provide approximately 500–600 mg of EPA and DHA, which is in line with population recommendations for heart disease risk reduction (Gebauer *et al.*, 2006). The government recommends 450–900 mg of the long-chain EPA and DHA per day, which can also be met with two portions of oily fish per week. The American Heart Association recommends 1000 mg daily. However, based on the most recent meta-analyses, supplements are unlikely to prevent cardiovascular disease.

ARE THERE ANY SIDE EFFECTS?

Very high doses (more than 3 g/day) may increase the risk of bleeding. This is due to fish oil's ability to break down blood clots.

Glutamine

WHAT IS IT?
Glutamine is a non-essential amino acid. It can be made in the muscle cells from other amino acids (glutamic acid, valine and isoleucine) and is the most abundant free amino acid in muscle cells. It is essential for cell growth and a critical source of energy for immune cells called lymphocytes. Many protein and meal replacement supplements contain glutamine.

WHAT DOES IT DO?
Glutamine is needed for cell growth, as well as serving as a fuel for the immune system. During periods of heavy training or stress, blood levels of glutamine fall, weakening your immune system and putting you at risk of infection. Muscle levels of glutamine also fall, which results in a loss of muscle tissue, despite continued training. Supplementation during intense training periods is thought to help offset the drop in glutamine, boost immunity, reduce the risk of overtraining syndrome and prevent upper respiratory tract infections.

Manufacturers claim that glutamine has a protein-sparing effect during intense training. This is based on the theory that glutamine helps draw water into the muscle cells, increasing the cell volume. This inhibits enzymes from breaking down muscle proteins and also counteracts the effects of stress hormones (such as cortisol), which are increased after intense exercise.

WHAT IS THE EVIDENCE?
The evidence for glutamine is divided. Some studies have suggested that supplements may reduce the risk of infection and promote muscle growth (Parry-Billings et al., 1992; Rowbottom et al., 1996). Researchers at Oxford University have shown that glutamine supplements taken immediately after running and again 2 hours later appeared to lower the risk of infection and boost immune cell activity in marathon runners (Castell & Newsholme, 1997). Only 19% of those taking glutamine became ill during the week following the run while 51% of those taking a placebo became ill. However, not all studies have managed to replicate these findings. A more recent review of studies concluded that while many athletes take glutamine supplements to protect against exercise-related impairment of the immune system, supplements do not prevent post-exercise changes in immune function or reduce the risk of infection (Gleeson, 2008).

Glutamine does not improve performance, body composition or muscle breakdown (Haub, 1998). According to a Canadian study, glutamine produces no increase in strength or muscle mass compared with a placebo (Candow et al., 2001). After 6 weeks of weight training, those taking glutamine achieved the same gains in strength and muscle mass as those taking a placebo.

DO I NEED IT?
The case for glutamine is not clear. It is unlikely to prevent immune-suppression or improve body composition or performance.

ARE THERE ANY SIDE EFFECTS?
No side effects have been found so far.

HMB

WHAT IS IT?
HMB (beta-hydroxy beta-methylbutyrate) is made in the body from the BCAA leucine. You

can also obtain it from a few foods such as grapefruit, alfalfa and catfish.

WHAT DOES IT DO?

No one knows exactly how HMB works, but it is thought to be involved in cellular repair. HMB is a precursor to an important component of cell membranes that helps with growth and repair of muscle tissue. HMB supplements claim to protect muscles from excessive breakdown during exercise, accelerate repair and build muscle.

WHAT IS THE EVIDENCE?

The evidence for HMB is divided. A review of studies published by the International Society of Sports Nutrition concluded that HMB promotes recovery, reduces exercise-induced muscle breakdown and damage, promotes muscle repair, and increases muscle mass (Wilson *et al.*, 2013). Researchers at Iowa State University have shown muscle mass gains of 1.2 kg and strength gains of 18% after 3 weeks with HMB, compared with 0.45 kg muscle gain and 8% strength gain from a placebo (Nissen *et al.*, 1996; Nissen *et al.*, 1997). One study suggests HMB may boost muscle mass more effectively when taken together with creatine (Jowko *et al.*, 2001).

However, this degree of improvement hasn't been found in all HMB studies. It appears to have little effect in experienced athletes (Kreider *et al.*, 2000). One study at the Australian Institute of Sport failed to find strength or mass improvements in 22 athletes taking 3 g per day for 6 weeks (Slater *et al.*, 2001). Researchers at the University of Queensland in Australia found no beneficial effect on reducing muscle damage or muscle soreness following resistance exercise (Paddon-Jones *et al.*, 2001).

There is some evidence that HMB combined with alpha-ketoisocaproic acid may reduce signs and symptoms of exercise-induced muscle damage in novice weight trainers (van Someren *et al.*, 2005).

DO I NEED IT?

If you're new to lifting weights, HMB may help to boost your strength and build muscle, but probably for only the first 2 months of training. Consuming sufficient calories, protein, carbohydrate and fat in conjunction with consistent resistance training is likely to produce better results. No long-term studies have been carried out to date – it is unlikely to benefit more experienced athletes.

ARE THERE ANY SIDE EFFECTS?

No side effects have yet been found.

Leucine

WHAT IS IT?

Leucine is an essential amino acid, and the most abundant of the three branched-chain amino acids (BCAAs) in muscles (the other two are isoleucine and valine).

WHAT DOES IT DO?

Leucine is an important trigger for protein synthesis. It acts as a signal to the muscle cells to make new muscle proteins, activating a compound called mTOR (mammalian target of rapamycin), a molecular switch that turns on the machinery that manufactures muscle proteins.

WHAT IS THE EVIDENCE?

Research suggests that leucine can stimulate protein synthesis (when consumed after exercise) and reduce protein breakdown (when consumed before exercise). In a study at the University of Maastricht, athletes who consumed a leucine/carbohydrate/protein drink after resistance training had less muscle protein breakdown and greater muscle protein synthesis than those who consumed a supplement without leucine (Koopman *et al.*, 2005). Similarly, another study found that consuming a leucine-enriched protein drink during endurance exercise resulted in less muscle breakdown and greater muscle synthesis (Pasiakos *et al.*, 2011). A study with canoeists found that 6 weeks of leucine supplementation improved endurance performance and upper body power (Crowe *et al.*, 2006). However, there is no benefit to taking extra leucine if you consume protein (as food or drink) before or after exercise. Researchers found that consuming more than 1.8 g leucine does not produce any additional benefit (Pasiakos & McClung, 2011)

DO I NEED IT?

Getting sufficient leucine is particularly important for those wanting to build strength and muscle mass. However, it isn't necessary to get leucine in the form of supplements. It is found widely in foods, the best sources being eggs, dairy products, meat, fish and poultry. It is also found in high concentrations in whey protein. You'll need around 2 g leucine to get maximum muscle-building benefits; that's the amount found in approximately 20 g of an animal protein source (*see* p. 85).

ARE THERE ANY SIDE EFFECTS?

There are no reported side effects.

Arginine/ Nitric Oxide Supplements

WHAT ARE THEY?

The active ingredient in nitric oxide (NO) supplements is L-arginine, a non-essential amino acid made naturally in the body. It is usually sold as arginine alpha keto-glutarate (A-AKG) and arginine keto iso-caproate (A-KIC). Supplements are marketed to bodybuilders for promoting and prolonging muscle pumps and increasing lean body mass and strength.

WHAT DO THEY DO?

Arginine is an amino acid that is readily converted to NO in the body. NO is a gas that is involved in vasodilation, which is the process that increases blood flow to muscles, allowing better delivery of nutrients and oxygen. The idea behind supplementation is to increase the muscle 'pump' when lifting weights, and promote recovery and muscle growth.

WHAT IS THE EVIDENCE?

Little research supports these assertions directly. An analysis of several studies concludes that NO supplements may produce a small benefit for beginners, but not for more highly trained athletes and not for females (Bescos *et al.*, 2012). Most studies suggest that arginine supplements have no effect on NO production or exercise performance in elite athletes (Liu *et al.*, 2009). In one study, there was no difference in NO levels, blood flow or performance in athletes taking A-AKG supplements or a placebo (Willoughby *et al.*, 2011).

DO I NEED THEM?

Arginine is unlikely to benefit your performance – it does not increase NO levels to an appreciable extent. Other NO boosters, such as beetroot juice, are likely to be more effective (*see* p. 113).

ARE THERE ANY SIDE EFFECTS?

Side effects are unlikely from the doses recommended on the supplement label.

Probiotics

WHAT ARE THEY?

Probiotics are the live micro-organisms (bacteria) that live in the gut and are crucial for optimal intestinal health, digestion and immunity. They are found in yoghurt and other cultured milk products as well as capsules, tablets and powders. The main commercially used species are Lactobacillus acidophilus, Bifidobacterium bifidum and L.casei imunitass® cultures.

WHAT DO THEY DO?

Probiotic supplements work by recolonising the small intestine and crowding out disease-causing bacteria, thereby strengthening or restoring the balance to the intestinal flora.

WHAT'S THE EVIDENCE?

Hard training can put a significant strain on your immune system, increasing the risk of catching infections such as upper respiratory tract infections (URTI). Studies show that various immune cell functions are impaired following prolonged intense training sessions. Probiotics have been shown to reduce the incidence of URTI in athletes during winter months, and may also reduce gastrointestinal distress often associated with longer bouts of training.

A study carried out by researchers at the Australian Institute of Sport found that probiotic supplementation can dramatically cut the risk and length of upper respiratory tract infections (URTI) in elite long-distance runners (Cox *et al.*, 2008). Those taking probiotic supplements experienced symptoms of URTI for 30 days during 4 months of intensive training compared with 72 days in the placebo group, and the severity of symptoms was less. This was attributed to higher levels of interferon (immune cells that fight viruses). In a follow-up study with competitive cyclists, 11 weeks of probiotic supplementation reduced the severity and duration of lower respiratory illness by 30% compared with a placebo (West, 2011). There was also a reduction in the severity of gastrointestinal symptoms and athletes used cold and flu medication less frequently.

A review of randomised controlled trials (the gold standard for studies) concluded that probiotics are effective for preventing URTIs and reducing antibiotic use compared with a placebo (Hao et al., 2011).

DO I NEED THEM?

They may enhance the immune system and help protect against and reduce symptoms of gastrointestinal and upper respiratory tract infections (URTI). They may also improve intestinal tract health and increase the bioavailability of nutrients.

ARE THERE ANY SIDE EFFECTS?

No adverse health effects have been reported.

Protein supplements

WHAT ARE THEY?

Protein supplements can be divided into three main categories: protein powders (which you mix with milk or water into a shake); ready-to-drink shakes; and high protein bars. They may contain whey protein, casein, egg, soya or other non-dairy sources (e.g. pea, brown rice and hemp protein) or a mixture of these.

WHAT DO THEY DO?

They provide a concentrated source of protein to supplement your usual food intake. Whey protein is derived from milk and contains high levels of the essential amino acids, which are readily digested, absorbed and retained by the body for muscle repair. Whey protein may also help enhance immune function. Casein, also derived from milk, provides a slower-digested protein, as well as high levels of amino acids. Soy protein is less widely used in supplements but is a good option for vegans and people with high cholesterol levels – 25 g of soya protein daily (as part of a diet low in saturated fat) can help reduce cholesterol levels. Other non-dairy proteins such as pea, brown rice and hemp are often combined so they provide the full range of essential amino acids.

WHAT IS THE EVIDENCE?

Studies have shown that consuming either a casein or whey supplement immediately after resistance training raises blood levels of amino acids and promotes muscle protein synthesis (Tipton *et al.*, 2004). Male volunteers who consumed a whey protein supplement (1.2 g/kg BW/day) during 6 weeks of resistance training achieved greater muscle mass and strength gains compared with those who took a placebo (Candow *et al.*, 2006),

but others have reported no or minimal effects (Campbell *et al.*, 1995; Haub, 2002).

In one study, those consuming 20 g of whey supplement before and after resistance exercise had greater increases in muscle mass and muscle strength over 10 weeks compared with those consuming a placebo (Willoughby *et al.*, 2007). Another study found that when athletes consumed a whey supplement immediately before and after a training session they could perform more reps and lift heavier weights 24 hours and 48 hours after the workout compared with those taking a placebo (Hoffman *et al.*, 2008).

However, consuming any high quality protein source immediately after resistance training will also promote muscle repair and growth (Tipton *et al.*, 2004). Compared with casein or soy, whey supplements may be a better option in the immediate post-exercise period as whey is absorbed quicker, but there is no evidence that it results in greater muscle growth over 24 hours (Tang *et al.*, 2009).

Whey may also help boost immunity. Researchers found that those who consumed whey supplements following a 40 km cycling time trial experienced a smaller drop in glutathione levels, which is linked with lowered immunity (Middleton & Bell, 2004).

However, in studies where athletes were already consuming adequate amounts of protein in their diet, taking additional protein in the form of supplements before and after their workouts made no difference to muscle synthesis or strength (Weisgarber *et al.*, 2012).

DO I NEED THEM?

It is undisputed that resistance training increases muscle protein turnover and therefore the daily protein requirement. But it remains controversial whether supplements are necessary to increase muscle mass and strength or whether you can get sufficient protein from food. The ACSM advise that protein requirements can be met from diet alone without the use of protein or amino acid supplements (Rodriguez *et al.*, 2009).

Foods such as milk, eggs, meat, poultry and fish supply all eight essential amino acids in amounts closely matched to the body's requirements and are also naturally rich in the amino acid leucine, an important trigger for MPS (*see* p. 132). If you are already consuming sufficient protein in your diet (1.2–2.0g/kg BW/day) and getting around 20–25g protein per meal, then additional protein from supplements is unlikely to produce further gains in muscle mass, strength or performance.

Whey vs. casein supplements

Most of the research on whey vs. casein shows there is no difference in muscle mass and strength gains between those taking whey or casein proteins (Dangin, 2001; Kreider, 2003; Candow *et al.*, 2004; Brown *et al.*, 2004), although some studies have suggested that whey produces greater gains in strength and muscle mass compared with casein (Cribb *et al.*, 2006).

Whey protein, the most popular protein ingredient, is derived from milk using either a process called micro-filtration (the whey proteins are physically extracted by a microscopic filter) or by ion-exchange (the whey proteins are extracted by taking advantage of their electrical charges). It has a higher biological value (BV) than milk (and other protein sources) and is digested and absorbed relatively rapidly, making it useful for promoting post-exercise recovery. It has a higher concentration of Essential Amino Acids (around 50%) than whole milk, about half of which are BCAAs (23–25%), which may help minimise muscle protein breakdown during and immediately after high intensity exercise. Research at McGill University in Canada suggests that the amino acids in whey protein also stimulate glutathione production in the body (Bounous & Gold, 1991). Glutathione is a powerful antioxidant and also helps support the immune system. This is particularly useful during periods of intense training, when the immune system is suppressed. Whey protein may also help to stimulate muscle growth by increasing insulin-like growth factor-1 (IGF-1) production – a powerful anabolic hormone made in the liver that enhances protein manufacture in muscles.

Casein, also derived from milk, comprises larger protein molecules, which are digested and absorbed more slowly than whey. It also has a high BV and a high content of the amino acid glutamine (around 20%) – a high glutamine intake may help spare muscle mass during intense exercise and prevent exercise-induced suppression of the immune system. As casein is a 'slow-acting' protein, it may be beneficial taken before sleep for promoting overnight recovery.

A study at Maastricht University in the Netherlands found that protein synthesis was 22% higher in resistance-trained males who consumed 40 g of protein in the form of a casein drink before sleep (Res *et al.*, 2012). Casein produced a sustained rise in amino acids throughout the night and increased whole body protein synthesis compared with a placebo.

However, protein supplements may benefit you if you have particularly high protein requirements (e.g. for athletes weighing 100 kg or more), you are on a calorie restricted diet or you cannot consume enough protein from food alone (e.g. a vegetarian or vegan diet). Estimate your daily protein intake from food and compare that with your protein requirement.

Perhaps the main benefit of protein supplements and the best-argued case for taking them is their convenience. Whether in the form of drinks, bars, flapjacks, cookies or gels, they are portable, easy-to-consume on the go and provide a defined quantity of protein.

ARE THERE ANY SIDE EFFECTS?

An excessive intake of protein, whether from food or supplements, is not harmful but offers no health or performance advantage. Concerns about excess protein harming the liver and kidneys or causing calcium loss from the bones have been disproved.

Pro-hormones/steroid precursors/testosterone boosters

WHAT ARE THEY?

Pro-hormone supplements include dehydro-epiandrosterone (DHEA), androstenedione ('andro') and norandrostenedione, weak androgenic steroid compounds. They are produced naturally in the body and converted into testosterone. Supplements are marketed to bodybuilders and other athletes for increased strength and muscle mass.

WHAT DO THEY DO?

Manufacturers claim the supplements will increase testosterone levels in the body and produce similar muscle-building effects to anabolic steroids, but without the side effects.

WHAT IS THE EVIDENCE?

Current research does not support supplement manufacturers' claims. Studies show that andro supplements and DHEA have no significant testosterone-raising effects, and no effect on muscle mass or strength (King *et al.*, 1999; Broeder *et al.*, 2000; Powers, 2002). A study at Iowa State University found that 8 weeks of supplementation with andro, DHEA, saw palmetto, *Tribulus terrestris* and chrysin, combined with a weight training programme, failed to raise testosterone levels or increase muscle strength or mass – despite of increased levels of androstenedione – compared with a placebo (Brown *et al.*, 2000).

DO I NEED THEM?

It is unlikely that pro-hormones work and they may produce unwanted side effects (see below). They are on the World Anti-Doping Agency's prohibited list (WADA, 2014). All athletic associations, including the International Olympic Committee (IOC), ban pro-hormones. Pro-hormones are highly controversial supplements and, despite the rigorous marketing, there is no research to prove the testosterone-building claims.

ARE THERE ANY SIDE EFFECTS?

Studies have found that pro-hormones increase oestrogen (which can lead to gynecomastia, male breast development) and decrease

HDL (high density lipoproteins or good cholesterol) levels (King *et al.*, 1999). Reduced HDL carries a greater heart disease risk. Other side effects include acne, enlarged prostate and water retention.

Some supplements include anti-oestrogen substances, such as chrysin (dihydroxyflavone), to counteract the side effects, but there is no evidence that they work either (Brown *et al.*, 2000).

Taurine

WHAT IS IT?

Taurine is a non-essential amino acid produced naturally in the body. It is also found in meat, fish, eggs and milk. It is the second most abundant amino acid in muscle tissue. Taurine is sold as a single supplement, but more commonly as an ingredient in certain protein drinks, creatine-based products and sports drinks. It is marketed to athletes for increasing muscle mass and reducing muscle tissue breakdown during intense exercise.

WHAT DOES IT DO?

Taurine has multiple roles in the body, including brain and nervous system function, blood pressure regulation, fat digestion, absorption of fat-soluble vitamins and control of blood cholesterol levels. It is used as a supplement because it is thought to decrease muscle breakdown during exercise. The theory behind taurine is that it may act in a similar way to insulin, transporting amino acids and sugar from the bloodstream into muscle cells. This would cause an increase in cell volume, triggering protein synthesis and decreasing protein breakdown.

WHAT IS THE EVIDENCE?

Intense exercise depletes taurine levels in the body, but there is no sound research to support the claims for taurine supplements. In a randomised double-blind crossover trial, US researchers found no difference in either strength or muscular endurance in athletes following consumption of 500 ml sugar-free Red Bull energy drink (containing taurine and caffeine) compared with a drink containing caffeine (without taurine) or a placebo (without caffeine or taurine) (Eckerson *et al.*, 2013).

DO I NEED IT?

As you can obtain taurine from food (animal protein sources), there appears to be no convincing reason to recommend taking the supplements for athletic performance or muscle gain.

ARE THERE ANY SIDE EFFECTS?

Taurine is harmless in the amounts found in protein and creatine supplements. Very high doses of single supplements may cause toxicity.

Testosterone boosters

WHAT ARE THEY?

These include *Tribulus terrestris* (a flowering plant), horny goat weed (a leafy plant), and zinc. They are marketed as natural alternatives to anabolic steroids.

WHAT DO THEY DO?

Manufacturers claim that the phytochemicals in the plants increase testosterone production and therefore increase muscle mass and strength as well as boosting libido.

WHAT IS THE EVIDENCE?

There is no evidence supporting the claims for *Tribulus terrestris* or horny goat weed. A 4-week study of 21 healthy young men failed to find any measurable differences in testosterone levels between those taking a *Tribulus terrestris* supplement and a placebo group (Neychev & Mitev, 2005). Similarly, a study of 22 Australian elite rugby players found no difference in testosterone levels or any improvement in strength or body composition after 5 weeks of supplementation with *Tribulus terrestris* compared with a placebo (Rogerson *et al.*, 2007).

Despite the manufacturers' claims, there have been no studies on horny goat weed and testosterone levels in humans – only studies with rats!

Zinc supplements do not raise testosterone levels unless you have a deficiency, i.e. abnormally low testosterone levels. By correcting the deficiency, you may notice a short-term improvement in strength and muscle mass.

ARE THERE ANY SIDE EFFECTS?

Tribulus supplements are unlikely to produce side effects. However, they are contraindicated for people with breast or prostate cancer.

DO I NEED THEM?

Despite the claims, testosterone boosters do not increase testosterone, improve muscle mass or enhance athletic performance. Although some manufacturers claim *Tribulus terrestris* will not lead to a positive drug test, others have suggested it may increase the urinary testosterone epitestosterone (T:E) ratio, which may place athletes at risk of a positive drug test. So you should avoid anything containing this supplement if you compete in a drug-tested sport.

ZMA

WHAT IS IT?

ZMA (zinc monomethionine aspartate and magnesium aspartate) is a supplement that combines zinc, magnesium, vitamin B_6 and aspartate in a specific formula. It is marketed to bodybuilders and strength athletes as a testosterone booster.

WHAT DOES IT DO?

Manufacturers claim that ZMA can boost testosterone production, strength, muscle mass and recovery after exercise. Zinc is needed for growth, cell reproduction and testosterone production. In theory, a deficiency may reduce the body's anabolic hormone levels and adversely affect muscle mass and strength. Magnesium helps reduce levels of the stress hormone cortisol (high levels are produced during periods of intense training), which would otherwise promote muscle breakdown. A magnesium deficiency may increase catabolism. ZMA supplements may therefore help increase anabolic hormone levels and keep high levels of cortisol at bay by correcting a zinc and magnesium deficiency.

WHAT IS THE EVIDENCE?

Both zinc and magnesium deficiencies can impair performance (Nielson & Lukaski, 2006). It is feasible that ZMA supplementation corrects underlying zinc and/or magnesium deficiencies, thus 'normalising' various body processes and improving testosterone levels. This is supported by one study, which found ZMA increased testosterone and strength in a group of football players (Brilla & Conte, 2000). However, this was a small study with a high drop-out rate and has not been replicated since.

A more rigorous randomised, double-blind study with 42 experienced weight-trainers found that supplementation with ZMA for 8 weeks failed to increase testosterone levels, strength, muscle mass, anaerobic capacity or muscular endurance compared with a placebo (Wilborn *et al.*, 2004).

DO I NEED IT?

Unless you are deficient in zinc or magnesium, taking ZMA won't help you gain muscle mass or get stronger. You can obtain zinc from whole grains, including wholemeal bread, nuts, beans and lentils. Magnesium is found in whole grains, vegetables, fruit and milk.

ARE THERE ANY SIDE EFFECTS?

Do not exceed the safe upper limit of 25 mg daily for zinc; 400 mg daily for magnesium. High levels of zinc – more than 50 mg – can interfere with the absorption of iron and other minerals, leading to iron deficiency. Check the zinc content of any other supplement you may be taking.

Summary of key points

	Endurance/ recovery	Muscle mass/ strength	Weight loss	General health
Strong evidence	• Caffeine • Carbohydrate drinks, bars and gels • Beta-alanine • Beetroot juice • Bicarbonate	• Creatine • Protein	• Calorie-reduced diet • Exercise	• Probiotics • Vitamin D
Moderate or emerging evidence	• Cherry juice • Blackcurrant extract • Glutamine	• Leucine • HMB • BCAAs		• Multivitamins • Fish oil/ omega-3s
Lack of evidence or prohibited by WADA	• Antioxidants • Vitamin C • Vitamin E • Arginine • Taurine	• Pro-hormones • ZMA • Colostrum • Testosterone boosters • *Tribulus terrestris* • Horny goat weed	• CLA • Fat burners • Ephedrine • Synephrine • Ma huang	• Colostrum

Hydration

Exercise is thirsty work.

Whenever you exercise you lose fluid, not only through sweating but also as water vapour in the air that you breathe out. During high intensity exercise in hot, humid conditions, your body's fluid losses can be very high and, if the fluid is not replaced quickly, dehydration will follow. This will have an adverse effect on your physical and mental performance, yet it can be avoided, or at least minimised, by appropriate drinking strategies.

This chapter explains the effects of dehydration on performance, how to reduce the risk of both dehydration and overhydration (hyponatraemia), when is the best time to drink, and how much to drink. It deals with the timing of fluid intake, before, during and after exercise, and considers the science behind the formulation of sports drinks. Do they offer an advantage over plain water and can they improve performance? Finally, this chapter looks at the effects of alcohol on performance and health, and gives a practical, sensible guide to drinking.

WHY DO I SWEAT?

First, let us consider what happens to your body when you exercise. When your muscles start exercising, they produce extra heat. In fact, about 75% of the energy you put into exercise is converted into heat, which is then lost. This is why exercise makes you feel warmer. Extra heat has to be dissipated to keep your inner body temperature within safe limits – around 37–38°C. If your temperature rises too high, normal body functions are upset and eventually heat stroke can result.

The main method of heat dispersal during exercise is sweating. Water from your body is carried to your skin via your blood capillaries and as it evaporates you lose heat. For every litre of sweat that evaporates, you will lose around 600 kcal of heat energy from your body. (You can lose some heat through convection and radiation, but it is not very much compared with sweating.)

HOW MUCH FLUID DO I LOSE?

The amount of sweat that you produce and, therefore, the amount of fluid that you lose, depends on:

- how hard you are exercising;
- how long you are exercising for;
- the temperature and humidity of your surroundings;
- individual body chemistry.

The harder and longer you exercise, and the hotter and more humid the environment, the more fluid you will lose. During exercise, an average person could lose anywhere between 0.5 and 2.5 litres/hour. In more extreme conditions of heat and humidity, sweat rates may be even higher.

Some people sweat more profusely than others, even when they are doing the same exercise in the same surroundings. This depends partly on body weight and size (a smaller body produces less sweat), your fitness level (the fitter and better acclimatised to warm conditions you are, the more readily you sweat due to better thermoregulation), and individual factors (some people simply sweat more than others!). In general, women tend to produce less sweat than men, due to their smaller body size and their greater economy in fluid loss. The more you sweat, the more care you should take to avoid dehydration.

You can estimate your sweat loss and, therefore, how much fluid you should drink by weighing yourself before and after exercise. Every 1 kg decrease in weight represents a loss of approximately 1 litre of fluid.

WHAT ARE THE DANGERS OF DEHYDRATION?

A body water deficit of 2% BW is generally defined as hypohydration or dehydration and can impair aerobic performance in warm and hot conditions (Below *et al.*, 1995; McConnell *et al.*, 1997). However, it has less impact on performance in cool conditions.

As blood volume decreases and body temperature rises, it places extra strain on the heart, lungs and circulatory system, which means the heart has to work harder to pump blood round your body. The strain on your body's systems means that exercise feels much harder, you will fatigue earlier and your performance drops. Hypohydration also leads to mental fatigue, a drop in concentration and low mood.

Although there is considerable difference between individuals, the scientific consensus is that fluid deficits greater than 2% body weight (BW) will affect your aerobic and cognitive performance, particularly in hot weather (Cheuvront *et al.*, 2003; Sawka, 1992). Maximal aerobic capacity may fall by 10–20% during endurance exercise lasting more than 90 minutes (Armstrong *et al.*, 1985). However, dehydration of up to 3% BW loss has little effect on strength, power and sprint exercise.

A drop in the performance of anaerobic or high intensity activities, sport-specific skills and aerobic performance in cool weather usually occurs once you have lost 3–5% of BW (Sawka *et al.*, 2007; Shirreffs & Sawka, 2011). If you lose 4%, you may experience nausea, vomiting and diarrhoea. At 5% your aerobic capacity will decrease by 30%, while an 8% drop will cause dizziness, laboured breathing, weakness and confusion (*see* Fig. 7.1). Greater drops have very serious consequences (ACSM, 2007; Montain & Coyle, 1992; Noakes, 1993). Figure 7.2 shows the danger of dehydration with progressively greater fluid losses.

Ironically, the more dehydrated you become, the less able your body is to sweat. This is because dehydration results in a smaller blood volume (due to excessive loss of fluid), and so a compromise has to be made between maintaining the blood flow to muscles and maintaining the blood flow to the surface of the skin to carry away heat. Usually the blood flow to the skin is reduced, causing your body temperature to rise.

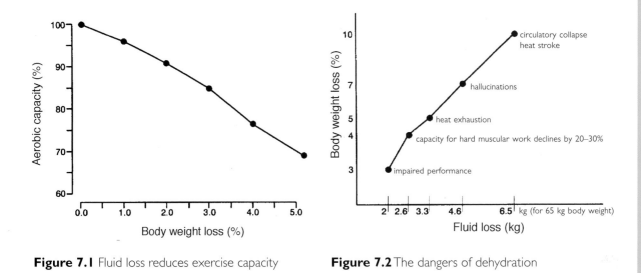

Figure 7.1 Fluid loss reduces exercise capacity

Figure 7.2 The dangers of dehydration

A CONTROVERSY: DEHYDRATION AND PERFORMANCE

For elite athletes, mild dehydration (<2% BW loss) may not impair performance. For example, an analysis of previous studies suggests that, contrary to popular dogma, exercise-induced dehydration up to 3 or 4% body weight loss can be well tolerated and does not affect performance in elite cyclists in outdoor (as opposed to lab) conditions (Goulet, 2011). In fact, researchers suggest that mild dehydration may actually be an advantage in elite runners as a lower body weight will lower the energy cost of running.

A study of elite Ethiopian distance runners found that they consumed comparatively little fluid (1.75 litres per day) and did not drink anything before or during training (Beis *et al.*, 2011). A 2006 study of Ironman triathletes in Australia found that quite large fluid losses of up to 3% of body mass had no adverse effect on performance (Laursen *et al.*, 2006). There was little change in core temperature and other

measures of dehydration stayed within normal ranges. Another study by researchers in France and South Africa weighed 643 marathon runners before and after a marathon and found that dehydration equivalent to a 3% body weight loss had no adverse effect on performance (Zouhal *et al.*, 2011). In fact, those completing the marathon in the fastest times had the greatest body weight loss and there was a clear inverse relationship between body weight loss and performance time.

The link between mild dehydration and decreased performance is based mainly on lab studies on US military research preparing soldiers for desert or jungle combat in the Second World War, which is not applicable to most real-life sporting situations. Also, these studies did not distinguish between thirst and dehydration, so it is possible that the unpleasant sensation of thirst slowed volunteers down, rather than a shortage of fluid in the body. Newer double-blind studies using intravenous drips to hydrate cyclists while they cycled, and where neither the cyclists nor researchers knew whether fluid was actually administered, have found that dehydration up to 3% BW loss did not affect performance. A study at Brock University, Canada, dehydrated 11 cyclists by 3% then measured their performance in a 20 km time trial with or without an IV drip (Cheung *et al.*, 2015). They showed no drop in performance. In other words, when athletes didn't know they are dehydrated they didn't perform any worse. What's more, even when thirst was taken out of the equation (cyclists were permitted to rinse their mouth with water then spit it out), mild dehydration did not affect cycling performance.

A similar study by Australian researchers found that 3% dehydration had no effect on performance in a 25 km cycling time trial when cyclists were blinded to their hydration status (Wall *et al.*, 2015).

CAN I MINIMISE MY FLUID LOSS?

You cannot prevent your body from losing fluid. After all, this is a natural and desirable way to regulate body temperature. On the other hand, you can prevent your body from becoming dehydrated by offsetting fluid losses as far as possible. The best way to do this is to make sure you are well hydrated before you start exercising, and to drink adequate fluids (according to your thirst) during and after exercise (*see* 'When, what and how much should I drink?', p. 146).

ARE YOU DEHYDRATED?

Many people, both athletes and non-athletes, suffer mild dehydration without realising it. Dehydration is cumulative, which means you can easily become dehydrated over successive days of training or competition if you fail to rehydrate fully between workouts or races. Symptoms of dehydration include sluggishness, a general sense of fatigue, headaches, loss of appetite, feeling excessively hot, lightheadedness and nausea.

The most simple method to assess hydration status is to look at urine colour. From a practical point of view, you should be producing a dilute, pale-coloured urine. Concentrated, dark-coloured urine of a small volume indicates you are dehydrated and is a signal that you should drink more before you exercise. Indeed, many coaches and trainers advise their players or athletes to monitor their urine output and colour because this is a surprisingly accurate way of assessing hydration status. University of Connecticut researchers found that urine colour correlated very accurately with hydration status – as good as measurements of specific gravity and osmolality of the urine (Armstrong *et al.*, 1998). Urine described as 'very pale yellow' or 'pale yellow' indicates you are within 1% of optimal hydration.

Hydration status may also be assessed by measuring urinary osmolality, which is the number of dissolved particles (such as electrolytes, urea, phosphates, proteins and glucose) per unit of water in the urine. If you are properly hydrated, urinary osmolality should be between 300 and 900 mOsmol/kg. Higher values indicate that you are dehydrated (ACSM/AND/DC, 2016).

HOW DO SWEATSUITS AFFECT FLUID LOSS?

Many athletes in weight-category sports use sweatsuits, plastic, neoprene and other clothing to 'make weight' for competition. By preventing sweat evaporation, the clothing prevents heat loss. This will cause the body temperature to rise more and more. In an attempt to expel this excess

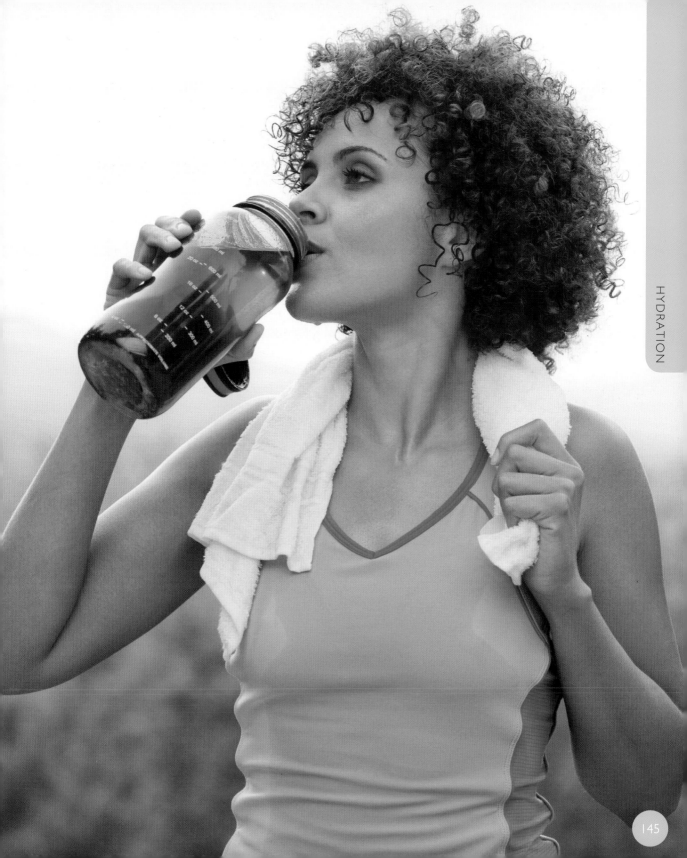

heat, your body will continue to produce more sweat, thus losing increasing amounts of fluid. You will become dehydrated, with the undesirable consequences this entails.

This is definitely not a good idea! While the idea is to restore the fluid deficit between weigh-in and the start of competition, in practice this is often difficult to achieve in a short time period. If you compete in a dehydrated state, as mentioned above, your ability to exercise will be impaired – you will suffer fatigue much sooner and will have to slow down or stop altogether. Obviously, this is not a good state in which to train or compete.

Losing weight through exercise in sweatsuits is not only potentially dangerous, but has no effect whatsoever on fat loss. Any weight loss will simply be fluid, which will be regained immediately when you next eat or drink. The exercise may seem harder because you will be sweating more, but this will not affect the body's rate of fat breakdown. If anything, you are likely to lose less fat, because you cannot exercise as hard or for as long when you wear a sweatsuit.

When, what and how much should I drink?

1. Before exercise

Your main priority is to ensure you are well hydrated before exercise. It is clear that if you begin a training session or competition in a dehydrated state, your performance will suffer and you will be at a competitive disadvantage (Shirreffs & Sawka, 2011). For example, in one study, runners performed a 5000 m run and a 10,000 m run in either a normally hydrated or slightly dehydrated condition (Armstrong et al., 1985).

Fluid calculator

Experts advise drinking to thirst but here's a rough guide to calculating your sweat rate and calculating how much to drink during exercise.

1. Weigh yourself before your workout.
2. Exercise for 1 hour, recording how much fluid you drink.
3. Weigh yourself immediately after your exercise session.
4. Calculate the difference between your pre- and post-workout weight. You can assume that almost all of your weight loss is sweat (although this is not strictly accurate as a small amount will come from the breakdown of carbohydrate and fat). So a weight loss of 1 kg represents a fluid loss of about 1 litre.
5. Add to this value the volume of fluid consumed. This is your hourly sweat rate.
6. Divide your hourly sweat rate by 4 to give you a guideline for how much to drink every 15 minutes under those particular environmental conditions.
7. Repeat the test for different environmental conditions.

When dehydrated by 2% of body weight, their running speed dropped substantially (6–7%) in both events.

Obviously, prevention is better than cure. Make sure you are well hydrated before you begin exercising, especially in hot and humid weather. The easiest way to check your hydration status is by monitoring the colour and volume of your urine. It should be pale yellow, not completely

Can you 'fluid load' before exercise?

'Loading up' or 'hyperhydrating' with fluid before an event seems advantageous for those competing in ultra-endurance events, activities during which there is little opportunity to drink, or in hot humid conditions. Unfortunately, you cannot achieve hyperhydration by consuming large volumes of water or sports drinks before the event. The body simply excretes surplus fluid and you will end up paying frequent visits to the toilet or bushes. However, there is a method of hyperhydration that involves the consumption of glycerol along with fluid 2 hours before exercise. Glycerol is a hyperhydrating agent, or a 'plasma expander', which, through its strong osmotic activity, drags water into both the extra-cellular and intra-cellular fluid. This results in an increase in total body fluid. In theory, you will be able to maintain blood volume, increase sweating and reduce the rise in core body temperature that occurs during exercise. Studies at the Australian Institute of Sport found that by doing this, athletes retained an extra 600 ml of fluid and improved performance in a time trial by 2.4% (Hitchins et al., 1999). A study at the University of Glasgow found that hyperhydrating with a combination of creatine and glycerol resulted in increased total body water but did not improve performance in a 16 km time trial compared with normal hydration (Easton et al., 2007). However, the use of glycerol and other plasma expanders is now prohibited by the World Anti-Doping Agency (WADA), so you should avoid them if you compete in a drug-tested sport.

clear. The American College of Sports Medicine (ACSM) recommends drinking 5–10 ml of fluid/kg BW slowly in the 2 to 4 hours before exercise to promote hydration and allow enough time for excretion of excess water (ACSM/AND/DC, 2016; Sawka et al., 2007). That's equivalent to 300–600 ml for a 60 kg person, or 350–700 ml for a 70 kg person. If this does not result in urine production within 2 hours or if your urine is dark coloured, you should continue drinking. But don't force yourself to drink so much that you gain weight. The 2010 International Olympic Committee (IOC) Consensus Conference on Nutrition and Sport and the 2007 consensus statement of the International Association of Athletic Federations (IAAF) both caution against overdrinking before and during exercise, because of the risk of water intoxication (hyponatraemia).

2. During exercise

There are no hard and fast rules about how much to drink, and old advice to 'drink before you feel thirsty' is no longer valid. The ACSM makes no specific recommendations about how much to drink because sweat rates and sweat composition vary considerably from one person to the next, depending on exercise intensity, duration, fitness, heat acclimatisation, altitude, heat and humidity.

A small net fluid loss, equivalent to less than 2% of your body weight, is unlikely to affect your performance. However, greater losses may result in a drop in performance for most (non-elite) athletes, so experts advise limiting dehydration to less than 2% of your body weight (Sawka, 2007; IOC, 2004; Coyle, 2004). You can work out how much fluid you lose through sweating by weighing yourself before and after a typical workout, then aim to drink sufficient to ensure a weight loss of no more than about 2–3% (see 'Fluid Calculator', p. 146). For example, this would mean 1 kg for a 50 kg person, 1.5 kg for a 75 kg person and 2 kg for a 100 kg person. However, in cold environments, dehydration greater than 2% is likely to be better tolerated.

HOW MUCH SHOULD I DRINK DURING EXERCISE?

Previous advice from the American College of Sports Medicine (ACSM, 1996; ACSM, 2000) to drink 'as much as possible' during exercise or 'to replace the weight lost during exercise' or *ad libitum* has been replaced with advice to drink according to thirst. It seems too simple to be true but the scientific evidence suggests that thirst will actually protect you from the risks of both underdrinking and overdrinking, particularly during prolonged exercise (IMMDA, 2006; Noakes, 2007; Noakes, 2010; Noakes, 2012). Drinking too much water during exercise dilutes the concentration of sodium in the blood and may lead to hyponatraemia, a potentially fatal condition.

We now know that drinking to thirst is at least as effective as drinking to prevent or limit body weight loss to 2% (Goulet, 2013). A Canadian study found that cyclists who drank according to thirst performed better than when they drank 'below' or 'above thirst' (Goulet, 2011). Drinking when you're not thirsty confers no advantage.

We also know that being mildly dehydrated (< 2–3% BW loss) does not harm performance or health, as was once believed to be the case, so there is no advantage to be gained by replacing all of your sweat losses during exercise.

The IAAF and the International Marathon Medical Directors Association (IMMDA) both recommend refraining from drinking if you are not thirsty, i.e. don't force yourself to drink. If you feel you cannot rely on thirst, then experiment in training with a planned fluid intake using the IMMDA guidelines in Table 7.1. Remember that individual requirements vary considerably and that one size doesn't fit all! Adjust the amount you drink to your exercise intensity and duration. The slower your pace, the slower your drinking rate should be. For example, for marathon runners with a finishing time over 5 hours (10–11 min/mile pace), the maximum

Table 7.1	FLUID GUIDELINES FOR MARATHON RUNNING	
Finish time (race pace)	**Rate of fluid intake**	**Total fluid intake**
< 4 hours (< 8 min/mile)	1000–1250 ml/h	3.4–4 l
4–5 hours (9–10 min/mile)	750 ml/h	3–3.5 l
> 5 hours (> 10 min/mile)	500–600 ml/h	2.5–3 l

Source: IMMDA, 2006.

intake should be 500–600ml/ hour. Those with quicker finishing times below 4 hours (< 8 minutes/mile pace) may drink 1000–1250 ml/ hour. However, for most athletes and events, an intake of 400–800 ml/hour prevents dehydration as well as overhydration, with the upper level being in warmer environments for faster and heavier athletes, and the lower level in cooler conditions for slower athletes (Sawka *et al.*, 2007; ACSM/AND/DC, 2016).

Monitor your weight during training: if you gain weight during your workout or event, you are drinking too much. If you lose more than 2–3% of your weight, increase your fluid intake. Checking urine colour before and after exercise

> ### Drinking according to thirst vs. planned fluid intake
>
> Some athletes prefer to drink according to thirst while others prefer to follow a planned fluid intake schedule that replaces fluid according to sweat losses (as calculated from body weight losses). As there is no evidence that one offers greater performance benefits over the other, you should experiment with both strategies to find out which works best for you. A study at the University of Sherbrooke, Canada, found that runners who completed a half-marathon on the treadmill drinking to a planned fluid intake aimed at maintaining < 2% BW loss drank considerably more (1380 ml/h vs. 385 ml/h) than those who drank to thirst but did not run any faster (Dion *et al.*, 2013). Performance times were no different between the two groups of runners.

will also give you a good indication of your hydration status (*see* p. 146).

IS IT POSSIBLE TO DRINK TOO MUCH DURING EXERCISE?

Athletes planning to spend longer than 4 hours exercising are at risk of developing fluid-overload hyponatraemia (abnormally low sodium levels in the blood) if they drink only water. However, it can also be caused by excessive sodium losses through sweating during prolonged high intensity events (Noakes, 2000; Speedy *et al.*, 1999; Barr *et al.*, 1989). During intense exercise, urine output is reduced, which further limits the body's ability to correct the imbalance. As the water content of the blood increases, the sodium content is diluted. Consequently, the body's water regulation mechanism becomes disrupted, and cellular swelling ensues.

Hyponatraemia is usually diagnosed when plasma sodium concentration falls below 135 mmol/litre. Symptoms include dizziness, nausea, bloating, puffiness, weight gain, muscle weakness, lapses in consciousness, cerebral oedema, and even seizures, coma and death due to swelling of the brain. However, some of these symptoms are also associated with dehydration so it's important not to confuse the two conditions and to be aware of how much you are drinking.

A study of 1089 triathletes who participated in the Ironman European Championships between 2005 and 2013 found that 115 (10.6%) had documented hyponatraemia: 95 had mild hyponatremia (8.7%), 17 severe hyponatraemia (1.6%), and 3 critical hyponatraemia (0.3%) (Danz *et al.*, 2016).

Women could be at greater risk for overhydrating because they tend to be smaller and have

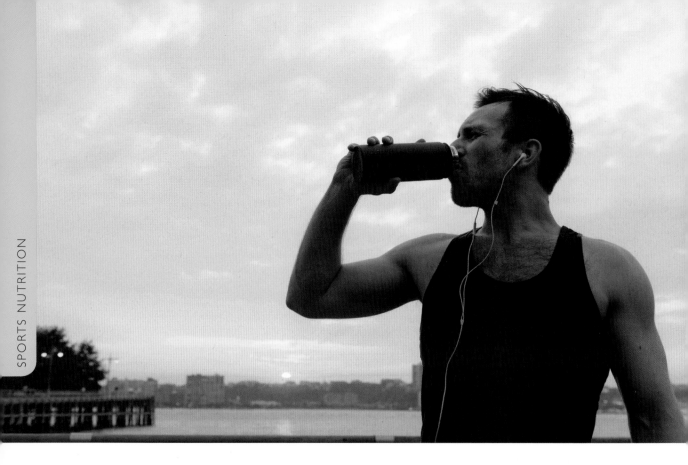

lower sweating rates. Slower runners who take longer to complete the race also are at higher risk because they tend to overestimate their water deficit and over-drink.

An advisory statement on fluid replacement in marathons written for the International Marathon Medical Directors Association advises endurance runners to drink to thirst, not to drink as much as possible, and for slower runners (> 10 minutes/ mile pace) to limit themselves to no more than 500–600 ml per hour (IMMDA, 2006). The notion that by the time you're thirsty you're already dehydrated is an old wives' tale. You can minimise your risk of hyponatraemia by ensuring that you drink only to the point at which you're maintaining your weight, not gaining weight. During endurance events, such as a marathon or triathlon, do not feel compelled to drink at every fluid station. Drink less if you begin to have a queasy, sloshy feeling in your stomach.

PRACTICAL CONSIDERATIONS

From a practical point of view, the ACSM recommend cool drinks (15–22°C). You will also be inclined to drink more if the drink is palatable and in a container that makes it easy to drink. Studies have shown that, during exercise, athletes voluntarily drink more of a flavoured sweetened drink than water, be it a sports drink, diluted fruit juice, or fruit squash (Passe *et al.*, 2004; Wilk & Bar-Or, 1996; Minehan, 2002). Drinks bottles with sports caps are probably the most popular containers. It is also important to make drinks readily accessible: for example, for swim training have drinks bottles at the poolside; for games played on a pitch or court (soccer, hockey, rugby, netball, tennis), have the bottles available adjacent to the pitch or court.

WHAT SHOULD I DRINK DURING EXERCISE?

During low or moderate intensity activities such as 'easy pace' swimming, cycling or power walking carried out for less than 45 minutes, fluid losses are likely to be relatively small and can be replaced fast enough with plain water. There is little benefit to be gained from consuming carbohydrate or drinking sports drinks compared with water during these types of activities.

For intense exercise lasting between 45 and 75 minutes, you may either consume an isotonic drink containing 40–80 g carbohydrate/litre or, if you are prone to gastrointestinal problems during exercise, try 'mouth rinsing' (swilling the drink in your mouth then spitting out, *see* p. 61). Both strategies may improve performance but through different mechanisms. With carbohydrate mouth rinsing, the performance enhancing effect is mediated by the central nervous system (the brain), and not by any increase in carbohydrate uptake (Carter, 2004; Burke *et al.*, 2011). Carbohydrates in the mouth stimulate oral sensors that act on the brain's pleasure and reward centres, thus reducing the perception of effort. Studies have shown that simply rinsing the mouth with a carbohydrate drink for 5–10 seconds improves performance. A systematic review of 11 studies found that mouth rinsing can increase performance by 1.5 to 11.6% during moderate to high intensity exercise lasting approximately 1 hour (de Ataide e Silva *et al.*, 2013).

During high intensity exercise lasting longer than 1 hour (e.g. half-marathon, football match), you require rapid fluid replacement, as well as fuel replacement. In other words, you need to avoid early glycogen depletion and low blood sugar, as well as dehydration, as all three can result in fatigue.

Table 7.2	SUMMARY OF RECOMMENDATIONS FOR CARBOHYDRATE INTAKE DURING EXERCISE	
Exercise duration	**Recommended amount of carbohydrate**	**Type of carbohydrate**
< 45 minutes	None	None
45–75 minutes	v. small amounts (mouth rinse)	Any
1–2 hours	Up to 30 g/h	Any
2–3 hours	Up to 60 g/h	Glucose, maltodextrin
3 hours	Up to 90 g/h	Multiple transportable carbohydrates (glucose + fructose or maltodextrin + fructose in 2:1 ratio)

Source: adapted from Burke *et al.*, 2011.

For high intensity exercise lasting 1–3 hours, the consensus recommendation is an intake of 30–60 g carbohydrate/h (IOC, 2011; Burke *et al.*, 2011; ACSM/AND/DC, 2016; Coggan and Coyle, 1991) to maintain blood sugar levels and delay fatigue. Generally speaking, 30 g/h is more appropriate for exercise lasting 1–2 hours, and 60 g/h is more appropriate for exercise lasting 2–3 hours. This range corresponds to the maximum rate at which fluid can be emptied from the stomach and the maximum rate at which glucose can be absorbed in the small intestines. You can get this by drinking 500 ml of a sports drink. Most commercial sports drinks contain 40–80 g carbohydrate/litre, so drinking 500 ml per hour would provide 20–40 g/h.

During hot and humid conditions, you may be losing more than 1 litre of sweat per hour. Therefore, you should increase your drink volume (although still be guided by your thirst), if possible, and use a more dilute drink (around 20–40 g/litre). More concentrated fluids take longer to absorb (ACSM, 1996).

For high intensity exercise lasting more than 3 hours, an intake of 90 g carbohydrate/h is recommended (Burke *et al.*, 2011). However, this can only be achieved by consuming dual energy source drinks that provide a 2:1 mixture of glucose and fructose ('multiple transportable carbohydrates') (IOC, 2011; Jeukendrup, 2008) (*see* p. 63). Ready-to-drink and powdered dual energy source sports drinks are now widely available.

Sports drinks based on maltodextrin (glucose polymers) may be a good choice if your sweat rate is low (e.g. during cold conditions) yet you are exercising hard, because they can provide more fuel than standard sports drinks as well as reasonable amounts of fluid. In practice, many athletes find that concentrated maltodextrin drinks cause stomach discomfort and that sports drinks containing 40–80 g carbohydrate do an equally good job.

The key to choosing the right drink during exercise is to experiment with different drinks in training to find one that suits you best (*see* Table 7.2, p. 151).

Why do I feel nauseous when I drink during exercise?

If you feel nauseous or experience other gastrointestinal symptoms when you drink during exercise, this may either indicate that you are dehydrated or be related to the fact you are exercising at a very high intensity for a prolonged period. In the former case, you need to be aware that even a fairly small degree of dehydration (around 2% of body weight) slows down stomach emptying and upsets the normal rhythmical movement of your gut. This can result in bloating, nausea and vomiting. Avoid this by ensuring you are well hydrated before exercise and then continue drinking little and often according to thirst during your workout. In the latter case, it is the nature of the training (i.e. high intensity prolonged exercise) that affects gut motility, causing discomfort and nausea. If you are prone to such symptoms during training or competition, ensure that you are well hydrated before exercise so the risk of dehydration and therefore the need to drink during exercise will be less. (See p. 285)

152

WHY DO SOME PEOPLE GET GI PROBLEMS FROM SPORTS DRINKS?

There are lots of anecdotal reports suggesting sports drinks can cause stomach discomfort or heaviness during exercise. Indeed, a study at the Gatorade Sports Science Institute, Illinois, found that athletes experienced greater stomach discomfort during circuit training after drinking an 8% sports drink compared with a 6% drink (Shi *et al.*, 2004). It is known that more concentrated drinks empty more slowly from the stomach and are absorbed more slowly from the intestines, which would explain the increased gastrointestinal discomfort. Many people find that diluting sports drinks helps alleviate these problems, but there's a balance to be struck between obtaining enough carbohydrate to fuel your exercise and avoiding gastrointestinal discomfort. If the drink is too dilute, you may not consume enough carbohydrate to achieve peak performance. A study at the Georgia Institute of Technology found that athletes performed equally after drinking a 6% or 8% drink (Millard-Stafford *et al.*, 2005). And researchers at the University of Iowa in the US found that diluting a 6% drink down to 3% (i.e. 3 g carbohydrate per 100 ml) had no effect on stomach emptying rate and resulted in a similar rate of water absorption (Rogers *et al.*, 2005). The bottom line is: work out from trial and error the concentration of sports drink that suits you best.

What causes cramps during exercise?

It is widely believed that cramps are due to dehydration or lack of salt. However, there is little evidence to support these theories. One study of 209 Ironman athletes found no significant difference in the levels of dehydration or sodium loss between those who developed cramp and those who didn't, thus challenging the prevailing electrolyte depletion hypothesis of cramps (Schwellnus *et al.*, 2011).

Instead, it is thought that cramps are due to neuromuscular alterations, which may occur during high intensity exercise or at the beginning of unaccustomed workouts (Minetto *et al.*, 2013). This is called the 'altered neuromuscular control hypothesis'. Researchers also believe that there is an element of genetic susceptibility, that some people are simply more prone to cramp than others. The remedy is to reduce your exercise intensity, stretch, and try to relax the affected muscle(s). Correcting any muscle imbalances and developing a more efficient technique for your sport may also help avoid cramp.

3. After exercise

Both water and sodium need to be replaced to restore normal fluid balance after exercise. This can be achieved by water plus accompanying food (if there is no urgency for recovery) or a sport drink (Shirreffs & Sawka, 2011). Researchers recommend you should consume about 1.2–1.5 times the weight of fluid lost during exercise (IAAF, 2007; Shirreffs *et al.*, 2004; Shirreffs *et al.*, 1996). The simplest way to work out how much you need to drink is to weigh yourself before and after training. Working on the basis that 1 litre of sweat is roughly equivalent to a 1 kg body weight loss, you need to drink 1.2–1.5 litres of fluid for each kg of weight lost during exercise.

You should not drink the whole amount straight away, as a rapid increase in blood volume promotes urination and increases the risk of hyponatraemia. Consume as much as you feel comfortable with, then drink the remainder in divided doses until you are fully hydrated.

Sports drinks that contain sodium and carbohydrate may be better than water for speeding recovery after exercise, particularly when fluid losses are high or for those athletes who train twice a day and need to recover rapidly. The problem with drinking water is that it causes a drop in blood osmolality (i.e. it dilutes sodium in the blood), reducing your thirst and increasing urine output, and so you may stop drinking before you are rehydrated (Maughan *et al.*, 1996; Gonzalez-Alonzo *et al.*, 1992). Sodium plays an important role in driving the thirst mechanism. A low sodium concentration in the blood signals to the brain a low thirst sensation. Conversely, a high sodium concentration in the blood signals greater thirst and thus drives you to drink. Hence, the popular strategy of putting salted peanuts and crisps at the bar to encourage customers to buy more drink to quench their thirst! Similarly, sports drinks, increase the urge to drink and decrease urine production.

But research at Loughborough University suggests that skimmed milk may be an even better option for promoting post-exercise rehydration (Shirreffs *et al.*, 2007). Volunteers who drank skimmed milk after exercise achieved net positive hydration throughout the recovery period, but returned to net negative fluid balance 1 hour after drinking either water or a sports drink. More recently, a study at Griffith University, Australia, showed that milk, soy milk and a milk-based supplement all rehydrated athletes more effectively than a sports drink following a workout that induced 2% dehydration (Desbrow *et al.*, 2014).

A UK study comparing the hydrating properties of 13 different drinks found that skimmed and whole milk, orange juice and an oral rehydration solution all resulted in better fluid retention after 2 hours, compared with water (Maughan *et al*, 2016). Contrary to popular belief, lager, coffee and tea did not have a significant diuretic effect and hydrated the body as well as water.

HOW MUCH SHOULD I DRINK ON NON-EXERCISING DAYS?

The current European Food Safety Authority (EFSA) dietary reference value for water intakes is 2.5 litres/day for men and 2.0 litre/day for women (EFSA, 2010). However, this is simply a guideline and the amount you need to drink depends on your fluid losses through sweating, breathing and urine. Most people can rely on their sense of thirst as a good indicator of when they should drink.

From a hydration point of view, it does not matter where you get your liquid from – coffee, tea, fruit juice, soup, squash and milk all count towards the total.

The science of sports drinks

WHAT TYPES OF SPORTS DRINKS ARE AVAILABLE?

Sports drinks can be divided into two main categories: fluid replacement drinks and carbohydrate (energy) drinks.

- Fluid replacement drinks are dilute solutions of electrolytes and sugars (carbohydrate). The sugars most commonly added are glucose, sucrose, fructose and glucose polymers (malto-dextrin). The main aim of these drinks is to replace fluid faster than plain water, although the extra sugars will also help maintain blood sugar levels and spare glycogen. These drinks may be either hypotonic or isotonic (*see right*).

- Carbohydrate (energy) drinks provide more carbohydrate per 100 ml than fluid replacement drinks. The carbohydrate is mainly in the form of glucose polymers (maltodextrin). The main aim is to provide larger amounts of carbohydrate but at an equal or lower osmolality than the same concentration of glucose. They will, of course, provide fluid as well. Ready-to-drink brands are generally isotonic. Powders that you make up into a drink may be made hypotonic or isotonic (*see right*).

WHAT IS THE DIFFERENCE BETWEEN HYPOTONIC, ISOTONIC AND HYPERTONIC DRINKS?

- A hypotonic drink – often marketed as a 'lite' sports drink – has a relatively low osmolality, which means it contains fewer particles (carbohydrate and electrolytes) per 100 ml than the body's own fluids. As it is more dilute, it is absorbed faster than plain water. Typically, a hypotonic drink contains less than 40 g carbohydrate/litre.
- An isotonic drink – a typical 'sports drink' – has the same osmolality as the body's fluids, which means it contains about the same number of particles (carbohydrate and electrolytes) per 100 ml and is therefore absorbed as fast as or faster than plain water. Most commercial

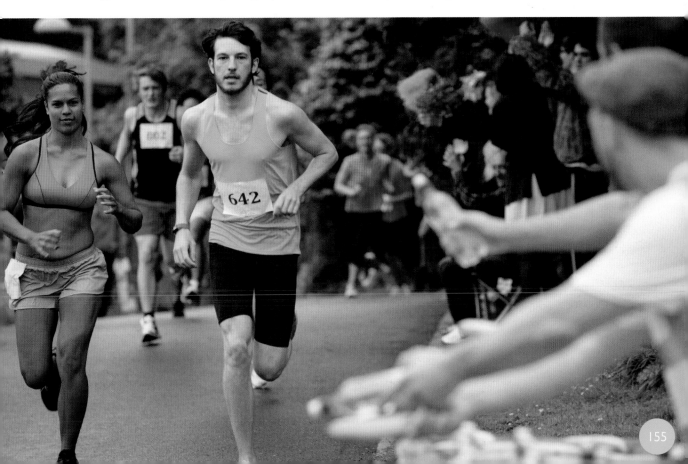

isotonic drinks contain between 40 and 80 g carbohydrate/litre. In theory, isotonic drinks provide the ideal compromise between rehydration and refuelling.

- A hypertonic drink – such as cola and other ready-to-drink soft drinks – has a higher osmolality than body fluids, as it contains more particles (carbohydrate and electrolytes) per 100 ml than the body's fluids, i.e. it is more concentrated. This means it is absorbed more slowly than plain water. A hypertonic drink usually contains more than 80g carbohydrate/litre.

WHEN SHOULD I OPT FOR A SPORTS DRINK INSTEAD OF WATER?

Opting for an isotonic sports drink would benefit your performance during any moderate or high intensity event lasting longer than about 1 hour. Numerous studies have shown that sports drinks containing about 40–80 g carbohydrate/litre promote both hydration and increased blood sugar levels, and enhance performance during intense and/or prolonged exercise (Coggan & Coyle, 1991; Coyle, 2004; Jeukendrup, 2004). If you are exercising longer than 2 hours or sweating very heavily, you should opt for a sports drink that also contains sodium (Coyle, 2007).

Researchers at the Medical School at the University of Aberdeen found that sports drinks containing glucose and sodium can delay fatigue (Galloway & Maughan, 2000). Cyclists given a dilute sports drink (2% carbohydrate) were able to keep going considerably longer (118 minutes) than those drinking plain water (71 minutes) or even a higher strength (15% carbohydrate) sports drink (84 minutes). The success of the more dilute drink may be due to the larger volume drunk.

Sports drinks and tooth enamel

Research at Birmingham University has found that sports drinks can dissolve tooth enamel and the hard dentine underneath, resulting in tooth erosion (Venables et al., 2005). Their high acidity levels means that they can erode up to 30 times more tooth enamel than water. A 2007 study comparing the 'buffering capacity' of various drinks found that popular sports drinks and energy drinks have a greater potential to cause tooth erosion than cola (Owens, 2007). Drinking them during exercise makes the effects worse because exercise reduces saliva needed to combat the drink's acidity. Similar erosive problems can occur when drinking soft drinks and fruit juice. In a survey of 302 athletes from 25 different sports competing at the 2012 Olympics, 55% had evidence of cavities, 45% had dental erosion and 18% said that their oral health had a negative impact on their training and performance (Needleman et al, 2014).

Best advice is to drink quickly to minimise contact with the teeth, use chilled drinks (they are less erosive) and rinse your mouth with water after drinking them. Researchers are hoping to produce a sports drink that is less harmful to the teeth.

For example, in a study carried out by researchers at Loughborough University, 7 endurance runners drank similar volumes of either water, a 5.5% sports drink (5.5 g carbohydrate/100 ml) or 6.9% sports drink (6.9 g carbohydrate/100 ml) before and during a 42 km treadmill run

(Tsintzas *et al.*, 1995). Those who drank the 5.5% sports drink produced running times on average 3.9 minutes faster compared with water, and 2.4 minutes faster compared with the 6.9% drink.

At Texas University, 8 cyclists performed a time trial lasting approximately 10 minutes after completing 50 minutes of high intensity cycling at 85% VO_2max. Those who drank a sports drink (6 g carbohydrate/100 ml) during the 50 minute cycle reduced the time taken to cycle the final trial by 6% compared with those who drank water (Below *et al.*, 1995).

In a study at the University of South Carolina, cyclists who consumed a sports drink containing 6 g carbohydrate/100 ml knocked 3 minutes off their time during a time trial, compared with those who drank plain water (Davis *et al.*, 1988).

What does 'osmolality' mean?

Osmolality is a measure of the number of dissolved particles in a fluid. A drink with a high osmolality means that it contains more particles per litre than one with a low osmolality. These particles may include sugars, glucose polymers, sodium or other electrolytes. The osmolality of the drink determines which way the fluid will move across a membrane (e.g. the gut wall). For example, if a drink with a relatively high osmolality is consumed, then water moves from the bloodstream and gut cells into the gut. This is called net secretion. If a drink with a relatively low osmolality is consumed, then water is absorbed from the gut (i.e. the drink) to the gut cells and bloodstream. Thus there is net water absorption.

WHAT ARE ELECTROLYTES?

Electrolytes are mineral salts dissolved in fluid, and carry an electrical charge. They include sodium, chloride, potassium and magnesium, and help to regulate the fluid balance between different body compartments (for example, the amount of fluid inside and outside a muscle cell) and the volume of fluid in the bloodstream. The water movement is controlled by the concentration of electrolytes on either side of the cell membrane. For example, an increase in the concentration of sodium outside a cell will cause water to move to it from inside the cell. Similarly, a drop in sodium concentration will cause water to move from the outside to the inside of the cell. Potassium draws water across a membrane, so a high potassium concentration inside cells increases the cell's water content.

WHY DO SPORTS DRINKS CONTAIN ELECTROLYTES?

Sodium is the only electrolyte that has a potential benefit but only for those exercising at a high intensity for longer than 2 hours. Electrolyte replacement is only beneficial when sweat losses are high and prolonged, and you lose around 3–4 g sodium (Coyle, 2004).

If you're exercising for less than 2 hours and sweat losses are not excessive, extra electrolytes will not speed fluid absorption or benefit performance (Shirreffs & Sawka, 2011). It was originally thought that sodium also speeds water absorption in the intestines. However, research at the University of Iowa has since shown that adding sodium to a sports drink does not enhance fluid absorption (Gisolphi *et al.*, 1995). Researchers discovered that after you have consumed any kind of drink, sodium passes from the blood plasma into the intestine, where it then stimulates water absorption. In other words, the body sorts out the sodium concentration of the liquid in your intestines all by itself, so the addition of sodium to sports drinks is unnecessary.

Sodium in sports drinks increases the urge to drink, improves palatability and promotes fluid retention. The increase in sodium concentration and decrease in blood volume that accompany exercise increase your natural thirst sensation, making you want to drink. If you drink plain water it effectively dilutes the sodium, thus reducing your urge to drink before you are fully hydrated. Therefore, consuming a small amount of sodium (0.23–0.69 g/litre) in a sports drink will encourage you to drink more fluid (Sawka et al., 2007).

WHY DO SPORTS DRINKS CONTAIN CARBOHYDRATES (SUGARS)?

Carbohydrate in sports drinks serves two purposes: speeding up water absorption (Gisolphi et al., 1992) and providing an additional source of energy (Coggan & Coyle, 1987).

Relatively dilute solutions of carbohydrate (hypotonic or isotonic) stimulate water absorption from the small intestine into the bloodstream. A carbohydrate concentration usually in the range 40–80 g/litre is used in isotonic sports drinks to accelerate water absorption. More concentrated drinks (hypertonic), above 80 g/litre, tend to slow down the stomach emptying and therefore reduce the speed of fluid replacement (Murray et al., 1999).

Studies have shown that consuming extra carbohydrate during exercise can improve performance because it helps maintain blood glucose levels (Febbraio et al., 2000; Bosch et al., 1994).

WHAT IS MALTODEXTRIN?

Between a sugar (1–2 units) and a starch (several 100,000 units), although closer to the former, is maltodextrin (glucose polymers). These are chains of between 4 and 20 glucose molecules produced from boiling corn starch under controlled commercial conditions.

The advantage of using maltodextrin instead of glucose or sucrose in a drink is that a higher

How does weather affect performance?

Air temperature and wind speed can both affect performance. The hotter and more humid the weather, and the less wind there is, the more fluid your body will lose and the greater the chance of dehydration occurring.

In one study, 6 athletes cycled on a stationary bike at a set resistance. When the surrounding temperature was 2°C they could cycle for 73 minutes before experiencing exhaustion. When the surrounding temperature increased to 33°C, they could only cycle for 35 minutes. When the athletes were given a carbohydrate drink, it was found that they could keep going for longer in the cold temperature. However, the drink made no difference in the hot temperature.

In hot conditions, the body's priority is to replace water rather than carbohydrate. So drink water or a dilute carbohydrate electrolyte drink rather than a more concentrated carbohydrate drink. If you exercise in cold weather and sweat only a little, you may find a more concentrated carbohydrate drink beneficial.

concentration of carbohydrate can be achieved (usually between 100 and 200 g/litre) at a lower osmolality. That's because each molecule contains several glucose units yet still exerts the same osmotic pressure as just one molecule of glucose. So an isotonic or hypotonic drink can be produced with a carbohydrate content greater than 80 g/litre.

Also, maltodextrin is less sweet than simple sugars, so you can achieve a fairly concentrated drink that does not taste too sickly. In fact, most maltodextrin drinks and gels are fairly tasteless unless they have added artificial flavours or sweeteners.

WHAT ARE 'MULTIPLE TRANSPORTABLE CARBOHYDRATES'?

This term refers to a mixture of carbohydrates (e.g. glucose and fructose; maltodextrin and fructose) in sports drinks. These carbohydrates are absorbed from the intestine by different transporters, and using a mixture rather than a single type of carbohydrate in a sports drink overcomes the usual limitation of gut uptake of glucose. Studies show that such mixtures increase muscle carbohydrate uptake and oxidation during exercise compared with glucose-only drinks (Jeukendrup, 2010; IOC, 2011; Jeukendrup, 2008).

It means that more concentrated drinks can be consumed, providing the body with 90 g carbohydrate/hour instead of 30–60 g/hour. These drinks would be appropriate only if you are exercising at a high intensity for 3 hours or longer.

SHOULD I CHOOSE STILL OR CARBONATED SPORTS DRINKS?

Experiments at East Carolina University and Ball State University found that carbonated and still sports drinks produced equal hydration in the body (Hickey *et al.*, 1994). However, the carbonated drinks tended to produce a higher incidence of mild heartburn and stomach discomfort. In practice, many athletes find that carbonated drinks make them feel full and 'gassy', which may well limit the amount they drink.

SHOULD I TAKE SALT TABLETS IN HOT WEATHER?

No, salt tablets are not a good idea, even if you are sweating heavily in hot weather. They produce a very concentrated sodium solution in your stomach (strongly hypertonic), which delays stomach emptying and rehydration as extra fluid must first be absorbed from your body into your stomach to dilute the sodium. The best way to replace fluid and electrolyte losses is by drinking a dilute sodium/carbohydrate drink (either hypotonic or isotonic) with a sodium concentration of 40–110 mg/100 ml.

CAN I MAKE MY OWN SPORTS DRINKS?

Definitely! Commercial sports drinks work out to be very expensive if you are drinking at least 1 litre per day to replace fluid losses during exercise. (If you need to drink less than 1 litre, you probably don't need a sports drink anyway.)

Table 7.3 includes some recipes for making your own sports drink.

Other non-alcoholic drinks

CAN ORDINARY SOFT DRINKS AND FRUIT JUICE IMPROVE PERFORMANCE?

Ordinary soft drinks (typically between 90 and 200 g carbohydrate/litre) and fruit juices (typically between 110 and 130 g carbohydrate/litre) are hypertonic; in other words, they are more concentrated than body fluids, so are not ideal as fluid replacers during exercise. They empty more slowly from the stomach than plain water because they must first be diluted with water from the body, thus causing a temporary net reduction in body fluid.

If you dilute one part fruit juice with one part water, you will get an isotonic drink, ideal for rehydrating and refuelling during or after exercise (see Table 7.3).

CAN 'LITE' SPORTS DRINKS IMPROVE PERFORMANCE?

These types of drinks are hypotonic, containing around 20 g sugar/litre along with artificial sweeteners, flavourings, and electrolytes. Their high sodium content means they may promote fluid retention and stimulate thirst more than plain water, and the flavours make the drinks palatable – but they don't deliver much carbohydrate energy. They would therefore not be advantageous for intense workouts lasting longer than 1 hour and, even for shorter workouts, offer few advantages over plain water, apart from improving palatability and encouraging you to drink more.

ARE 'DIET' DRINKS SUITABLE DURING EXERCISE?

'Diet' or low calorie drinks contain artificial sweeteners in place of sugars and have a very low sodium concentration. They will help replace fluid at approximately the same speed as plain water but offer no performance advantage. Artificial sweeteners have no known advantage or disadvantage on performance. Choose these types of drink only if you dislike the taste of water, and under the same circumstances that you would normally choose water, i.e. for low to moderate intensity exercise lasting less than 1 hour.

CAN CAFFEINE-CONTAINING ENERGY DRINKS IMPROVE MY PERFORMANCE?

A number of energy drinks containing caffeine claim to improve some aspect of performance,

Table 7.3 DIY SPORTS DRINKS	
Hypotonic	**Isotonic**
• 20–40 g sucrose • 1 litre warm water • 1–1.5 g (¼ tsp) salt (optional) • Sugar-free/low-calorie squash for flavouring (optional)	• 40–80 g sucrose • 1 litre warm water • 1–1.5 g (¼ tsp) salt (optional) • Sugar-free/low-calorie squash for flavouring (optional)
• 100 ml fruit squash • 900 ml water • 1–1.5 g (¼ tsp) salt (optional)	• 200 ml fruit squash • 800 ml water • 1–1.5 g (¼ tsp) salt (optional)
• 250 ml fruit juice • 750 ml water • 1–1.5 g (¼ tsp) salt (optional)	• 500 ml fruit juice • 500 ml water • 1–1.5 g (¼ tsp) salt (optional)

such as alertness, endurance or concentration during exercise. The exact mechanism is not clear, but it is thought that caffeine at doses of 1–3 mg/kg reduces the perception of fatigue and allows you to continue exercising at a higher intensity for a longer period (Graham & Spriet, 1995) (*see* p. 117). For a 70 kg person, this would be 210 mg, equivalent to about 2 cups of coffee or 2 cans of caffeinated energy drink. Performance benefits occur soon after consumption so caffeine may be consumed just before exercise, spread throughout exercise, or late in exercise as fatigue is beginning to occur. As individual responses vary, you should experiment during training to find the dose and protocol that suits you.

A study at the University of Saskatchewan tested the effects of Red Bull energy drink on weight training performance (Forbes *et al.*, 2007). They found that consuming Red Bull (in amounts equivalent to 2 mg caffeine per kg body weight; each can contains 80 mg caffeine) 1 hour before exercise significantly increased bench press muscle endurance.

SHOULD I AVOID REHYDRATING WITH CAFFEINATED DRINKS?

It is a myth that you should completely avoid rehydrating with caffeinated drinks such as tea, coffee or cola. Researchers at the University of Maastricht found that cyclists were able to rehydrate after a long cycle equally well with water or a caffeine-containing cola drink (Brouns, 1998). Urine output was the same after both drinks. However, large doses of caffeine – over 600 mg, enough to cause a marked ergogenic effect – may result in a larger fluid loss. A study at the University of Connecticut, US, found that both caffeine-containing cola and caffeine-free cola

Table 7.4	CAFFEINE CONTENT OF VARIOUS DRINKS AND FOODS
Drink	**mg caffeine/cup**
Ground coffee	80–90
Instant coffee	60
Decaffeinated coffee	3
Tea	40
Energy/sports drinks	Up to 100 (per can)
Can of cola	40
Energy gel (1 sachet)	40
Chocolate (54 g bar)	40

maintained hydration in athletes (during the non-exercise periods) over 3 successive days of training (Fiala *et al.*, 2004). The athletes drank water during training sessions but rehydrated with either caffeinated or caffeine-free drinks. A further study by the same researchers confirmed that moderate caffeine intakes (up to 452 mg caffeine/kg body weight/day) did not increase urine output compared with a placebo and concluded that caffeine does not cause a fluid electrolyte balance in the body (Armstrong *et al.*, 2005).

Alcohol

HOW DOES ALCOHOL AFFECT PERFORMANCE?

Drinking alcohol before exercise may appear to make you more alert and confident but, even in small amounts, it will certainly have the following negative effects:

- reduce coordination, reaction time, balance and judgement;
- reduce strength, power, speed and endurance;
- reduce your ability to regulate body temperature;
- reduce blood sugar levels and increase the risk of hypoglycaemia;
- increase water excretion (urination) and the risk of dehydration;
- increase the risk of accident or injury.

CAN I DRINK ALCOHOL ON NON-TRAINING DAYS?

There is no reason why you cannot enjoy alcohol in moderation on non-training days. The government recommends 14 units a week as a safe upper limit (see Table 7.5 for 1 unit equivalent measures). Ideally, this should be spread evenly over 3 days or more and you should try to have alcohol-free days. Pregnant women should avoid drinking altogether. However, research has shown that alcohol drunk in moderation reduces the risk of heart disease. Moderate drinkers have a lower risk of death from heart disease than teetotallers or heavy drinkers. The exact mechanism is not certain, but it may work by increasing HDL cholesterol levels, the protective type of cholesterol in the blood. HDL transports cholesterol back to the liver for excretion, thereby reducing the chance of it sticking to artery walls. It may also reduce the stickiness of blood platelets, thus reducing the risk of blood clots (thrombosis). Red wine, in particular, may be especially good for the heart. Studies have shown that drinking up to 2 glasses a day can lower heart disease

Table 7.5	ALCOHOLIC AND CALORIE CONTENTS OF DRINKS	
Drink equivalent to 1 unit	% alcohol by volume	Calories
250 ml standard beer/lager	4	90
25 ml spirits	40	50
250 ml alcopop	14	155
76 ml wine	13	75
50 ml sherry	17.5	75
25 ml liqueur	40	85

risk by 30–70%. It contains flavonoids from the grape skin, which have an antioxidant effect and thus protect the LDL cholesterol from free radical damage.

WHAT EXACTLY HAPPENS TO ALCOHOL IN THE BODY?

When you drink alcohol, about 20% is absorbed into the bloodstream through the stomach and the remainder through the small intestine. Most of this alcohol is then broken down in the liver (it cannot be stored, as it is toxic) into a substance called acetyl CoA and then, ultimately, into ATP (adenosine triphosphate or energy). Obviously, while this is occurring, less glycogen and fat are used to produce ATP in other parts of the body.

However, the liver can carry out this job only at a fixed rate of approximately 1 unit alcohol/ hour. If you drink more alcohol than this, it is dealt with by a different enzyme system in the liver (the microsomal ethanol oxidising system, MEO) to make it less toxic to the body. The more alcohol you drink on a regular basis, the more MEO enzymes are produced, which is why you can develop an increased tolerance to alcohol – you need to drink more to experience the same physiological effects.

Initially, alcohol reduces inhibitions, increases self-confidence and makes you feel more at ease. However, it is actually a depressant rather than a stimulant, reducing your psychomotor (coordination) skills. It is potentially toxic to all of the cells and organs in your body and, if it builds up to high concentrations, it can cause damage to the liver, stomach and brain.

Too much alcohol causes hangovers – headache, thirst, nausea, vomiting and heartburn. These symptoms are due partly to dehydration and a swelling of the blood vessels in the head. Congeners, substances found mainly in darker alcoholic drinks such as rum and red wine, are also responsible for many of the hangover symptoms. Prevention is better than cure, so make sure you follow the guidelines on p. 162. The best way to deal with a hangover is to drink plenty of water or, better still, a sports drink. Do not attempt to train or compete with a hangover!

Summary of key points

- Dehydration causes cardiovascular stress, increases core body temperature and impairs performance.
- Fluid losses during exercise depend on exercise duration and intensity; temperature and humidity; body size; fitness level and the individual. They can be as high as 1–2 litres/hour.
- Always start exercise well hydrated.
- During exercise, drink only to the point at which you are maintaining, not gaining weight, to avoid the risk of hyponatraemia.
- After exercise, replace by 150% any body weight deficit.
- Water is a suitable fluid replacement drink for low or moderate intensity exercise lasting less than 1 hour.
- For intense exercise between 1 and 3 hours duration, a sports drink containing up to 80 g carbohydrate/litre can speed up water absorption, provide additional fuel, delay fatigue and improve performance.
- Consuming 30–60 g carbohydrate/hour can maintain blood sugar levels and improve performance in intense exercise lasting more than 1 hour. For high intensity exercise longer than 3 hours, consuming up to 90 g carbohydrate/hour in the form of multiple transportable carbohydrates will help increase endurance.
- Hypotonic (< 40g/litre and isotonic (40–80 g/litre) sports drinks are most suitable when rapid fluid replacement is the main priority.
- Carbohydrate drinks based on maltodextrin also replace fluids, but provide greater amounts of carbohydrate (100–200g/litre) at a lower osmolality. They are most suitable for prolonged intense exercise (> 90 minutes), when fuel replacement is a major priority or fluid losses are small.
- The main purpose of sodium in a sports drink is to increase the urge to drink, promote fluid retention and increase palatability.
- Alcohol before exercise has a negative effect on strength, endurance, coordination, power and speed, and increases injury risk.
- Men and women should not regularly drink more than 14 units of alcohol a week.

Body fat and dietary fat

As athletes in almost every sport strive to get leaner and competitive standards get higher, the relationship between body fat, health and performance becomes increasingly important. However, the optimal body composition for fitness or sports performance is not necessarily a desirable one from a health point of view. This chapter covers the different methods for measuring body fat percentage and body fat distribution, and considers their relevance to performance. It highlights the dangers of attaining very low body fat levels, as well as the risks associated with a very low fat diet. It gives realistic guidance on recommended body fat ranges and fat intakes, and explains the difference between the various types of fats found in the diet.

DOES BODY FAT AFFECT PERFORMANCE?

Carrying around excess body weight in the form of fat is a distinct disadvantage in almost every sport. It can adversely affect strength, speed and endurance. Surplus fat is basically surplus baggage. Carrying around this extra weight is not only unnecessary, but also costly in terms of energy expenditure. There are three main categories of sports where body fat can have a detrimental effect on performance:

1. Gravitational sports, where excess body fat impairs performance for gravitational reasons. For example, in long distance running and road cycling, surplus fat can reduce speed and increase fatigue. It is like carrying a couple of shopping bags with you as you run; they make it harder for you to get up speed, slow you down and cause you to tire quickly. It is best to leave your shopping bags at home, or at least to lighten the load. In explosive sports (e.g. sprinting/jumping), where you must transfer or lift the weight of your whole body very quickly, extra fat again is non-functional weight, slowing you down, reducing your power and decreasing your mechanical efficiency. Muscle is useful weight, whereas excess fat is not.
2. Weight-category sports (e.g. boxing, karate, judo, lightweight rowing), where greater emphasis is put on body weight, particularly during the competitive season. The person with the greatest percentage of muscle and the smallest percentage of fat has the advantage.
3. Aesthetic sports, such as figure skating, artistic and rhythmic gymnastics, diving and synchro-

nised swimming, where success depends on body shape and composition as well as physical skill.

In virtually every sport, it is the leanest body that wins. Reducing your body fat while maintaining lean mass and health will result in improved performance.

IS BODY FAT AN ADVANTAGE IN CERTAIN SPORTS?

Until recently, it was believed that extra weight – even in the form of fat – was an advantage for certain sports in which momentum is important (e.g. discus, hammer throwing, judo, wrestling).

A heavy body can generate more momentum to throw an object or knock over an opponent, but there is no reason why this weight should be fat. It would be better if it were in the form of muscle. Muscle is stronger and more powerful than fat – although, admittedly, it is harder to acquire! If two athletes both weighed 100 kg, but one comprised 90 kg lean (10 kg fat) mass, and the other 70 kg lean (30 kg fat) mass, the leaner one would obviously have the advantage. Perhaps the only sport where fat could be considered a necessary advantage is sumo wrestling – it would be almost impossible to acquire a very large body mass without fat gain.

HOW CAN I TELL IF I AM TOO FAT?

Looking in the mirror is the quickest and simplest way to see if you are too fat by everyday standards, but this will not give the accurate

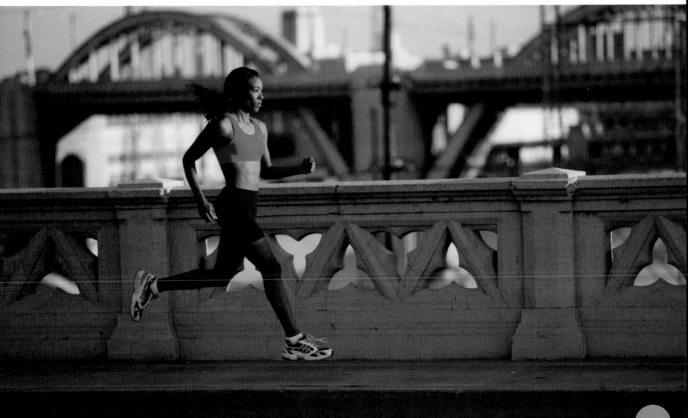

information that you need for your sport. Many people also tend to perceive themselves as fatter or thinner than they really are. It is useful, therefore, to employ some sort of measurement system so that you can work towards a definite goal.

Standing on a set of scales, reading your weight and comparing it to standard weight and height charts is simple. However, it has several drawbacks. Weights and heights given in charts are based on average weights of a sample population. They are only *average* weights for *average* people, not ideal weights, and give no indication of body composition or health risk.

To get a general picture of your health risk, you can calculate your Body Mass Index (BMI) from your weight and height measurements.

WHAT IS THE BODY MASS INDEX?

Doctors and researchers often use a measurement called the Body Mass Index (BMI) to classify different grades of body weight and to assess health risk. It is sometimes referred to as the Quetelet Index after the Belgian statistician Adolphe Quetelet, who observed that for normal weight people there is more or less a constant ratio between weight and the square of height. The BMI assumes that there is no single ideal weight for a person of a certain height, and that there is a healthy weight range for any given height.

The BMI is calculated by dividing a person's weight (in kg) by the square of his or her height (in m). For example, if your weight is 60 kg and height 1.7 m, your BMI is 21.

$$\frac{60}{1.7 \times 1.7} = 21$$

For a quick online BMI calculator and detailed BMI charts in imperial and metric measurements, log on to www.whathealth.com. or www.nhs.uk/Tools/Pages/Healthyweightcalculator.aspx

HOW USEFUL IS THE BMI?

Researchers and doctors use BMI measurements to assess a person's risk of acquiring certain health-related conditions, such as heart disease. Studies have shown that people with a BMI of between 18.5 and 25 have the lowest risk of developing diseases that are linked to obesity, e.g. cardiovascular disease, gall bladder disease, hypertension (high blood pressure) and type 2 diabetes. People with a BMI of between 25 and 29.9 are at increased risk, while those with a BMI above 30 are at a greater risk.

It is not true that the lower a person's BMI the better, however (*see* Table 8.1). A very low BMI is also not desirable; people with a BMI below 20 have a higher risk of other health problems, such as respiratory disease, certain cancers and metabolic complications.

Both those with a BMI below 18.5 and those above 30 have an increased risk of premature death (*see* Fig. 8.1).

Table 8.1	BMI CATEGORIES
Category	**BMI**
Underweight	< 18.5
Ideal	18.5–24.9
Overweight	25–29.9
Obese	30–39.9
Very obese	40+

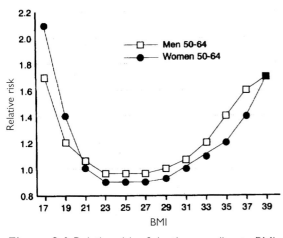

Figure 8.1 Relative risk of death according to BMI

WHAT ARE THE LIMITATIONS OF THE BMI?

BMI does not give information about body composition, i.e. how much weight is fat and how much lean tissue. It simply gives an indication of the health risk for *average* people – not *sportspeople*!

When you stand on the scales, you weigh everything – bone, muscle and water, as well as fat. Therefore you do not know how fat you actually are. Individuals who are athletic and/or have a muscular build may be categorised as overweight. For example, bodybuilders and rugby players with a high percentage of lean body mass and a low percentage body fat would be erroneously categorised as overweight or obese. Body fat can be underestimated in individuals who have little muscle or who are very overweight.

Also, BMI doesn't take into account *where* fat is stored in your body. This is important because it affects your health risk as well as your body shape.

IS THE DISTRIBUTION OF BODY FAT IMPORTANT?

Scientists believe that the distribution of your body fat is more important than the total amount of fat. This gives a more accurate assessment of your risk of metabolic disorders such as heart disease, type 2 diabetes, high blood pressure and gall bladder disease. Fat stored mostly around the abdomen (visceral fat) gives rise to an 'apple' or 'barrel' shape, and this carries a much bigger health risk than fat stored mostly around the hips and thighs (peripheral or gynecoid obesity) in a pear shape. For most people, visceral fat is the largest store and is one of the first places where excess fat is laid down. When the store gets too large, it begins to pump out inflammatory and clot-producing compounds. This means that a man with a 'beer belly' but slim limbs may be at greater risk of heart disease and diabetes than a pear-shaped person with the same BMI but less visceral fat.

The way we distribute fat on our body is determined partly by our genetic make-up and partly by our natural hormonal balance. Men, for example, have higher levels of testosterone, which favours fat deposition around the abdomen, between the shoulder blades and close to the internal organs. Women have higher levels of oestrogen, which favours fat deposition around the hips, thighs, breasts and triceps. After the menopause, however, when oestrogen levels fall, fat tends to transfer from the hips and thighs to the abdomen, giving women more of an apple shape and pushing up their chances of heart disease.

Excess fat in the abdomen is a health risk. This is partly to do with the close proximity of the intra-abdominal fat to the liver. Fatty acids from the adipose tissue are delivered into the portal vein that goes directly to the liver. The liver thus receives a continuous supply of fat-rich blood and this stimulates increased cholesterol synthesis. A high blood cholesterol level is a major risk factor for heart disease. Visceral fat also reduces the body's sensitivity to insulin, which increases the risk of developing type 2 diabetes.

HOW CAN I MEASURE MY BODY FAT DISTRIBUTION?

You can assess your body fat distribution by two methods:

1. *Waist circumference*: Scientists at the Royal Infirmary, Glasgow, have found that waist circumference measurement correlates well with intra-abdominal fat and total body fat percentage (Lean *et al.*, 1995) and is more accurate than body weight or BMI in predicting type 2 diabetes (Wang *et al.*, 2005). A waist circum-

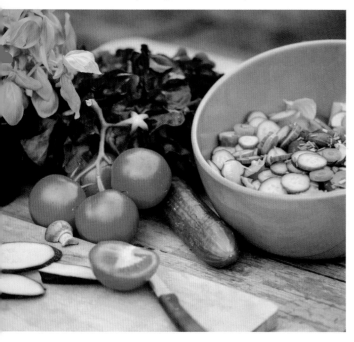

ference of 94 cm or more in men or 80 cm or more in women indicates excess abdominal fat.

2. *Waist-to-height ratio* This is a more accurate method than BMI for assessing health risk (Ashwell *et al.*, 2011). Divide your waist measurement by your height. It should be no more than half your height. If your waist measures more than half your height then your health risks are higher and your life expectancy lower. For example, if you are 1.72m (5ft 8in/68in) tall, your waist size should be 86cm (34in) or less.

WHAT DOES BODY COMPOSITION MEAN?

Body composition can be defined as the proportion of fat and fat-free mass (FFM) in the body. FFM includes muscles, organs, bones and blood. Fat mass includes fat that is stored as an energy source and fat in the central nervous system, bone marrow and the fat surrounding your organs, known as essential fat. The proportion of these two components in the body is called body composition. This is more important than total body weight. Body composition is typically expressed as % body fat and FFM.

For example, two people may weigh the same, but have a different body composition. Athletes usually have a smaller percentage of body fat and a higher percentage of lean weight than less physically active people. Lean body tissue is functional (or useful) weight, whereas fat is non-functional in terms of sports performance.

HOW CAN I MEASURE BODY COMPOSITION?

Clearly, height and weight measurements are not very accurate for assessing your body composition.

To give you a more accurate idea of how much fat and how much muscle you have, there are a number of techniques for measuring body composition. These will tell you how much of your weight is muscle or fat as a percentage of your total weight.

The only method that is 100% accurate is cadaver analysis. Clearly this is impractical, so indirect methods must be used.

Underwater weighing

For a long time, this method was judged to be the most accurate. Its accuracy rate averages 97–98%. However, there are other methods, such as dual energy x-ray absorptiometry and magnetic resonance imaging, which produce similar, if not more accurate, results.

Underwater weighing works on the Archimedes' principle, which states that when an object is submerged under water it creates a buoyant counter force equal to the weight of water that it has displaced. Since bone and muscle are more dense than water, a person with a higher percentage of lean mass will weigh more in water, indicating a lower percentage of fat. Since fat is less dense than water, a person with a high fat percentage will weigh less in water than on land.

In this test, the person sits on a swing-seat and is then submerged into a water tank. After expelling as much air as possible from the lungs, the person's weight is recorded. This figure is then compared with the person's weight on dry land, using standard equations on a computer, and the fat percentage calculated.

The disadvantage of this method is that the specialised equipment is expensive and bulky and found only at research institutions or laboratories,

i.e. it is not readily available to the public. The person also needs to be water-confident.

BOD POD (air displacement plethysmography)

A newer method is the BOD POD, which is similar to the principle behind underwater weighing but uses air displacement rather than weight under water. But, like underwater weighing, it is available only through university exercise science departments and is relatively expensive.

Skinfold callipers

The skinfold measurement method is widely available and in many gyms, health clubs, clinics and practices. The callipers measure in millimetres the layer of fat just underneath the skin at various places on the body. This is done on three to seven specific places (such as the triceps, biceps, hip bone area, lower back, abdomen, thigh and below the shoulder blade). Using these measurements, scientists have developed mathematical equations that account for age, sex, known body densities and estimated hidden fat that the callipers cannot measure. These equations produce a body density value, which another equation then changes into a body fat percentage.

The accuracy of this method depends almost entirely on the skill of the person taking the measurements. Also, it assumes that everyone has a predictable pattern of fat distribution as they age. Therefore, it becomes less accurate with elite athletes, as they tend to have a different pattern of fat distribution compared with sedentary people, and for very lean and obese people. There are different sets of equations to use, which take account of these factors. For the general population (over 15% body fat), the Durnin and

Womersley (1974) equations are more suitable. The Jackson–Pollock (1984) equations apply best to lean and athletic people.

Kinanthropometry is the term for the recording of skinfold thickness measurements and body girth measurements (e.g. arms, chest, legs etc.) in order to monitor changes in body composition over time. The sites of girth measurements are shown in Figure 9.2 (*see* p. 193).

An alternative is to present the body fat measurement as a 'sum of skinfolds'. This is the sum of the individual skinfold thicknesses from the seven specific sites.

Bioelectrical impedance analysis

Most body fat monitors and scales work using bioelectrical impedance analysis (BIA). These are widely available and used in gyms, sports centres and clinics. Here, a mild electrical current is sent through the body between electrodes attached to two specific points of the body (either between the hand and opposite foot, or from one foot to the other). The principle is that lean tissue (such as muscle and blood) contains high levels of water and electrolytes and is therefore a good conductor of electricity, whereas fat creates a resistance. Increasing levels of fat mass result in a higher impedance value and correspond to higher levels of body fat.

The advantages are the machine is portable, simple to operate and testing takes less than one minute. The disadvantage is the poor degree of accuracy compared with other methods. For example, changes in body fluid levels and skin temperature will affect the passage of the current and therefore the body fat reading. It tends to overestimate the body fat percentage of lean muscular people by 2–5% and underestimate the

body fat percentage of overweight people by the same amount (Sun *et al.*, 2005). It is important that you are well-hydrated when having a BIA measurement; if you are dehydrated, the current will not be conducted through your lean mass so well, giving you a higher body fat percentage reading.

Dual energy x-ray absorptiometry

Dual energy x-ray absorptiometry (DEXA) was originally developed for measuring bone density and diagnosing osteoporosis. However, it can also be used to measure total body fat. It produces an accurate body composition map, showing exactly where your fat is distributed around the body. In this method, two types of x-rays are scanned over the whole body to measure fat, bone and muscle. The procedure takes about 5–20 minutes, depending on the type of machine.

It is one of the most accurate methods for assessing body fat, although less reliable for lean athletes. The disadvantages are the cost and size of the machine and lack of accessibility. DEXA machines are found in hospitals and research institutions. It may be possible to request a body fat analysis at your nearest site, but be prepared to pay considerably more than you would for the other methods.

Near-infrared interactance

In near-infrared interactance, an infrared beam is shone perpendicularly through the upper arm. The amount of light reflected back to the analyser from the bone depends on the amount of fat located there, which is correlated to the body fat percentage. Age, weight, height, sex and activity level are all taken into account in the calculations.

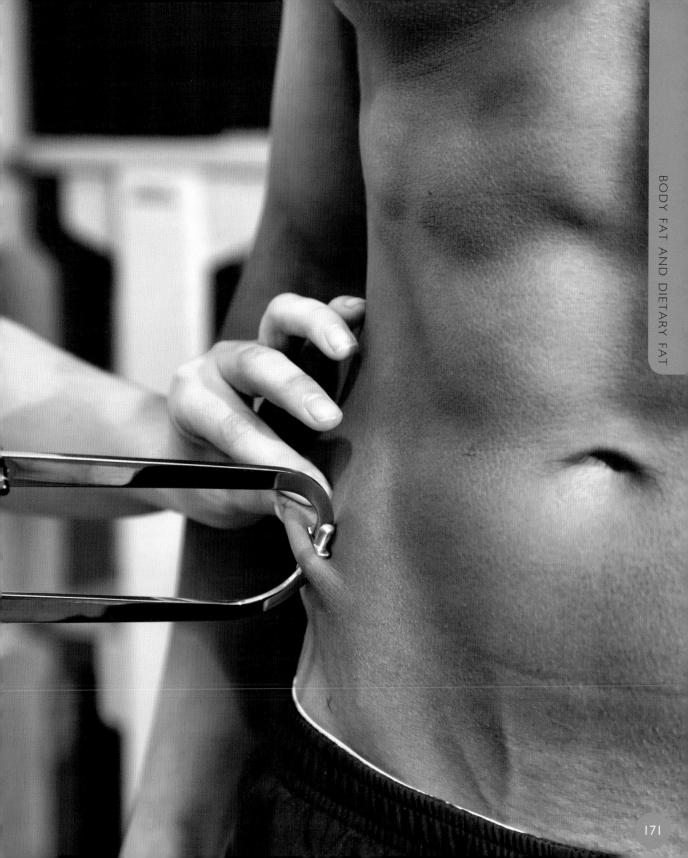

The obvious disadvantage of this method is the assumption that fat in the arm is proportional to total body fat. However, it is a very fast, easy and cheap method. The equipment is portable, and anyone can operate it.

HOW ACCURATE ARE THESE METHODS?

Table 8.2 summarises studies that have assessed the accuracy of the various methods. DEXA and underwater weighing are regarded as the most accurate methods. Skinfold and BIA measurements – provided they are carefully carried out – can estimate body fat percentages with a 3–4% error (Houtkooper, 2000; Lohman, 1992). For example, if the actual body fat percentage is 15%, then predicted values could range from 12 to 18% (assuming a 3% error). But if poor measurement techniques or incorrectly calibrated instruments are used, then the margin of error could be greater. Since a relatively high degree of error is associated with these indirect body fat assessment methods, it is not recommended to set a specific body fat goal for athletes (ACSM, 2000). Instead, a range of target body fat values would be more realistic.

WHAT IS THE MINIMUM BODY FAT I NEED?

A fat-free body would not survive. It is important to realise that a certain amount of body fat is absolutely vital. In fact, there are two components of body fat: essential fat and storage fat. *Essential fat* includes the fat that forms part of your cell membranes, brain tissue, nerve sheaths, bone marrow and the fat surrounding your organs (e.g. heart, liver, kidneys). Here it provides insulation, protection and cushioning against physical damage. In a healthy person, this accounts for about 3% of body weight.

Women have an additional essential fat requirement called sex-specific fat, which is stored mostly in the breasts and around the hips. This fat accounts for a further 5–9% of a woman's body weight and is involved in oestrogen production as well as the conversion of inactive oestrogen into its active form. So, this fat ensures normal hormonal balance and menstrual function. If stores fall too low, hormonal imbalance and menstrual irregularities result, although these can be reversed once body fat increases. There is some recent evidence that a certain amount of body fat in men is necessary for normal hormone production too. It is commonly suggested that 5% body fat for men and 12% for women is the minimum required for healthy endocrine and immune function (Lohman, 1992).

The second component of body fat, *storage fat*, is an important energy reserve that

Table 8.2	ACCURACY OF BODY FAT MEASUREMENT METHODS
Method	**Degree of inaccuracy**
DEXA	< 2%
Skinfold measurement	3–4%
BOD POD	2–3.5%
Underwater weighing	2–3%
Bioelectrical impedance	3–5%
Near-infrared interactance	5–10%

Source: Ackland et al., 2012.

Table 8.3	AVERAGE BODY FAT PERCENTAGES IN VARIOUS SPORTS				
Sport	Male	Female	Sport	Male	Female
Baseball	12–15%	12–18%	Shot put	16–20%	20–28%
Basketball	6–12%	20–27%	Skiing (X country)	7–12%	16–22%
Bodybuilding	5–8%	10–15%	Sprinting	8–10%	12–20%
Cycling	5–15%	15–20%	Swimming	9–12%	14–24%
Gymnastics	5–12%	10–16%	Tennis	12–16%	16–24%
High/long jumping	7–12%	10–18%	Triathlon	5–12%	10–15%
Ice/field hockey	8–15%	12–18%	Volleyball	11–14%	16–25%
Racquetball	8–13%	15–22%	Weightlifting	9–16%	No data
Rowing	6–14%	12–18%	Wrestling	5–16%	No data

Source: Ackland et al., 2012.

takes the form of fat (adipose) cells under the skin (subcutaneous fat) and around the organs (intra-abdominal fat). Fat is used virtually all the time during any aerobic activity: while sleeping, sitting, standing and walking, as well as in most types of exercise. It is impossible to spot reduce fat selectively from adipose tissue sites by specific exercises or diets. The body generally uses fat from all sites, although the exact pattern of fat utilisation (and storage) is determined by your genetic make-up and hormonal balance. An average person has enough fat for 3 days and 3 nights of continuous running – although, in practice, you would experience fatigue long before your fat reserves ran out. So, your fat stores are certainly not a redundant depot of unwanted energy!

WHAT IS A DESIRABLE BODY FAT PERCENTAGE FOR ATHLETES?

There is no 'one size fits all' recommendation. Body fat percentages for athletes vary depending on the particular sport. According to scientists at the University of Arizona, the ideal body fat percentage, in terms of performance, for most male athletes lies between 6 and 15%, and for female athletes, 12 and 18% (Wilmore, J. H., 1983). In general, for men, middle- and long-distance runners and bodybuilders have the lowest body fat levels (less than 6%) while cyclists, gymnasts, sprinters, triathletes and basketball players average between 6 and 15% body fat (Sinning, 1998). In female athletes, the lowest body fat levels (6–15%) are observed in bodybuilders, cyclists, gymnasts, runners and triathletes (Sinning, 1998).

Physiologists recommend a minimum of 5% fat for men and 12% fat for women to cover the most basic functions associated with good health (Lohman, 1992). However, optimal body fat levels may be much higher than these minimums. The percentage of fat associated with lowest health risk is 13–18% for men and 18–25% for women. Figure 8.2 gives the body fat percentages for standard (non-athletic) adults.

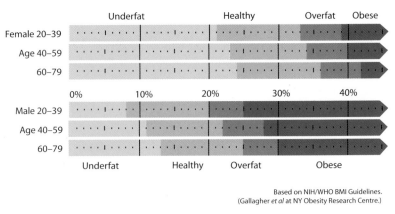

Based on NIH/WHO BMI Guidelines.
(Gallagher *et al* at NY Obesity Research Centre.)

Figure 8.2 Healthy body ranges for adults

Clearly, there is no ideal body fat percentage for any particular sport. Each individual athlete has an optimal fat range at which their performance improves yet their health does not suffer. For this reason, sports scientists believe that a range of values for body fat percentage should be established, outside of which your performance and/or health is likely to be impaired. Staying below the upper limit should be your target but lower is not necessarily better.

LOWER IS NOT NECESSARILY BETTER

Reducing your body fat may lead to improvements in performance but if the loss is too rapid or too severe, then your performance and health may suffer. Women and men who try to attain very low body fat levels, or a level that is unnatural for their genetic make-up, encounter problems. These problems can be serious, particularly for women, who may suffer long-term effects. Collectively known as 'Relative Energy Deficiency in Sport (RED-S)', these problems are discussed in greater detail in Chapter 11: The Female Athlete.

WHAT ARE THE DANGERS FOR WOMEN WITH VERY LOW BODY FAT LEVELS?

One of the biggest problems for women with very low body fat levels is the resulting hormonal imbalance and amenorrhoea (absence of periods).

As explained in more detail in Chapter 11, this tends to be triggered once body fat levels fall below 15–20% – the threshold level varies from one person to another. This fall in body fat, together with other factors such as low calorie intake and heavy training, is sensed by the hypothalamus of the brain, which then decreases its production of the hormone (gonadotrophin-releasing hormone) that acts on the pituitary gland. This, in turn, reduces the production of important hormones that act on the ovaries (luteinising hormone and follicle-stimulating hormone), causing them to produce less oestrogen and progesterone. The end result is a deficiency of oestrogen and progesterone and a cessation of menstrual periods (*see* Fig. 8.3).

Amenorrhoea can lead to more serious problems such as bone loss, because low oestrogen levels result in loss of bone minerals and, therefore,

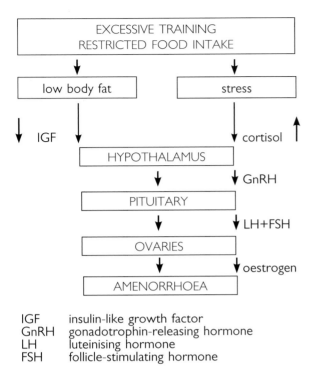

IGF	insulin-like growth factor
GnRH	gonadotrophin-releasing hormone
LH	luteinising hormone
FSH	follicle-stimulating hormone

Figure 8.3 The development of amenorrhoea

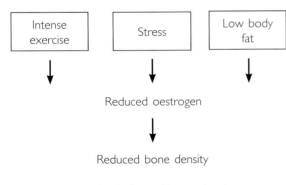

Figure 8.4 Low body fat and bone density

is similar to the osteoporosis that affects post-menopausal women, where bones become thinner, lighter and more fragile. Amenorrhoeic athletes, therefore, run a greater risk of stress fractures. The British Olympic Medical Centre has reported cases of athletes in their twenties and thirties with osteoporotic-type fractures.

Low body fat levels also upset the metabolism of the sex hormones, reducing their potency and thus fertility. Therefore, a very low body fat level drastically reduces a woman's chances of getting pregnant. However, the good news is that once your body fat level increases over your threshold and your training volume is reduced, your hormonal balance, periods and fertility generally return to normal.

WHAT ARE THE DANGERS FOR MEN WITH VERY LOW BODY FAT LEVELS?

Studies on competitive male wrestlers 'making weight' for contests found that once body fat levels fell below 5%, testosterone levels decreased, causing a drastic fall in sperm count, libido and sexual activity. Studies on male runners found similar changes. However, testosterone levels and libido return to normal once body fat increases. Team doctors in the US recommend a minimum of 7% fat before allowing wrestlers to compete.

Thyroid hormone, growth hormone, IGF-1, metabolic rate, and the immune system are all severely reduced when body fat levels drop too low. Cortisol levels rise drastically, especially during periods of intense training.

WHAT ARE THE PROBLEMS WITH LOW-FAT DIETS?

It is recommended that athletes should consume a minimum of 20% energy from fat (ACSM/

bone density (*see* Fig. 8.4). In younger (premenopausal) women, this is called osteopoenia (i.e. lower bone density than normal for age), which

AND/DC, 2016). Lower fat intakes can leave you deficient in a variety of nutrients and lead to several health problems. You will certainly be missing out on the essential fatty acids (linoleic acid and linolenic acid) found in vegetable oils, seeds, nuts and oily fish (*see* pp 179–182), and will therefore be susceptible to dull, flaky skin and other dermatological problems; cold extremities; prostaglandin (hormone) imbalance; poor control of inflammation, blood pressure, vasoconstriction and blood clotting.

Low fat diets will be low in fat-soluble vitamins A, D and E. More importantly, fat is needed to enable your body to absorb and transport them, and to convert beta-carotene into vitamin A in the body. Although you can get vitamin D from UV light and vitamin A from beta-carotene in brightly coloured fruit and vegetables, getting enough vitamin E can be much more of a problem. It is found in significant quantities only in vegetable oils, seeds, nuts and egg yolk. Vitamin E is an important antioxidant that protects our cells from harmful free radical attack (*see* Chapter 5, p. 96). It is thought to help prevent heart disease and certain cancers and even retard aging. It may also help reduce muscle soreness after hard exercise. So, cutting out oils, nuts and seeds means you are increasing your risk of free radical damage.

Chronically low fat diets often result in a low calorie and low nutrient intake overall. Low calorie diets quickly lead to depleted glycogen (carbohydrate) stores, resulting in poor energy levels, reduced capacity for exercise, fatigue, poor recovery between workouts and eventual burnout. They can also increase protein breakdown – causing loss of muscle mass and strength or a lack of muscular development. This is just the opposite of what you should be achieving in your fitness programme.

Fat in your diet

HOW MUCH FAT SHOULD I EAT?

The ACSM/AND/DC position statement, IOC and IAAF currently make no specific recommendation for fat intake. The focus should be on meeting carbohydrate and protein goals with fat making up the calorie balance. It is recommended that athletes follow the public health guidelines for fat intake, which are less than 35% of daily energy intake, but adapt their intake according to individual training and body composition goals (ACSM/AND/DC, 2016). The emphasis should be on obtaining adequate energy, essential fatty acids and fat soluble vitamins.

For example, an athlete consuming 3000 kcal a day and meeting their requirement for carbohydrate and protein could consume 66–117g fat:

- $(3000 \times 20\%) \div 9 = 66$ g
- $(3000 \times 35\%) \div 9 = 117$g
  i.e. between 66 and 117g fat a day.

Although athletes need to focus on obtaining adequate carbohydrate and protein, this does not mean eating a low fat diet. There is evidence that restricting fat too much may reduce your performance. Conversely, eating more than the recommended maximum of 35% calories from fat intake does not appear to have any adverse effect on heart disease risk factors in athletes. In one study, runners who consumed a 42% fat diet had higher levels of HDL ('good') cholesterol and lower cardiovascular risk factors than those consuming a 16% fat diet (Leddy *et al.*, 2007).

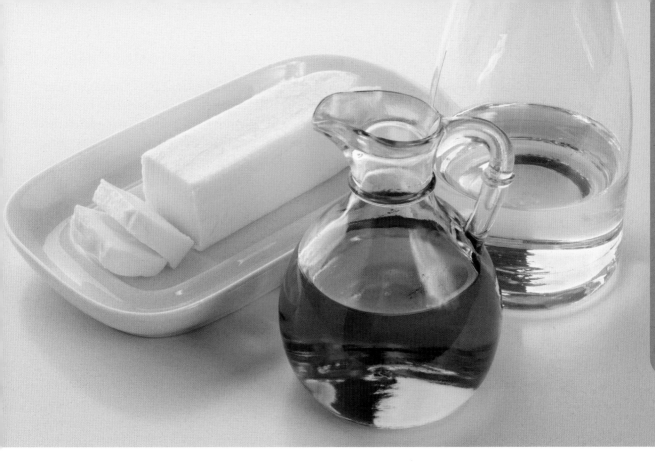

Another study by New Zealand researchers found that during periods of hard endurance training when energy requirements are high, increasing the percentage of fat in the diet to 50% of energy did not have an adverse effect on blood fats or cardiovascular risk (Brown & Cox, 1998).

The link between fat and cardiovascular disease is based mainly on Ancel Keys's Seven Countries study, which suggested that heart disease was caused by eating too much fat (Keys, 1980). More recently, the link has been shown to be weak and diets containing moderate amounts of fat (such as the traditional Mediterranean diet) may be more effective than low fat diets for protecting against heart disease, stroke and type 2 diabetes (Estruch *et al*., 2013). Researchers suggest it's the *type* of fat you eat that is more important than the *amount* you eat when it comes to cardiovascular risk. Artificial trans fatty acids appear to raise cardiovascular risk; unsaturated fatty acids (especially omega-3s) lower the risk; while saturated fatty acids are thought to be neutral.

WHAT ARE FATS?

Fats and oils found in food consist mainly of *triglycerides*. These are made up of a unit of glycerol and three fatty acids. Each fatty acid is a chain of carbon and hydrogen atoms with a carboxyl group (–COOH) at one end and a methyl group at the other end (–CH3) – chain lengths between 14 and 22 carbon atoms are most common. These fatty acids are classified in three different groups, according to their chemical structure: saturated, monounsaturated and poly-unsaturated. In food, the proportions of each group determine whether the fat is hard or liquid, how it is handled by the body and how it affects your health.

WHAT ARE SATURATED FATS?

Saturated fatty acids are fully saturated with the maximum amount of hydrogen; in other words, all of their carbon atoms are linked with a single bond to hydrogen atoms. Fats containing a high proportion of saturates are hard at room temperature and mostly come from animal products such as butter, lard, cheese and meat fat, as well as processed foods made from these fats (biscuits, cakes and pastries). Palm oil and coconut oil are also highly saturated, and are commonly used in spreads, as well as in biscuits and bakery products.

Saturated fats and health

Saturated fatty acids have long been considered the culprit fat in heart disease because they can increase total cholesterol and the more harmful low density lipoprotein (LDL) cholesterol in the blood. The Department of Health (DoH) recommends a saturated fatty acid intake of no more than 11% of total calorie intake.

However, more recent studies have shown that the link between saturated fat and heart disease risk is not as clear cut as once thought (Chowdhury *et al.*, 2014; de Oliveira Otto *et al.*, 2012; German *et al.*, 2009). While it is true that saturated fat increases blood cholesterol levels, scientists are not certain how this affects cardio-vascular risk. Some studies show that saturated fats increase the risk, while others do not. We also know that not all saturated fatty acids behave in the same way. Excess lauric, myristic and palmitic

acid are shown to decrease LDL cholesterol clearance, which increases heart disease risk, but other fatty acids do not. Research also suggests that the saturated fats found in dairy products, meat and eggs not only raise LDL cholesterol but they also raise levels of 'good' HDL (high-density lipoprotein) cholesterol, so the overall effect on cardiovascular disease risk is probably neutral (Mensink, 2003; Toth, 2005).

What you replace saturated fats with is important. If you replace saturated fats with highly refined carbohydrates, LDL cholesterol levels and heart disease risk increase. This may explain why some studies have found little benefit to reducing saturated fat since most people tend to replace them with equally unhealthy carbohydrates.

Most recent studies suggest that you should replace some of the saturated fats in your diet with unsaturated fats (found in vegetable oils, nuts, seeds and oily fish) (Hooper *et al.*, 2015; Astrup *et al.*, 2010; Jakobsen *et al.*, 2009). These healthy fats raise HDL and lower harmful LDL levels. They also improve the ratio of total cholesterol to HDL cholesterol, lowering the risk of cardiovascular disease. A 2012 review of studies from the Cochrane Collaboration found that people who did this for at least 2 years reduced their risk of heart attacks, angina and stroke by 14% (Hooper *et al.*, 2012).

Scientists from Harvard T.H. Chan School of Public Health analysed data from two large populations: 84,628 women in the Nurses' Health Study and 42,908 men in the Health Professionals Follow-Up Study, who were followed from the 1980s to 2010 (Li *et al.*, 2015). People who ate more saturated fat had a higher risk of heart disease compared to those who ate less. Also, people who ate more unsaturated fats and more wholegrain carbohydrates lowered their risk of heart disease compared to people who included less of these nutrients in their diet. They estimated that replacing 5% energy intake from saturated fats with an equivalent energy intake from either polyunsaturated fats, monounsaturated fats, or carbohydrates from whole grains was associated with 25%, 15% and 9% lower risk of heart disease, respectively.

The consensus recommendation is to consume no more than 11% daily calories from saturated fat and to replace some of the saturated fat in your diet with unsaturated fat, not refined carbohydrates. Do not aim for a 'low fat diet'; eat a 'moderate fat' diet that includes mostly mono- and polyunsaturated fats.

WHAT ARE MONOUNSATURATED FATS?

Monounsaturated fatty acids have slightly less hydrogen because their carbon chains contain one double or unsaturated bond (hence 'mono'). Oils rich in monounsaturates are usually liquid at room temperature, but may solidify at cold temperatures. The richest sources include olive, rapeseed, groundnut, hazelnut and almond oil, avocados, olives, nuts and seeds.

Monounsaturated fatty acids are thought to have the greatest health benefits. They can reduce total cholesterol, in particular LDL cholesterol, without affecting the beneficial high density lipoprotein (HDL) cholesterol. The DoH recommends a monounsaturated fatty acid intake of up to 12% of total calorie intake.

WHAT ARE POLYUNSATURATED FATS?

Polyunsaturated fatty acids have the least hydrogen – the carbon chains contain two or more double bonds (hence 'poly'). Oils rich in poly-unsaturates are liquid at both room and cold temperatures. Rich sources include most vegetable oils, nuts, seeds and oily fish (and their oils).

Numerous studies have found that eating polyunsaturated fat can reduce LDL blood cholesterol levels and lower the risk of heart disease (Mozaffarian *et al.*, 2011). However, they can also lower the good HDL cholesterol slightly. It is a good idea to replace some with monounsaturates, if you eat a lot of them. For this reason, the DoH recommends a maximum intake of 10% of total calorie intake.

WHAT ARE THE ESSENTIAL FATTY ACIDS?

A subcategory of polyunsaturated fats, called essential fatty acids, cannot be made in your body, so they have to come from the food you eat. They are grouped into two series:

- the omega-3 series, derived from alphalinolenic acid (ALA);
- the omega-6 series, derived from linoleic acid.

The series are called omega-3 and omega-6 because the last double bond is 3 and 6 carbon atoms from the last carbon in the chain respectively.

The omega-3 fatty acids can be further divided into two groups: long chain and short chain. The long-chain omega-3 fatty acids are eicosapentanoic acid (EPA) and docosahexanoic acid (DHA). They are found in oily fish and can also be formed in the body from ALA – the short-chain omega-3 fatty acid. EPA and DHA are then converted into hormone-like substances called prostaglandins, thromboxanes and leukotrienes. These control many key functions, such as blood clotting (making the blood less likely to form unwanted clots), inflammation (improving the ability to respond to injury or bacterial attack), the tone of blood vessel walls (widening and constriction of blood vessels) and the immune system.

Studies show that people with the highest intake of omega-3 fatty acids have a lower risk of heart attacks. This is because the prostaglandins reduce the ability of red blood cells to clot and reduce blood pressure. Omega-3s also help protect against heart disease and stroke and, according to recent research, may also help improve brain function, prevent Alzheimer's disease, treat depression, and help improve the behaviour of children with dyslexia, dyspraxia and ADHD.

The omega-6 fatty acids include linoleic acid, gamma-linolenic acid (GLA) and docosapentanoic acid (DPA) (*see* Fig. 8.5) and are important for healthy functioning of cell membranes. They are especially important for healthy skin. People on very low fat diets, who are deficient in linoleic acid, often develop extremely dry, flaky skin. Omega-6 fatty acids reduce LDL cholesterol, but a very high intake may also reduce HDL cholesterol. A high intake may also encourage increased free radical damage and, therefore, cancer risk. A moderate intake is recommended. Figure 8.5 shows how the body converts the two series of fatty acids.

WHAT ARE THE BEST FOOD SOURCES OF ESSENTIAL FATTY ACIDS?

Oily fish such as mackerel, fresh tuna (not tinned), salmon and sardines are undoubtedly the richest sources of DHA and EPA, but don't worry if you are a vegetarian or do not eat fish, because you can also get reasonably good amounts of ALA from certain plant sources. The richest plant sources include flaxseeds, flaxseed oil, pumpkin seeds, walnuts, chia seeds, rapeseed oil and soybeans. The dark green leaves of leafy vegetables (e.g. spinach, kale) also contain small amounts. There is an increasing range of omega-3 enriched foods, including omega-3 eggs (achieved by feeding hens on omega-3 enriched feed), bread and spreads. It is easier to meet your requirement for omega-6 fatty acids because they are found in more commonly eaten foods: vegetable oils, polyunsaturated margarine and many dishes and processed foods made from these oils and fats (e.g. fried foods, cakes, stir-fry, sandwiches spread with margarine, biscuits, crisps, cakes).

HOW MUCH DO I NEED?

We need both omega-3s and omega-6s to be healthy, but our diets are more often deficient in omega-3s. Most people have a far greater intake of omega-6 compared with omega-3; we tend to get most of our omega-6s from spreads and

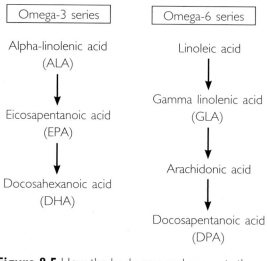

Figure 8.5 How the body uses and converts the omega-3 and omega-6 fatty acids

Table 8.4	OMEGA-3 FATTY ACID CONTENT OF SOME FISH	
Weight	**Source**	
0.5 g or less	Cod, haddock, mullet, halibut, skipjack tuna, clams, scallops, crab, prawns	
0.6–1 g	Red snapper, yellow fin tuna, turbot, swordfish, mussels, oysters	
1 g or more	Rainbow trout, mackerel, herring, sardines, salmon, blue fin tuna	

vegetable oils. Experts recommend shifting this balance in favour of omega-3s.

The right balance between omega-3 and omega-6 fatty acids is the most important factor if you are to get enough EPA and DHA. That's because both ALA (omega-3) and linoleic acid (omega-6) compete for the same enzymes to metabolise them. You should also aim to achieve an LA to ALA ratio of around 5:1 or even lower, i.e. at least 1 g omega-3s for every 5 g of omega-6s (Simopoulos & Robinson, 1998). A high intake of LA interferes with the conversion process of LA to EPA and DHA. The best way to correct this is to eat more oily fish or other ALA-rich foods (*see above*) or take supplements.

There is no recommended intake in the UK for omega-3 and omega-6 fatty acids but the DoH recommends a minimum of 450–900 mg EPA and DHA per day, and advises people to eat at least 2 portions of fish a week, one of which should be oily fish. This will supply about 2–3 g omega-3 fatty acids per week. To get 900 mg a day, you can eat one of the following:

- 32 g mackerel
- 45 g (half a small tin) tuna in oil (0.45 g) plus 1 small (120 g) chicken leg portion (0.45 g)
- 2 tbsp (30 g) flaxseeds
- 4 tbsp (40 g) pumpkin seeds
- 12–15 g walnuts
- 1 level tbsp flaxseed oil
- 6 omega-3 eggs*
  * from hens fed an omega-3-rich diet

Most fish-oil-based supplements supply 0.1 g omega-3 fatty acids. Taking 9 supplements a day may be unrealistic, so get as close as possible to the recommended intake from food and then top up with a supplement if you need to (*see* Table 8.4 for fish sources of omega-3).

HOW CAN OMEGA-3 FATTY ACIDS HELP ATHLETIC PERFORMANCE?

Studies have shown that omega-3 fatty acids can lead to improvements in strength and endurance by enhancing aerobic metabolism (Brilla & Landerholm, 1990; Bucci, 1993) – a critical energy system for all types of activities. Omega-3 fats have been shown to minimise post-exercise soreness (Jouris *et al.*, 2011). A study at Saint Louis University, US, found that women who consumed 3 g/day of DHA for 7 days experienced less muscle soreness and stiffness following eccentric exercise compared with a placebo (Corder *et al.*, 2016). The benefits of omega-3 fatty acids can be summarised as follows:

- improved delivery of oxygen and nutrients to cells because of reduced blood viscosity
- more flexible red blood cell membranes and improved oxygen delivery
- enhanced aerobic metabolism
- increased energy levels and stamina
- increased exercise duration and intensity
- improved release of growth hormone in response to sleep and exercise, improving recovery and promoting anabolic (or anticatabolic) environment
- anti-inflammatory, preventing joint, tendon, ligament strains
- reduction of inflammation caused by overtraining, assisting injury healing.

WHAT ARE TRANS FATTY ACIDS?

Small amounts of trans fatty acids are found naturally in meat and dairy products, but most come from processed fats. These are produced by hydrogenation, a process that changes liquid oils into solid or spreadable fats. During this highly pressurised heat treatment, the geometrical arrangement of the atoms changes. Technically speaking, one or more of the unsaturated double bonds in the fatty acid is altered from the usual *cis* form to the unusual *trans* form. This means the two hydrogen atoms are on opposite sides of the double bond.

Artificially produced trans fats may be found in foods made from hydrogenated vegetable oils such as certain snack products, bakery products, fried foods and takeaway foods. The exact effect of trans fatty acids on the body is not certain, but it is thought that they may be worse than saturates: they could lower HDL and raise LDL levels. They may also increase levels of a substance that promotes blood clot forma-

tion and stops your body using essential fatty acids properly. A US meta-analysis of 41 previous studies by researchers at McMaster University, Canada, found that people eating more trans fats had a 34% higher risk of dying from any cause compared with those eating less, a 28% higher risk of dying from heart disease, and a 21% greater risk of having heart-related health issues (de Souza *et al.*, 2015). In a review of prospective studies, for every 2% increase in calorie intake from trans fats a person's heart disease risk increases by 23% (Mozaffarian et al., 2006). Adverse effects were observed when trans fats contributed as little as 3% of total calories.

This is why all major public health organisations are trying to phase trans fats out of the food supply. The World Health Organization recommends 'virtual elimination' of trans fats from the food supply (Uauy *et al.*, 2009). The UK Scientific Advisory Committee on Nutrition recommends that trans fatty acids make up no more than 2% of total calorie intake – roughly 5 g per day. The average intake is estimated to be around 0.7% of calories, so most people are within the recommended maximum.

As there is no law requiring trans fats to be listed on food labels, the best advice is to avoid any foods that list hydrogenated or partially hydrogenated oils on the label. Reformulation in recent years means that hydrogenated fats have been removed from many foods and replaced with palm oil and other fats. For example, they are no longer used in major brands of fat spreads.

WHAT IS CHOLESTEROL?

Cholesterol is an essential part of our bodies; it makes up part of all cell membranes and helps produce several hormones. Some cholesterol

Table 8.5	SOURCES OF OMEGA-3 FATTY ACIDS		
	g/100 g	Portion	g/portion
Salmon	2.5 g	100 g	2.5 g
Mackerel	2.8 g	160 g	4.5 g
Sardines (tinned)	2.0 g	100 g	2.0 g
Trout	1.3 g	230 g	2.9 g
Tuna (canned in oil, drained)	1.1 g	100 g	1.1 g
Cod liver oil	24 g	1 tsp	1.2 g
Flaxseed oil	57 g	1 tbsp (15 g)	8.6 g
Flaxseeds (ground)	16 g	1 tbsp (15 g)	2.4 g
Rapeseed oil	9.6 g	1 tbsp (15 g)	1.4 g
Walnuts	7.5 g	1 tbsp (15 g)	1.1 g
Walnut oil	11.5 g	1 tbsp (14 g)	1.7 g
Peanuts	0.4 g	Handful (50 g)	0.2 g
Broccoli	0.2 g	3 florets (100 g)	0.2 g
Pumpkin seeds	8.5 g	2 tbsp (30 g)	2.6 g
Omega-3 eggs	0.2 g	One egg	0.1 g
Typical omega-3 supplement		1 capsule	0.1–0.3 g

Source: MAFF/RSC (1991); British Nutrition Foundation (1999).

comes from our diet, but most is made in the liver from saturated fats. In fact, the cholesterol we eat has only a small effect on our LDL cholesterol; if we eat more cholesterol (from meat, offal, eggs, dairy products, seafood) the liver compensates by making less, and vice versa. This keeps a steady level of cholesterol in the bloodstream.

Several factors can push up blood cholesterol levels. The major ones are obesity (especially android or central obesity), lack of exercise and the amount of saturated fatty acids we eat. Studies have shown that replacing saturated fatty acids with carbohydrates or unsaturated fatty acids can lower total and LDL cholesterol levels.

SO, WHICH ARE THE BEST TYPES OF FATS TO EAT?

Fats should make up 20–35% of your total calorie intake. Use all spreading fats sparingly; opt for a spread with a high content of olive oil and avoid those containing hydrogenated vegetable oil or partially hydrogenated oil. Avoid hard margarines and vegetable fats because they have the highest content of hydrogenated fats and trans fatty acids.

For cooking and salad dressings, choose oils that are high in omega-3 fatty acids or monounsaturated fatty acids – olive, rapeseed, flax and nut oils are good choices for health as well as taste. These are healthier than oils rich in omega-6 fats, such as sunflower and corn oil, which disrupt the formation of EPA and DHA. Include nuts and seeds in your daily diet; they provide many valuable nutrients apart from omega-3 fatty acids and monounsaturates. If you eat fish, include one to two portions of oily fish (e.g. mackerel, herring, salmon) per week. Vegetarians should make sure they include plant sources of omega-3 fatty acids in their daily diet.

Summary of key points

- Excess body fat is a disadvantage in almost all sports and fitness programmes, reducing power, speed and performance.
- Very low body fat does not guarantee improved performance either. There appears to be an optimal fat range for each individual, which cannot be predicted by a standard linear relationship.
- There are three main components of body fat: essential fat (for tissue structure); sex-specific fat (for hormonal function); and storage fat (for energy).
- The minimum percentage of fat recommended for men is 5% and for women, 10%. However, for normal health, the recommended ranges are 13–18% and 18–25% respectively. In practice, many athletes fall below these recommended ranges.
- Very low body fat levels are associated with hormonal imbalance in both sexes, and amenorrhoea, infertility, reduced bone density and increased risk of osteoporosis in women.
- Very low fat diets can lead to deficient intakes of essential fatty acids and fat-soluble vitamins.
- A fat intake of 20–35% of energy is recommended for athletes and active people.
- Unsaturated fatty acids should make up the majority of your fat intake, with saturated fatty acids making up no more than 11% energy and trans fatty acids kept as close to zero as possible.
- There are health benefits from replacing saturated fats with unsaturated fats.
- Greater emphasis should be placed on omega-3 fatty acids to improve the omega-3:omega-6 ratio. Include oily fish 1–2 times a week or consume 1–3 tbsp of linseed oil, pumpkin seeds, walnuts and rapeseed oil a day.
- Omega-3 fatty acids can enhance oxygen delivery to cells and therefore improve athletic performance.

//Weight loss

Many athletes and fitness participants wish to lose weight, either for health or performance reasons, or in order to make a competitive weight category. However, rapid weight loss can have serious health consequences, leading to a marked reduction in performance. A knowledge of safe weight loss methods is, therefore, essential. Since 95% of dieters fail to maintain their weight loss within a 5-year period, lifestyle management is the key to long-term weight management.

This chapter examines the effects of weight loss on performance and health, and highlights the health risks of rapid weight loss methods.

It considers the evidence for low carbohydrate and low fat diets and what is the most effective strategy for weight loss. Up-to-date research on appetite control and metabolism is presented, along with guidance for losing fat and retaining muscle mass. It explodes many of the myths and fallacies about metabolic rates and, finally, gives evidence-based and simple step-by-step strategies for successful fat loss.

To lose body fat, you have to expend more energy (calories) than you consume. In other words, you have to achieve a negative energy balance (see Fig. 9.1).

Energy Balance

Energy intake   =   Energy expenditure
(Food and drink)   (Resting metabolism, dietary
                                                      thermogenesis, physical activity)

Positive Energy Balance
Energy intake   >   Energy expenditure

Negative Energy Balance
Energy intake   <   Energy expenditure

(< = less than; > = more than)

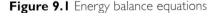

Figure 9.1 Energy balance equations

Research has shown that a combination of diet and activity is more likely to result in long-term success than diet or exercise alone. Unfortunately, there are no miracle solutions or short cuts. The objectives of a healthy diet and exercise programme are to:

- achieve a modest negative energy (calorie) balance
- maintain (or even increase) lean tissue
- gradually reduce body fat percentage
- avoid a significant reduction in your resting metabolic rate (see definition opposite)
- achieve an optimal intake of vitamins and minerals.

WILL DIETING AFFECT MY HEALTH OR PERFORMANCE?

Reducing body fat levels can be advantageous to performance in many sports (*see* 'Does body fat affect performance?' on p. 164). However, it is important to achieve this through scientifically proven methods.

Unfortunately, rapid weight loss can have serious health consequences, leading to a marked reduction in performance. The two most common are crash dieting and dehydration. Clearly, an athlete may achieve a desirable appearance, but to the detriment of his or her performance.

Rapid weight loss results in a diminished aerobic capacity (Fogelholm, 1994). A drop of up to 5% has been measured in athletes who had lost just 2–3% of body weight through dehydration. A loss of 10% can occur in those who lose weight through strict dieting. Anaerobic performance, strength and muscular endurance are also decreased, although researchers have found that strength (expressed against body weight)

Rapid weight loss

To make weight for a competition (e.g. boxing, bodybuilding, judo), athletes may resort to rapid weight loss methods, such as fasting, dehydration, exercising in sweatsuits, saunas, diet pills, laxatives, diuretics or self-induced vomiting. Weight losses of 4.5 kg in 3 days are not uncommon. In a study of 180 female athletes, 32% admitted they used more than one of these methods (Rosen *et al.*, 1986). In another, 15% of young female swimmers said they had tried one of these methods (Drummer *et al.*, 1987).

can actually improve after gradual weight loss (Tipton, 1987).

Prolonged dieting can have more serious health consequences. In female athletes, low body weight and body fat have been linked with menstrual irregularities, amenorrhoea and stress fractures; in male athletes, with reduced testosterone production. It has also been suggested that the combination of intense training, food restriction and the psychological pressure for extreme leanness may precipitate disordered eating and clinical eating disorders in some susceptible athletes (Sundgot-Borgen 1994 (a) and (b)).

There is a fine line between dieting and obsessive eating behaviour, and many female athletes, in particular, are under pressure to be thin and improve their performance. The warning signs and health consequences of eating disorders are discussed in Chapter 11.

WHAT HAPPENS TO THE BODY DURING RAPID WEIGHT LOSS BY DEHYDRATION?

Dehydration results in a reduced cardiac output and stroke volume, reduced plasma volume, slower nutrient exchange and slower waste removal, all of which have an impact on health and performance (Fogelholm, 1994; Fleck & Reimers, 1994). In moderate intensity exercise lasting more than 30 seconds, even dehydration of less than 5% body weight will diminish strength or performance, although it does not appear to affect exercise lasting less than 30 seconds. So, for athletes relying on pure strength (e.g. weightlifting), rapid weight loss may not be as detrimental.

IS REPEATED WEIGHT LOSS HARMFUL?

Repeated weight fluctuations, or yo-yo dieting, have been linked with an increased risk of heart disease, secondary diabetes, gall bladder disease and premature death. However, researchers are divided as to the exact reason. One explanation is that fat tends to be redeposited intra-abdominally, closer to the liver, rather than in the peripheral regions of the body, such as the hips, thighs and arms, and thus poses a greater heart disease risk. Another explanation is that repeated severe dieting can lead to a loss of lean tissue (including organ tissue) and nutritional deficiencies that can damage heart muscle. Contrary to popular belief, there is no evidence that yo-yo dieting permanently slows your metabolism (it returns to its original levels once normal eating is resumed). But yo-yo dieting can be bad for your psychological health. Each time you regain weight, you experience a sense of failure, which can lower your confidence and self-esteem.

WHAT MAKES YOUR RESTING METABOLIC RATE HIGH OR LOW?

The most important factor that determines your RMR is your body weight. The more you weigh, the higher your RMR, because the larger your body the more calories it needs for basic maintenance. The amount of fat-free mass you have (muscle, bone and vital organs) also affects RMR. This is calorie-burning tissue, so the more fat-free mass you have, the higher your RMR will be. However, the oft-quoted statistic that a pound of muscle burns 30–50 kcal/day has no scientific basis. The actual figure is 6 kcal/day.

High intensity exercise temporarily raises your RMR as your body pays off the oxygen debt, replenishes its energy reserves (PC and ATP) and repairs muscle tissue. The longer and more intense the workout, the greater this 'after-burn' will be. This post-exercise increase in RMR is called the excess post-exercise oxygen consumption (EPOC) and comes chiefly from the body's fat stores.

Metabolic rate

Metabolism is the term given to all processes by which your body converts food into energy. The *metabolic rate* is the rate at which your body burns calories. Your *basal metabolic rate (BMR)* is the rate at which you burn calories on essential body functions, such as breathing and blood circulation during sleep. In practice, the *resting metabolic rate (RMR)* is used, and is measured while you are awake and in a non-fasting state. It accounts for 60–75% of the calories you burn daily.

It is a myth that overweight people have a lower RMR (except in clinical conditions such as hypothyroidism or Cushing's syndrome). Numerous studies have shown a linear relationship between total weight and metabolic rate, i.e. the RMR increases proportionally with increasing body weight. Genetics undoubtedly play a role – some people are simply born with a more 'revved-up' metabolism than others.

CAN DIETING SLOW DOWN MY RMR?

Strict dieting will sabotage long-term efforts at weight control because it sends the body into 'famine' mode. When you restrict your calories, your RMR slows down as your body becomes more energy efficient. You need fewer calories just to maintain your weight. The more severe the calorie drop, the greater the decrease in your RMR. Generally, the decrease is between 10 and 30%. However, the effect is not permanent because the RMR returns to its original level once normal eating is resumed.

Avoid a big drop in your RMR by cutting your calories as modestly as possible (15% is recommended) and always consume more calories than your RMR. For example, if your maintenance calorie intake is 2500 kcal, you should reduce this to 2125 kcal.

HOW CAN I LOSE BODY FAT WITHOUT LOSING MUSCLE?

The key to losing body fat while retaining muscle is to reduce your usual calorie intake by 10–20%. This relatively modest reduction in calories will avoid the metabolic slowdown that is associated with more severe calorie reductions. The body will recognise and react to a smaller deficit by oxidising more body fat. If you cut

calories more drastically, it will not make you shed fat faster. Instead, it will cause your body to lower its metabolic rate in an attempt to conserve energy stores. This is called 'adaptive thermogenesis' (Rosenbaum & Leibel, 2010). Essentially it's your body's way of conserving energy when energy is in short supply (Tremblay et al., 2013). One study found that when people were put on a restricted calorie diet, they had a lower metabolic rate than could be explained by their weight loss (Heilbronn et al., 2006). Also, when you create a large calorie deficit, protein oxidation increases and this can lead to loss of lean muscle tissue, low energy levels, and extreme hunger.

In theory, 0.45 kg (1lb) of fat can be shed when a deficit of 3500 kcal is created, since 1 g fat yields 9 kcal ($9 \times 500 = 4500$ kcal). However, in practice, it may not work exactly like this because it depends on your initial calorie intake. For example, athlete A (male) normally eats 3000 kcal/day and athlete B (female) normally eats 2000 kcal/day. If both athletes reduced their calorie intake by 643 kcal/day (equivalent to 4500 kcal/week), athlete A now eats 2357 kcal/day and athlete B now eats 1357 kcal/day. The two athletes will, in practice, get very different results in terms of their body composition. Athlete A will almost certainly lose around 0.5 kg fat/week because his deficit is a 15% (modest) reduction. Athlete B will probably lose 0.5 kg fat/week for the first week or two, but after that she will lose significant amounts of muscle tissue. That's because she cut her calories by 32%, which is too severe. In general, calorie reductions of greater than 15% will lead to a metabolic slowdown and muscle loss, making fat loss slower.

So, for fat loss, aim for a reduction of calories as a percentage of your maintenance calorie intake. Reducing calorie intake by approximately 15% (or 10–20%) will lead to fat loss without slowing the metabolism. It may not allow you to lose 0.5 kg of fat/week – it may be 0.5 kg/10 days – but at least it will be fat, not muscle. Athlete B should eat 1700 kcal a day. This will produce a loss of 0.5 kg fat every 11 or 12 days.

Chapter 16, 'Your Personal Nutrition Plan', shows you how to calculate your calorie, carbohydrate, protein and fat requirements to lose body fat at an effective rate.

WILL I STILL BE ABLE TO TRAIN HARD WHILE LOSING WEIGHT?

The problem with most weight-loss diets is they do not provide enough calories or carbohydrate to support intense training. They can leave you with depleted muscle glycogen stores, which results in lethargy, fatigue and poor perfor-mance, as well as loss of lean body mass. If you compete in a weight-category or weight-sensitive sport (such as running, cycling or triathlon), you should aim to lose any excess weight during the base phase of training rather than during the build or competition phase, when training intensity is higher. It is possible to continue training hard provided you reduce your calorie intake by no more than 10–20%. This modest change should produce weight loss in the region of 0.5 kg per week without you feeling deprived, tired or overly hungry. One consistent finding from studies is that an adequate carbohydrate intake (> 3g/kg BW/day) is critical for preserving muscular strength, endurance, and both aerobic and anaerobic capacity. A lower intake can result in glycogen depletion and increased protein oxidation (muscle loss). Retaining lean mass is also vital for losing fat. The less muscle you have, the lower your resting metabolic rate and the harder it is to lose fat.

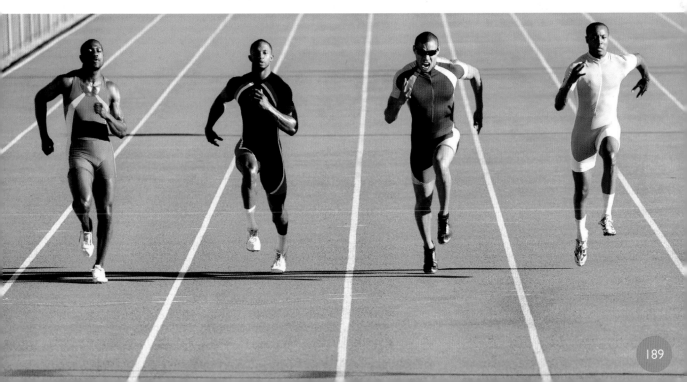

ARE LOW CARBOHYDRATE OR LOW FAT DIETS BETTER FOR WEIGHT LOSS?

Most diets work in the short term, but not all are healthy and most are not sustainable in the long term. The more extreme the diet, the lower the chance of adhering to it. Proponents of low carbohydrate diets claim that people lose weight more effectively when insulin levels are kept as low as possible. According to the 'insulin theory', carbohydrate causes a rise in blood insulin levels, which in turn, encourages the body to store fat. Over time, body cells become unresponsive to the actions of insulin ('insulin resistance') and, as a result, the pancreas produces more of it, further pushing the body into fat-storage mode. The solution, according to low carbohydrate proponents, is to cut carbohydrate intake dramatically and force the body to go into ketosis, i.e. fat is broken down in a different way to release ketones.

However, low carbohydrate diets have been criticised by eminent researchers who state that it is not the insulin that makes people put on weight; the opposite is more likely to be true. In most cases, it's being fat that makes people insulin resistant. When you lose weight, resistance returns to normal.

Low carbohydrate diets may work in the short term, partly due to depletion of glycogen stores (and the accompanying water), partly because you eat fewer calories. If you cut out virtually all carbohydrate, you automatically restrict the foods you can eat. It's difficult to overeat high protein foods like meat and eggs and with so few choices most people end up consuming fewer calories. Also, protein and fat are more satiating than carbohydrate so you feel less hungry and spontaneously eat less. It's a simple negative energy balance explanation.

Several studies have compared low carbohydrate diets with other diets but there is yet to be overwhelming evidence to support them. According to a rigorous study at the National Institutes of Health, US, calorie for calorie, cutting dietary fat results in more body fat loss than carbohydrate restriction (Hall *et al.*, 2015). In the study, 19 obese adults were confined to a metabolic ward for two 2-week periods and given diets that cut their calorie intake by a third, by reducing either carbohydrates or fat. Researchers analysed the amount of oxygen and carbon dioxide breathed out to calculate precisely the chemical processes taking place inside the body. After 6 days on each diet, those on the low fat diet lost 80% more body fat than those on the low carbohydrate diet.

According to a Harvard University systematic review of 53 studies comparing low fat and low carbohydrate diets in 68,000 people, those on low-carbohydrate diets lost just 1.1 kg more weight over a year than those on low fat diets. (Tobias *et al*, 2015).

Another scientific analysis examining the effectiveness of the Atkins, South Beach, Weight Watchers and Zone diets found that all methods – whether low fat or low carbohydrate – produced almost identical weight loss (2–4kg) after 12 months (Atallah *et al.*, 2014).

A randomised trial involving 300 women on either low carbohydrate, high carbohydrate, or low fat diets found that, while women on a low carbohydrate diet (specifically Atkins) lost a little more, weight loss through this diet was 'likely to be at least as large as for any other dietary pattern' (Gardner *et al.*, 2007).

A year-long study at the Tufts-New England Medical Centre in the US compared four different diets (Atkins diet, Ornish low fat diet, Weight Watchers and the Zone diet) and found that all produced a similar, albeit small, weight loss (three-quarters of them lost less than 5% of their body weight in a year) but that few dieters could stick to them for long enough to make a permanent difference (Dansinger *et al.*, 2005). They found that most dieters reduced their calorie intake initially but levels crept back up again. Of the diets tested, the low carbohydrate Atkins diet achieved the lowest weight loss over 12 months and had the lowest adherence.

A 2008 UK study compared the effectiveness and nutritional content of four commercial slimming programmes: Slim Fast, Atkins, Weight Watchers and Rosemary Conley's Eat Yourself Slim diet (Truby *et al.*, 2008). The researchers found that all the diets resulted in a reduced calorie intake and an average weight loss of between 3.7 kg and 5.2 kg after 8 weeks. There was no significant difference in weight loss between the diets themselves.

On balance, provided you eat fewer calories, all diets produce similar weight loss results in the long run. It is unimportant whether the calorie deficit comes from carbohydrate or fat. In other words, the most effective diet is one people can stick to. The key to losing weight and keeping it off is to eat more healthily, increase your activity and make sustainable changes to your lifestyle that you are comfortable with and will be able to adopt long term. Failing to keep to a diet can not only affect your health and metabolism but can cause psychological problems. A 2-year study at the University of California found that overweight women who did not follow a set diet, but who simply ate more healthily and listened to hunger and satiety cues, improved their health

Can alcohol make me fat?

Unsurprisingly, alcohol is the diet downfall of many people. It provides 7 kcal/g, which can significantly increase your total calorie intake if you consume large quantities. Also, many alcoholic drinks contain sugars, which increase the calorie content further. A glass (175 ml) of wine provides about 160 calories and a pint of beer about 200 calories. Indirectly, alcohol can encourage fat storage. Alcohol calories can't be stored and have to be used as they are consumed – and this means that calories excess to requirements from other foods get stored as fat instead.

(e.g. blood pressure and cholesterol levels) and had higher self-esteem (Bacon *et al.*, 2005). In contrast, those who dieted for 6 months regained their weight and reported significant drops in confidence and self-esteem.

WEIGHT LOSS STRATEGY
Step 1: Set realistic goals
Before embarking on a weight loss plan, write down your goals. Research has proven that by writing down your intentions, you are far more likely to turn them into actions.

These goals should be specific, positive and realistic ('I will lose 5 kg of body fat') rather than hopeful ('I would like to lose some weight'). Try to allow a suitable time frame (*see* Step 3): to lose 15 kg one month before a summer holiday is, obviously, unrealistic! Tracking your progress, for example by using an app that logs your food and exercise, will help to maintain your motivation and increase the chances of success.

Step 2: Monitor your progress

You can track your progress by measuring your waist circumference and weight once a week. Avoid too frequent weighing because this can lead to an obsession with weight. Bear in mind that weight loss in the first week may be as much as 2 kg, especially if your carbohydrate intake drops drastically, but this is mostly glycogen and its accompanying fluid (0.5 kg glycogen is stored with up to 1.5–2 kg water). Afterwards, aim to lose no more than 0.5 kg fat/week. Faster weight loss usually suggests a loss of lean tissue.

The best way to ensure you are losing fat not muscle is to measure your body composition regularly, e.g. once a week. The simplest method is to use a combination of girth or circumference measurements (e.g. chest, waist, hips, arms, legs), as shown in Figure 9.2, and skinfold thickness measurements, obtained by callipers (*see* Chapter 8, p. 169). Exercise physiologists recommend keeping a record of the skinfold thickness measurements themselves rather than converting them into body fat percentages. This is because the conversion charts are based on equations for the average, sedentary person and may not be appropriate for sportspeople or very lean or fat individuals. Monitoring changes in measurements at specific sites of the body allows you to see how your shape is changing and where most fat is being lost. This is a far better motivator than weighing scales! Alternatively, you can use one of the other methods of body composition measurement described in Chapter 8.

Step 3: Cut your calorie intake by 15%

As explained previously, reducing your calorie intake by approximately 15% (or 10–20%) will allow you to lose body fat without appreciably

The psychology of dieting

Researchers believe that a psychological difference exists between restrained eaters and non-dieters. In restrained eaters, the normal regulation of food intake becomes undermined as normal appetite and hunger cues are ignored. This leads to periods of restraint and semi-starvation, followed by overindulgence and guilt, followed by restraint, and so on.

Psychologists have shown that habitual dieters tend to have a more emotional personality than those who are not preoccupied with weight. They also tend to be more obsessive about food and weight.

At the University of Toronto, dieters and non-dieters were given a high calorie milkshake, followed by free access to ice cream (Herman & Polivy, 1991). The dieters actually went on to eat more ice cream than the non-dieters. This is due to a phenomenon known as 'counter regulation'; having lost the inbuilt regulation system of non-dieters, they were unable to detect and thus compensate for the calorie pre-load.

Researchers at Penn State University demonstrated that 'weight worriers' appear to lack the internal 'calorie counter' possessed by people who don't worry about their weight (Rolls & Shide, 1992). When given a yoghurt half an hour before lunch, those who worried about their weight ate more for lunch than those who were not weight concerned. It appears that such dieters have poor appetite control and are unable to compensate for previous food intake.

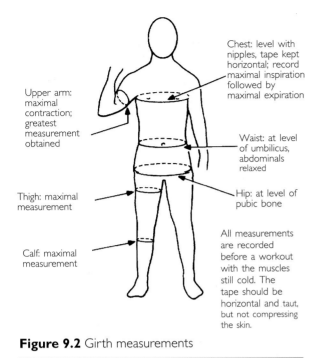

Upper arm: maximal contraction; greatest measurement obtained

Chest: level with nipples, tape kept horizontal; record maximal inspiration followed by maximal expiration

Waist: at level of umbilicus, abdominals relaxed

Thigh: maximal measurement

Hip: at level of pubic bone

Calf: maximal measurement

All measurements are recorded before a workout with the muscles still cold. The tape should be horizontal and taut, but not compressing the skin.

Figure 9.2 Girth measurements

slowing your metabolic rate. It will also help prevent loss of lean body mass. Although it may be tempting to cut calories further, a calorie deficit greater than 20% increases the risk of losing excessive lean tissue, severely depleting your glycogen stores and not getting enough vitamins and minerals in your diet. A sudden drop in calories sends a message to the body that starvation might be imminent, causing it to conserve energy. As your body goes into survival mode, adapting to a lower calorie intake, the rate at which you burn energy slows down. To compensate for the low calorie intake, your body will break down muscle tissue for fuel.

Step 4: Keep a food log

A food log or diary is a record of your daily food and drink intake. It is a very good way to evaluate your present eating habits and to find out exactly what, why and when you are eating. It will allow you to check whether your diet is well balanced or lacking in any important nutrients, and to take a more careful look at your usual meal patterns and lifestyle.

Weigh and write down everything you eat and drink for at least 3 consecutive days – ideally 7. This period should include at least one weekend day. It is important not to change your usual diet at this time and to be completely honest! Every spoonful of sugar in tea, every scrape of butter on bread should be recorded.

Use your food diary to evaluate:

- the nutrient-poor foods in your diet, which you need to eliminate – these are likely to be highly processed foods and drinks, high in sugar (e.g. biscuits, soft drinks, chocolate, crisps and snacks);
- your fibre intake – try to eat more fibre-rich foods such as lentils, oats, whole grains, nuts, seeds, fruit and vegetables in place of highly refined carbohydrates (e.g. white bread, pasta, rice and breakfast cereals);
- the timing of your meals and snacks – eat regularly spaced meals, avoid snacking if not genuinely hungry, and plan your meals around your workout.

Step 5: Match your carbohydrate intake to your training load

To create a calorie deficit of 15%, you will need to reduce your overall carbohydrate intake. This does not mean embarking on a low carbohydrate diet; rather reducing carbohydrate to a level that still allows you to train hard but not too low to cause fatigue or a drop in performance. A chronic low carbohydrate diet combined with high intensity training can result in symptoms of overtraining, lowered immunity and reduced performance.

The best way to achieve this is by matching your carbohydrate intake to your training load. So, on days when your carbohydrate needs are higher, for example when performing high intensity endurance training, aim to consume most of your daily carbohydrate in the 2–4 hour time period before exercise and the 2–4 hour time period after exercise so that your performance won't suffer and you will have enough energy to train hard. Remember, you cannot fuel high intensity exercise (more than 70% of maximal aerobic capacity) from fat alone (*see* p. 26). Aim for around 50–100 g of carbohydrate pre-exercise, depending on how close your meal is to your workout, and also how long and hard you plan to train. After exercise, consume 1–1.2 g/kg BW, equivalent to 70–84 g for a 70 kg person, but adjust this according to the duration and intensity of your workout. If you have exercised hard for longer than 2 hours you may need more than this, as your glycogen stores will be depleted. If you have exercised for less than an hour, then you will need less. Adding 15–25 g protein to your post-exercise recovery drinks and meals will promote optimal muscle recovery after hard training (*see* p. 82).

On days when carbohydrate needs are lower, for example when doing low intensity sessions (less than 70% of maximal aerobic capacity), training with lower muscle glycogen levels should not adversely affect your performance. Performing low intensity sessions with low carbohydrate availability not only helps to reduce body fat but also promotes endurance training adaptations, increases rates of fat oxidation and, in some cases, improves exercise capacity (*see* p. 43).

In general, keep sugar and highly processed foods to a minimum as they provide lots of calories for relatively few nutrients. Listed opposite are a number of ways to reduce sugar.

Step 6: Don't cut fats too drastically

Fat may be more calorie dense than carbohydrate or protein (9 kcal/g versus 4 kcal/g) but don't cut it out of your diet completely. You need a certain amount each day to provide essential fatty acids, stimulate hormone production, keep your skin healthy, and absorb and transport fat-soluble vitamins. It is also satiating so it gives the body the feeling of being full. Very low fat diets can lead to deficient intakes of essential fatty acids and fat-soluble vitamins. Aim to consume 20–35% of energy from fat. Unsaturated fatty acids should make up the majority of your fat intake, with saturated fatty acids making up no more than 11% energy and trans fatty acids kept as close to zero as possible.

Cut down on highly processed foods that are high in saturated fats, such as sausages, burgers, pastry and pies, cakes, biscuits, puddings and chocolate. Choose leaner meats, poultry and fish instead of fatty meat, and use less oil in cooking.

Step 7: Increase protein to offset muscle loss

A higher protein intake can offset some of the potential loss of muscle when losing weight. Studies suggest that increasing your protein intake to 1.8–2.7 g/kg BW/day (or 2.3–3.1 g/kg fat-free mass) while cutting your daily energy intake by a modest 10–20% can prevent muscle mass loss (Murphy *et al.*, 2015; Helms *et al.*,

How to reduce sugar

Get accustomed to less sweetness: Give your palate time to adjust. Instead of banning sugar, reduce the amount of sugar you add to foods and drinks a little at a time. Over time, you'll get accustomed to the taste of less-sweet foods.

Limit sugary drinks including fruit juice and sports drinks: They are not only a source of empty calories but sugary drinks also show the strongest relationship with tooth decay, obesity and type 2 diabetes. The problem is that it's easier to over-consume calories in liquid form than solid foods. Although fruit juice contains natural sugar, the juicing process means the sugars in the cell wall of the plant are released as 'free sugars', which damage teeth, raise blood sugar levels quickly and provide additional calories. Replace soft drinks, fruit juice and energy drinks with water, low fat milk or unsweetened tea or coffee.

Minimise highly processed foods: Replace highly processed sugary foods (sweets, chocolate, cakes, biscuits and desserts) in your diet with natural ones found in fruit and vegetables, which have a less drastic effect on your blood sugar levels. Processed foods also stimulate hunger and make it harder to control appetite and body weight.

Don't ban fruit: The sugars that occur naturally in fruit are much less concentrated and they're consumed along with fibre, which helps slow their absorption. Most varieties of fresh fruit have a low GI (see Appendix 1). Fruit is also a valuable source of vitamins, minerals and phytochemicals.

Read the label: There are many types of sugar so check labels for sucrose, glucose syrup, invert sugar, fructose, dextrose, maltodextrin, fruit syrup, raw sugar, cane sugar and glucose. Even foods disguised as health foods can be loaded with added sugars – agave nectar, honey, organic cane sugar and maple syrup all fall into the same category.

Go for natural sweetness: Opt for fresh fruit instead of sweets, cakes, biscuits and pastries. Add fruit to plain yoghurt or porridge/breakfast cereal instead of sugar. Swap puddings for fresh berries and plain yoghurt or baked bananas. But go easy on dried fruit – it's a concentrated source of sugar and easy to overeat.

Beware of 'low fat' foods: These often contain more sugar than their 'full fat' equivalents, since manufacturers replace the fat with other ingredients, including sugar, to improve their taste. These foods may not always satisfy your taste expectations so you may end up eating more of them.

Rethink your breakfast: Many breakfast cereals are loaded with sugar. Opt for porridge, eggs on toast, or yoghurt with fresh fruit and nuts – a higher protein breakfast will keep you feeling fuller for longer.

Alter recipes: As a rule, you can cut the sugar in most cakes and desserts by one-third without compromising flavour or texture. Try adding sweeter spices like cinnamon, nutmeg, vanilla, almond extract, ginger or lemon to improve flavour. For cakes, substitute puréed apple or mashed banana for some of the sugar.

2014; Phillips & Van Loon, 2011). This equates to 144–216 g protein/day for an athlete weighing 80 kg. You should distribute your daily protein evenly between meals and snacks, aiming to consume 0.25–0.3 g/kg BW/day or about 20–24 g per meal in order to maximise MPS.

One study found that when athletes ate 1.6 g or 2.4 g protein/kg BW (twice and three times the RNI respectively) they lost more fat and less muscle compared with those who just ate the RNI for protein, 0.8 g/kg body weight (Pasiakos *et al.*, 2013). All three groups lost the same amount of weight but those eating extra protein lost more fat and retained more muscle at the end of the dieting period.

Protein can also help control appetite and reduce hunger. Researchers have shown that it is more effective than carbohydrate and fat for switching off hunger signals and promoting satiety (Westerterp-Plantenga *et al.*, 2012). Protein triggers appetite-regulating hormones in the gut, which tell the appetite control centre in the brain that you are satiated (*see* p. 80). The higher the protein intake, the greater the level of satiety produced (Belza *et al.*, 2013).

A study at the University of Illinois found that women who exercised regularly (5 × 30-minute walking sessions; 2 × 30-minute weight training sessions per week) while eating a high protein diet lost more weight compared with those who ate a high carbohydrate diet containing the same number of calories (Layman *et al.*, 2005). Almost 100% of the weight loss in the high protein dieters was fat, and much of that was from the abdominal region. In contrast, in the high-carbohydrate group, up to a third of the weight loss was muscle. Researchers suggest that the high protein diet worked better because it contained

Can I gain muscle while losing fat?

Conventional dogma suggests that you cannot lose fat and gain muscle simultaneously. However, a study at McMaster University found that you can – if you combine a low calorie and high protein intake with a very high intensity training programme (Longland *et al.*, 2016). The study involved 40 overweight men who performed an intense resistance training programme (6 days a week, including 2 days of circuit resistance training, 2 days of high intensity intervals on a bike, one day of bike time trial and one day of plyometric body weight circuits) for 4 weeks while consuming 40% fewer calories than their calculated requirements. Those who consumed a high protein diet (2.4 g/kg BW/day) lost significantly more body fat (4.8 kg vs. 3.5 kg) and gained significantly more muscle (1.2 kg vs. 0.1 kg) than those who consumed 1.2 g protein/kg BW, which was close to what the volunteers typically consumed (but still higher than the recommended daily intake). However, the exercise regime was exceptionally tough and the weight loss benefits may not be sustainable.

a high level of leucine, which works with insulin to stimulate fat-burning while preserving muscle.

Step 8: Blood glucose control
This can be achieved by eating low GI meals – a balanced combination of carbohydrate, protein and fat, with a focus on high fibre foods (such

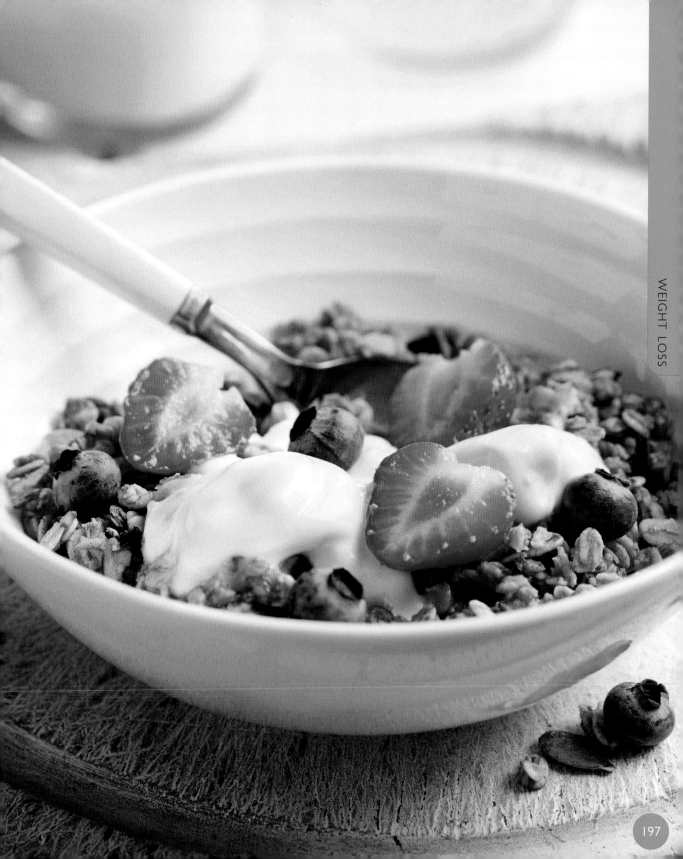

as whole grains, fruit and vegetables). This helps improve appetite regulation, increases feelings of fullness and delays hunger between meals. Remember that adding protein, fat or soluble fibre to carbohydrate always reduces the speed of absorption and produces a lower blood sugar rise. In practice, this is easy to achieve if you plan to eat a carbohydrate source (e.g. potatoes) with a high-protein source (e.g. fish) and add vegetables. Better still, include low GI carbohydrates, such as lentils and beans, in your meals.

Does skipping breakfast increase weight loss?

Studies show that people who skip breakfast are more likely to eat highly palatable high-calorie foods later on (Goldstone *et al.*, 2009) and also eat more at lunchtime (Chowdhury *et al.*, 2015). However, contrary to popular belief, they do not fully compensate for the calories saved at breakfast and generally still go on to consume fewer calories over the course of the day (Levitsky & Pacanowski, 2013).

A study from the University of Bath, UK, found that people who eat breakfast burn 442 more calories by being active, mainly in the morning after eating, than those who skip breakfast (Betts *et al.*, 2014). They suggest that people who skip breakfast burn fewer calories because they do less spontaneous physical activity.

While occasionally skipping breakfast may help reduce your daily calorie intake (Clayton & James, 2015), it is not a good weight loss strategy if you want to train hard later in the day. Researchers from Loughborough University, UK, found that those who omitted breakfast experienced a 4.5% drop in their performance in a cycling time trial (after lunch but before dinner) (Clayton *et al.*, 2015).

Step 9: Eat more fibre

Apart from reducing your risk of certain cancers and heart disease, fibre slows down the emptying of food from your stomach, reduces hunger and helps to keep you feeling full. Fibre also gives food more texture so you need to chew your food more. This slows down your eating speed, reducing the chances of overeating and increases satiety.

Fibre also slows the digestion and absorption of carbohydrates, resulting in a slow steady energy uptake and stable insulin levels. Non-fluctuating glucose and insulin levels will encourage the use of food for energy rather than for storage as body fat; it also reduces hunger and satisfies the appetite.

The most filling foods are those with a high volume per calorie. Water and fibre add bulk to foods, so load up on foods naturally high in these components. Fruit, vegetables, pulses and wholegrain foods give maximum fill for minimum calories. If you can eat a plate of food that is low in calories relative to its volume, you're likely to feel just as satisfied as eating smaller amounts of high-calorie food.

Step 10: Do not ban foods

Studies have shown that not banning foods and enjoying the occasional indulgence without feeling guilty is a successful strategy for maintaining weight loss. Many people find that a 'day off' from healthy eating or dieting once a week satisfies their cravings and keeps them motivated to eat well week after week. This means you can allow yourself to have chocolate, or your favourite ice cream or hamburger, without feeling guilty. If you know you can eat a little of your favourite food every week, you'll stop thinking of it as a forbidden food and won't want to overeat it.

Step 11: Make gradual lifestyle changes that are sustainable

Long-term weight management can only be achieved by making changes to your eating and exercise habits that you are comfortable with and can stick to. If you make too drastic a change, such as cutting out an entire food group or replacing meals with shakes, then it is very unlikely that you will be able to sustain it long term. A weight loss plan should be one that is sensible and sustainable. However, one of

Shrink your portions

Use smaller plates and opt for smaller packages. US researchers have found that the bigger the portion or serving size, the more calories are consumed (Wansink, 2005; Wansink et al., 2005). People who were given large containers of popcorn or soup consumed 45% and 73% more calories respectively than those given smaller containers.

the biggest barriers to this is an unwillingness to commit to a few necessary changes in lifestyle. Table 9.1 lists some of the common reasons why many people fail to manage their weight in the long term, together with some suggestions as to how to overcome them.

Table 9.1	LIFESTYLE CHANGES
Lifestyle	**Suggestion**
Not enough time to prepare healthy meals	Plan meals in advance so all ingredients are at hand. Make meals in bulk and refrigerate/freeze portions.
Work shifts	Plan regular meal breaks and take your own healthy food with you.
Work involves lots of travelling	Take portable healthy snacks (e.g. sandwiches, fruit, nuts, protein bars, dried fruit, yoghurt, milk, protein drinks).
Need to cook for rest of family	Adapt favourite family meals (e.g. spaghetti bolognese) to make them healthier. Add extra vegetables and high-fibre ingredients (e.g. beans, wholemeal pasta).
Overeat when stressed	Use stress management and relaxation techniques.
Eat out frequently	Choose healthier options in restaurants (e.g. salads, fish, vegetable-based dishes).

Step 12: Do the right type of exercise

Anyone on a calorie-reduced programme will lose both muscle and fat. On a severe calorie-reduced programme, muscle loss can account for up to 50% of weight loss. However, muscle loss can be minimised by the right choice of exercise.

Resistance exercise

Resistance exercise should be included in your fat-loss programme for two reasons. Firstly, your RMR will be elevated for up to 15 hours post-exercise, due to the oxidation of body fat (Melby *et al.*, 1993). You won't necessarily burn more calories lifting weights than doing cardiovascular exercise, but the increased muscle mass you develop as a result will make your body burn more calories during rest and exercise. One study found that people who did a combination of cardiovascular and resistance exercise lost more fat than those doing cardio-only exercise but also gained more muscle (Willis *et al.*, 2012).

Secondly, when resistance exercise is added to a weight-loss programme, more muscle is preserved and a greater proportion of weight loss is fat loss. Resistance training acts as a stimulus for muscle retention.

The American College of Sports Medicine recommends 2–3 days a week for beginners, progressing to 4–5 times a week for the more advanced (Garber C. E., 2009). In general, train each muscle group for 2–4 sets of exercises with a weight you can lift only 8–12 times, taking 30 seconds' rest between sets.

Cardiovascular (CV) exercise

The American College of Sports Medicine recommends 150 minutes per week to improve your health (Donnelly *et al.*, 2009) or 200–300 minutes to lose weight. That's equivalent to 5 sessions of 30 minutes (for health) or 5 sessions of 60 minutes (weight loss).

A sensible target would be 20–40 minutes per session, 3–5 times per week, but don't overdo it. Increase the intensity and duration of your sessions gradually, aiming for 60 minutes 5 times a week. Adding CV exercise to your fat-loss programme will burn more calories and offset some of the muscle wastage, but don't rely on aerobic exercise exclusively. You could still lose substantial amounts of muscle tissue with aerobic exercise – some studies have estimated as much as 40% (Aceto, 1997). This is because aerobic exercise does not act as sufficient stimulus to ensure muscle retention while you are in calorie deficit. Muscle loss will subsequently result in a lowering of your metabolic rate.

Despite what many people believe, low intensity, long duration aerobic exercise is not the best method for shedding fat. Research indicates that not only does high intensity aerobic exercise burn fat more effectively but it also speeds up your metabolism and keeps it revved up for a while after your workout. What actually counts is the number of calories burned per unit of time. The more calories you expend, the more fat you break down. For example, walking (i.e. low intensity aerobic exercise) for 60 minutes burns 270 kcal, of which 160 kcal (60% calories) comes from fat. Running (i.e. high intensity aerobic exercise) for the same amount of time burns 680 kcal, of which 270 kcal (40% calories) comes from fat. Therefore, high intensity aerobic exercise results in greater fat loss over the same time period. This principle applies to everyone, no matter what your level of fitness – exercise intensity is always relative to the individual. Walking at 6 km/h may represent high intensity exercise for an unconditioned individual; running at 10 km/h may represent low intensity exercise for a well-conditioned athlete.

High Intensity Interval Training (HIIT)
High intensity interval training (HIIT) has been shown to be more effective than steady-state training for promoting fat loss as well as for improving cardiovascular fitness. The basic concept of HIIT is to train at different speeds for a number of intervals. Researchers at Laval University in Quebec, Canada, found that 9 times more fat was lost in the group that used HIIT, compared to the group that used tradi-tional steady intensity cardio (Tremblay *et al.*, 1994). It also increases your metabolic rate for the following 24 hours. In other words, your body's fat-burning process continues long after your workout, even when you are at rest.

HIIT can be performed with a variety of activities or machines – running, swimming, treadmills, bikes, elliptical trainers or skipping ropes. Pick your equipment of choice, and make sure to warm up properly to prevent injury. Be aware of your own limits, and work out accordingly. After a 10-minute warm up, try 30–45 seconds of high intensity alternating with 1 minute of recovery. Repeat the interval 4 or 5 more times and then cool down for 10 minutes.

HOW SHOULD I CONSTRUCT MY FAT-BURNING EXERCISE PROGRAMME?

You have two parts to your fat-burning exercise programme:

1. weight training
2. high intensity aerobic exercise

Ideally, they should be performed on alternate days so you will have adequate time for recuperation between workouts and maximum energy for each workout. Here is a plan to achieve effective fat loss, and preservation (or building) of muscle mass and the metabolic rate:

- Perform your weight training workout 3 times a week on alternate days (e.g. Monday, Wednesday, Friday). Training sessions should be intense, causing you to reach muscular failure (maximum rating of intensity or perceived exertion on the last set of each exercise).

Table 9.2	SAMPLE FAT-BURNING EXERCISE PLAN						
Monday	**Tuesday**	**Wednesday**	**Thursday**	**Friday**		**Saturday**	**Sunday**
Week 1							
UBWT: Chest, back, shoulders, arms	AT: 20–25 minutes on stationary bike	LBWT: Legs, calves, abdominals	AT: 20–25 minute run	UBWT: Chest, back, shoulders, arms		AT: 20–25 minute swim	No training
Week 2							
LBWT: Legs, calves, abdominals	AT: 20–25 minutes on stationary bike	UBWT: Chest, back, shoulders, arms	AT: 20–25 minute run	LBWT: Legs, calves, abdominals		AT: 20–25 minute swim	No training

Key: UBWT = Upper body weight training LBWT = Lower body weight training AT = Aerobic training

- Each weight training session should last 40–45 minutes.
- Alternate training the muscles of the upper and lower body (i.e. a two-way split). For example, train upper body on Monday, lower body on Wednesday, upper body on Friday, etc.
- Perform a total of 6 sets for each muscle group, choosing one or two different exercises that target that muscle group. (*See* Table 9.2.)
- Maintain super-strict form and focus on each repetition, keeping the weight fully in control. The importance of technique cannot be stressed enough.
- Lift and lower for a count of two on each part of the movement, and aim to hold the fully contracted position for a count of one.
- Perform your aerobic training sessions three times a week on alternate days (e.g. Tuesday, Thursday, Saturday). Each session should take approximately 20–25 minutes.
- Suitable activities include running, cycling (stationary bike or outdoor cycling), stepping, swimming, rowing or any cardiovascular apparatus. The important factor is that the activity is continuous and you are able to vary your intensity.
- Start with a 3–5 minute warm-up phase. Increase the intensity gradually over the next 4 minutes until you have reached a high intensity effort. Maintain for 1 minute then reduce the intensity back to a moderate level for 1 minute. Repeat that pattern 4 times. Finish with a gradual reduction in intensity over 2–3 minutes.

Note: For a full description of the exercises in Tables 9.3 and 9.4, see *The Complete Guide to Strength Training* (5th edition) by Anita Bean.

Summary of key points

- To lose body fat, you have to expend more energy (calories) than you consume.
- The most important factor that determines your RMR is your body weight.

Table 9.3	SAMPLE WEIGHT TRAINING PLAN (UPPER BODY WORKOUT)	
Muscle group	**Exercise**	**Reps**
Chest	• Bench press (warm-up) • Bench press • Dumb-bell flyes	1 × 12–15 3 × 8–10 3 × 8–10
Back	• Lat pulldown (warm-up) • Lat pulldown • Seated row	1 × 12–15 3 × 8–10 3 × 8–10
Shoulders	• Dumb-bell shoulder press (warm-up) • Dumb-bell shoulder press • Lateral raise	1 × 12–15 3 × 8–10 3 × 8–10
Arms	• Barbell curl (warm-up) • Barbell curl • Lying tricep extension (warm-up) • Lying tricep extension	1 × 12–15 3 × 8–10 1 × 12–15 3 × 8–10

Table 9.4	SAMPLE WEIGHT TRAINING PLAN (LOWER BODY WORKOUT)	
Muscle group	**Exercise**	**Reps**
Legs	• Squat (warm-up) • Squat • Lunges • Calf raise (warm-up) • Calf raise	1 × 12–15 3 × 8–10 3 × 8–10 1 × 12–15 3 × 8–10
Abdominals	• Crunches • Oblique crunches • Reverse curl-ups	2 × 10–15 2 × 10–15 2 × 10–15

- Rapid weight loss methods can have an adverse effect on performance and health.
- Effective fat loss can be achieved by reducing calorie intake by 10–20%; this will minimise both lean tissue loss and resting metabolic rate (RMR) reduction.
- A higher protein intake of 1.8–2.7 g/kg BW/day (or 2.3–3.1 g/kg fat-free mass) can offset some of the potential loss of muscle when training with a calorie deficit.

- Protein can help control appetite and reduce hunger.
- The recommended rate of fat loss is no more than 0.5 kg/week.
- A variety of diets can lead to weight loss and what matters most is consistently eating fewer calories.
- Ultimately, for successful long-term weight loss, a diet plan needs to be sustainable and help you lose fat without compromising your performance.
- The main elements of an effective fat loss strategy include setting realistic goals, monitoring your progress, achieving a calorie reduction of 10–20%, adjusting carbohydrate according to training goals, minimising highly processed foods, including healthy fats, eating fibre-rich foods, not banning any food, making gradual lifestyle changes and including both cardiovascular and resistance training.

//Weight gain

There are two ways to gain weight: either by increasing your lean mass or by increasing your fat mass. Both will register as weight gain on the scales but result in a very different body composition and appearance!

Lean weight gain can be achieved by combining a consistent well-planned resistance training programme with a balanced diet. Resistance training provides the stimulus for muscle growth while your diet provides the right amount of energy (calories) and nutrients to enable your muscles to grow at the optimal rate. One without the other would result in only minimal lean weight gain.

WHAT TYPE OF TRAINING IS BEST FOR GAINING WEIGHT?

Resistance training (weight training) is the best way to stimulate muscle growth. Research shows that the fastest gains in size and strength are achieved using relatively heavy weights that can be lifted strictly for 6–10 repetitions per set (Bompa & Cornacchia, 2013). If you can do more than 10–12 repetitions at a particular weight, your size gains will be less, but you may still achieve improvements in muscular endurance, strength and power.

Concentrate on the 'compound' exercises, such as bench press, squat, shoulder press and lat pull-down, as these work the largest muscle groups of the body together with neighbouring muscles that act as 'assistors' or 'synergists'. These types of exercises stimulate the largest number of muscle fibres in one movement and are therefore the most effective and quickest way to gain muscle mass. Keep the smaller isolation exercises, such as biceps concentration curls or tricep kickbacks, to a minimum; these produce slower mass gains and should be added to your workout only occasionally for variety.

HOW MUCH WEIGHT CAN I EXPECT TO GAIN?

The amount of muscle weight you can expect to gain depends on several genetic factors, including your body type, muscle fibre mix, the arrangement of your motor units and your hormonal balance, as well as your training programme and diet.

Your genetic make-up determines the proportion of different types of fibres in your muscles. The fast-twitch (type II) fibres generate power and increase in size more readily than the slow-twitch (type I or endurance) fibres. So, if you naturally have plenty of fast-twitch fibres in your muscles, you will probably respond faster to a strength training programme than someone who has a higher proportion of slow-twitch fibres. Unfortunately, you cannot convert slow-twitch into fast-twitch fibres – hence two people can follow exactly the same training programme, yet the one with lots of fast-twitch muscle fibres will naturally gain weight faster than the other.

Your natural body type also affects how fast you gain lean weight. An ectomorph (naturally slim build with long lean limbs, narrow shoulders and hips) will find it harder to gain weight than a mesomorph (muscular, athletic build with wide shoulders and narrow hips) who tends to gain muscle readily. An endomorph (stocky, rounded build with wide shoulders and hips and an even distribution of fat) gains both fat and muscle readily.

People with a higher natural level of the male (anabolic) sex hormones, such as testosterone, will also gain muscle faster. That is why women cannot achieve the muscle mass or size of men unless they take anabolic steroids.

However, no matter what your genetics, natural build and hormonal balance, everyone can gain muscle and improve their shape with strength training. It is just that it takes some people longer than others.

HOW FAST CAN I EXPECT TO GAIN WEIGHT?

Mass gains of 20% of starting body weight are common after the first year of training. However, the rate of weight gain will gradually drop off over the years as you approach your genetic potential. Men can expect to gain 0.5–1 kg per month (GSSI, 1995). Women usually experience about

Training for muscle gain

Certain compound exercises, such as dead lifts, clean and jerks, snatches and squats, not only stimulate the 'prime mover' muscles, but also have a powerful anabolic ('systemic') effect on the whole body and the central nervous system. These are the classic mass builders and should be included once a week in any serious muscle/strength training programme.

To stimulate the maximal number of muscle fibres in a muscle group, select one to three basic exercises and aim to do 4–12 total sets for that muscle group. Latest research suggests that doing fewer sets (4–8) but using heavier weights (80–90% of your one-rep maximum – i.e. the maximum weight which can be lifted through one complete repetition) results in faster size and strength gains. If you exercise that muscle group to exhaustion, you will need to allow up to 7 days for recuperation before repeating the same workout. So, aim to train each muscle group once a week (on average). In practice, divide your body parts (e.g. chest, legs, shoulders, back, arms) into three or four, and train one part per workout.

Always use strict training form and, ideally, have a partner to 'spot' for you so that you can use near-maximal weights safely. Always remember to warm up each muscle group beforehand with light aerobic training (e.g. exercise bike) and some relevant stretches. Ensure you also stretch the muscles after (and, ideally, in between each part of) the workout to help relieve soreness.

50–75% of the gains of men – i.e. 0.25–0.75 kg/month – partly due to their smaller initial body weight and smaller muscle mass, and partly due to lower levels of anabolic hormones. Monitor your body composition rather than simply your weight. If you gain much more than 1 kg per month on an established programme, then you are likely to be gaining fat!

HOW MUCH SHOULD I EAT?

To gain lean weight and muscle strength at the optimal rate, you need to be in a positive energy balance, i.e. consuming more calories than you need for maintenance. This cannot be stressed too much. These additional calories should come from a balanced ratio of carbohydrate, protein and fat.

1. Calories

Estimate your maintenance calorie intake using the formulae in Steps 1–4, Chapter 16, p. 290–92. To gain muscle, increase your calorie intake by 20%, i.e. multiply your maintenance calories by 1.2 (120%).

Example:
If your maintenance calorie requirement is 2700 kcal, you will need to eat 2700 × 1.2 = 3240 kcal.

In practice, most athletes will need to add roughly an extra 500 kcal to their daily diet. Not all of these extra calories are converted into muscle – some will be used for digestion and absorption, given off as heat or used for physical activity. Increase your calorie intake gradually, say 200 a day for a while, then after a week or two, increase it by a further 200 kcal. Slow gainers may need to increase their calorie intake by as much as 1000 kcal a day.

2. Carbohydrate

In order to gain muscle, you need to train very hard, and that requires a lot of fuel. The key fuel for this type of exercise is, of course, muscle glycogen. Therefore, you must consume enough carbohydrate to achieve high muscle glycogen levels. If you train with low levels of muscle glycogen, you risk excessive protein (muscle) breakdown, which is just the opposite of what you are aiming for.

In a 24-hour period during low or moderate intensity training days, you should get 5–7 g/kg of body weight. During moderate to heavy endurance training, 7–10 g/kg is recommended. As your calorie needs increase by 20%, so should your usual carbohydrate intake. In practice, aim to eat an extra 50–100 g carbohydrate.

3. Protein

Your protein requirements are higher than those for endurance athletes. As explained in Chapter 4, dietary protein provides an enhanced stimulus for muscle growth (Phillips *et al.*, 2011; Phillips, 2012). To build muscle, you must be in 'positive nitrogen balance', which means your body retains more dietary protein than is excreted or used as fuel. A suboptimal intake of protein will result in slower gains in strength, size and mass, or even muscle loss, despite hard training.

The recommendation for athletes generally is 1.2–2.0 g/kg BW/day and an intake at the higher end of the range (between 1.4 and 2.0 g/kg BW/day) is generally recommended for those doing mostly strength and power exercise (ACSM/AND/DC, 2016 Phillips *et al.*, 2007; Tipton *et al.*, 2007; Williams, 1998). This level of protein intake should support muscle growth – studies show that increasing your intake above 2.0 g/kg body weight produces no further benefit. For example, if you weigh 80 kg you would need between 112 and 160 g protein a day.

4. Fat

Fat should comprise between 20 and 35% of total calories, or the balance of calories once you have met your needs for carbohydrate and protein. Most of your fat should come from unsaturated sources, such as olive oil and other vegetable oils, avocado, oily fish, nuts and seeds.

Example:

If you consume 3000 kcal a day, your fat intake should be:

- (3000 × 20%) ÷ 9 = 66 g
- (3000 × 35%) ÷ 9 = 117 g
  i.e. between 66 and 117 g fat a day.

NUTRIENT TIMING

The timing of your food intake around exercise is important. You can optimise glycogen recovery after training by consuming 1–1.2 g carbohydrate/kg BW during the 2-hour post exercise period (Burke *et al*, 2011). So, for example, if you weigh 80 kg you need to consume 80–96 g carbohydrate within 2 hours after exercise.

However, it's not only carbohydrate that aids recovery after training: several studies suggest that taking carbohydrate combined with protein after exercise helps create the ideal hormonal environment for glycogen storage and muscle building (Zawadzki *et al*., 1992; Bloomer *et al*., 2000; Gibala, 2000; Kreider *et al*., 1996). Both trigger the release of insulin and growth hormone in your body. These are powerful anabolic hormones. Insulin transports amino acids into cells, reassembles them into proteins, and prevents muscle breakdown. It also transports glucose into muscle cells and stimulates glycogen storage. Growth hormone increases protein manufacture and muscle building.

There is much evidence that protein consumed early in the post-exercise recovery phase increases the rate of MPS and promotes muscle repair (Van Loon, 2014). The optimal post-exercise protein intake is 0.25 g/kg BW, equivalent to 20 g for an athlete weighing 80 kg (ACSM/AND/DC, 2016; Phillips & Van Loon, 2011; Moore *et al*., 2009; IOC, 2011; Rodriguez *et al*., 2009). When athletes consumed less than 20 g they gained less muscle; when they consumed more than this amount they experienced no further muscle gains.

The window for muscle recovery and protein consumption is longer than once thought. It is now known that the anabolic effect of exercise

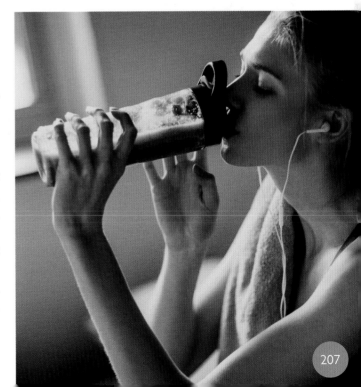

lasts up to 24 hours so the benefits of consuming protein may extend for many hours. In other words, consuming protein immediately after training will increase MPS, but so will protein consumption at any time over the subsequent 24 hours.

For optimal MPS throughout the day, you should consume 0.25–0.3 g protein/kg body weight at each meal. For an 80 kg athlete, this equates to 20–24 g per meal. Consuming less than this amount may result in a suboptimal rate of MPS; consuming more will not produce greater strength or mass gains. Excess protein will be oxidised and used as a fuel source. It is better to evenly distribute your protein throughout the day, consuming similar amounts at breakfast, lunch and dinner, rather than eating most of your protein at dinner (Mamerow *et al.*, 2014; Areta *et al.*, 2013).

Consuming some of your protein before sleep may also increase MPS and muscle mass gains. A study at Maastricht University found that athletes who consumed a pre-bed protein drink containing 28 g protein had greater increases in strength and muscle mass after 12 weeks compared with those who did not (Snijders *et al.*, 2015).

WHICH TYPE OF PROTEIN IS BEST FOR MUSCLE GAIN?

Milk, whey, casein, egg, meat, poultry and fish provide all the essential amino acids at levels that closely match the body's needs. Studies have shown that these types of protein stimulate muscle growth more than other types of protein.

These foods are also rich in the amino acid leucine, which has been shown to be a critical element in regulating protein manufacture in the body as well as playing a key role in muscle recovery after exercise (*see* p. 85). In combination with the other EAAs, it triggers protein manufacture, which in turn leads to increased muscle size and strength.

However, plant protein sources, such as beans, lentils, nuts, soya and (to a smaller degree) grains, also contribute amino acids to your diet and will count towards your total daily protein intake.

Liquid forms of protein (such as milk and whey protein drinks) are particularly beneficial for MPS immediately after exercise as they are digested and absorbed more rapidly than solid foods (Burke *et al.*, 2012). Milk consumed immediately after resistance exercise has been shown to increase muscle growth and repair, reduce post-exercise muscle soreness, improve body composition and rehydrate the body better than commercial sports drinks (Elliot, 2006; Hartman *et al.*, 2007; Wilkinson, 2007; Karp *et al.*, 2006).

Milk and whey protein are particularly rich sources of leucine so both represent ideal post-workout foods for promoting muscle growth. You can get 20 g protein from 500–600 ml of milk. This volume of milk also provides 30 g of carbohydrate, which will help replenish muscle glycogen stores and build muscle. The type of milk (skimmed or whole milk) is unimportant as far as MPS is concerned. Milkshake, hot chocolate, coffee latte and other drinks made with milk are also suitable recovery options.

WILL WEIGHT GAIN SUPPLEMENTS HELP?

There are literally dozens of supplements on the market that claim to enhance muscle mass, although many of the claims are not supported by scientific research, lack safety data and some have

Post-workout snacks

The following options provide around 20 g of high quality protein:

- 600 ml milk. Any type of milk will provide the protein needed to maximise muscle adaptation after strength and power training. It also contains the optimal amount of the branched-chain amino acid leucine to promote muscle building after exercise.
- 500 ml recovery milkshake. Use 500 ml of milk plus yoghurt and fresh fruit (in general, bananas, strawberries, pears, mango and pineapple give the best results) for an excellent mixture of protein, carbohydrate and those all-important antioxidants.
- 450 ml yoghurt. Choose plain yoghurt after a strength workout, or fruit yoghurt after an endurance session lasting an hour or more. Both contain high quality proteins that will accelerate muscle repair; fruit yoghurt has added sugar so it has the ideal 3:1 carbohydrate:protein ratio for speedy glycogen refuelling.
- 330–500 ml whey protein shake. Shakes made up with milk or water are an easy and convenient mini-meal in a glass. Opt for one containing 20 g protein. Powders and ready-to-drink versions generally contain a balanced mixture of carbohydrate (usually as maltodextrin and sugar), protein (usually whey), vitamins and minerals.
- 50 g of almonds or cashews plus 250 ml yoghurt – nuts provide not only 10 g of protein but also B vitamins, vitamin E, iron, zinc, phytonutrients and fibre. Yoghurt supplies another 10 g of protein. The fat in the nuts may reduce insulin a little, but will not affect muscle building.
- 250 ml strained Greek yoghurt. This is also perfect after a strength workout, because strained Greek yoghurt is more concentrated, containing about twice the protein of ordinary yoghurt.
- 500 ml ready-to-drink milkshake – opt for a shake that contains around 20 g protein for convenient refuelling after exercise. Alternatively, make your own speedy version by mixing 3 tsp of milkshake powder with 500 ml of milk.
- A 'protein' bar. Bars containing a mixture of carbohydrate and whey protein are a convenient option after workouts. Opt for one containing around 20 g protein.

even been found to contain illegal substances! For more information on supplements, *see* Chapter 6. However, some supplements may be worth considering for weight gain:

- Creatine may help increase performance, strength and muscle mass. Dozens of studies since the mid 1990s show significant increases in lean mass and total mass, typically 1–3% lean body weight (approx. 0.8–3 kg) after a 5-day loading dose, compared with controls. *See also* Chapter 6, pp. 122–25.

For example, in a study carried out at Pennsylvania State University, 13 weight trainers gained an average 1.3 kg body mass after taking creatine supplements for 7 days (Volek,

1997). The same team of researchers measured total weight gain of 1.7 kg and muscle mass gain of 1.5 kg after one week of creatine supplementation among 19 weight trainers (Volek, 1999). After 12 weeks, total weight gain averaged 4.8 kg and muscle gain averaged 4.3 kg. The observed gains in weight are due partly to an increase in cell fluid volume and partly to muscle synthesis. However, not all studies have shown a positive effect on muscle mass; some have found gains in total body weight only.

- All-in-one supplements containing protein, maltodextrin, vitamins and minerals provide a convenient alternative to solid food. They will not necessarily improve your performance but can be a helpful and convenient addition (rather than replacement) to your diet if you struggle to eat enough real food, you need to eat on the move or you need the extra nutrients they provide.

- Protein supplements may benefit you if you have particularly high protein requirements or cannot consume enough protein from food alone (e.g. a vegetarian or vegan diet).

Weight gain tips

Put more total eating time into your daily routine. This may mean rescheduling other activities. Plan your meal and snack times in advance and never skip or rush them, no matter how busy you are.

- Increase your meal frequency – eat at least three meals and three snacks daily.
- Eat regularly – every 2–3 hours – and avoid gaps longer than 3 hours.
- Plan nutritious high calorie, low bulk snacks

How does creatine cause weight gain?

Weight gain is due partly to water retention in the muscle cells and partly to increased muscle growth. Researchers have found that urine volume is reduced markedly during the initial days of supplementation with creatine, which indicates the body is retaining extra water (Hultman, 1996).

Creatine draws water into the muscle cells, thus increasing cell volume. In one study with cross-trained athletes, thigh muscle volume increased 6.6% and intra-cellular volume increased 2–3% after a creatine-loading dose (Ziegenfuss et al., 1997). It is thought that the greater cell volume caused by creatine supplementation acts as an anabolic signal for protein synthesis and therefore muscle growth (Haussinger et al., 1996). It also reduces protein breakdown during intense exercise.

The fact that studies show a substantially greater muscle mass even after long-term creatine supplementation indicates that creatine must have a direct effect on muscle growth. In studies at the University of Memphis, athletes taking creatine gained more body mass than those taking the placebo, yet both groups ended up with the same body water content (Kreider et al., 1996). If creatine allows you to train more intensely, it follows that you will gain more muscle mass. For more details on creatine supplement doses, see Chapter 6, pp. 122–25.

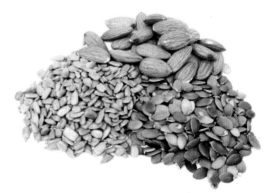

High calorie, nutrient dense snacks for hard gainers

- Nuts and dried fruit
- Milk-based drinks
- Smoothies
- Whole milk or Greek yoghurt
- Porridge
- Sandwiches, bagels, rolls and pitta with high protein fillings
- Granola or oat-based bar
- Flapjack
- All-in-one or protein shake
- Protein bar

– e.g. shakes, smoothies, yoghurt, nuts, dried fruit, protein bars.

- Eat larger portions but avoid overfilling!
- If you are finding it hard to eat enough food, try liquid meals such as milk, milk-based drinks, meal replacement or protein supplements or yoghurt-based smoothies once or twice a day to help bring up your calorie, carbohydrate and protein intake.
- Use whole milk rather than skimmed; Greek yoghurt or whole milk yoghurt instead of low fat varieties.
- Use more olive (or rapeseed) oil for cooking and drizzling on salads; scatter extra grated cheese on dishes; be generous with spreads on toast and sandwiches.
- Boost the calorie and nutritional content of your meals – e.g. add dried fruit, bananas, honey, chopped nuts or seeds to porridge, breakfast cereal or yoghurt. This is more nutritious than the common practice of adding sugar or jam ('empty calories').

Summary of key points

- To build muscle, a consistent weight training programme must be combined with a balanced intake of calories, carbohydrate, protein and fat.
- The amount of lean weight you gain depends on your genetic make-up, body type and hormonal balance.
- To gain lean weight, increase your maintenance calorie intake by 20%, or about 500 kcal daily.
- A protein intake of 1.4–2.0 g/kg body weight will meet your protein needs. As your calorie needs increase by 20%, so should your usual carbohydrate intake.
- Consume 1–1.2 g carbohydrate/kg body weight immediately after training, ideally combined with protein.
- Consume 0.25 g protein/kg BW immediately after training and include 0.25–0.3 g/kg BW in each meal.
- Proteins containing all 8 essential amino acids and high levels of leucine are particularly beneficial for promoting MPS, e.g. milk and milk-based products.
- To gain weight, put more total eating time into your daily routine, increase meal frequency and include more high calorie, nutrient dense foods e.g. milk-based drinks, smoothies, yoghurt, nuts, dried fruit, protein bars.
- There are very few supplements that are supported by good evidence; these include protein supplements and creatine.

The female athlete

This chapter covers the issues that relate specifically to female athletes. These centre around the syndrome previously called the 'Female Athlete Triad': Relative Energy Deficiency in Sport (RED-S), characterised by impaired menstrual function, metabolic rate, bone health, immunity, protein synthesis and cardiovascular health.

RED-S is relatively common among female athletes participating in sports where emphasis is placed on being lean or attaining a very low body weight. To achieve this goal, many female athletes undertake an intense and excessive training programme and combine it with a restrictive diet. However, in some athletes, this can lead to an obsessive preoccupation with body weight and calorie intake, and eventually disordered eating. This chapter examines why female athletes are more prone to disordered eating and gives some of the warning signs to look out for. It considers the effects on health and how to help someone suspected of having an eating disorder.

This chapter also considers the causes and treatment of amenorrhoea and explains the effect it has on health and performance. One of the most serious effects is the reduction in bone density and increased risk of bone loss, osteoporosis and stress fractures.

Female athletes are more prone than non-athletes to iron-deficiency anaemia, due to increased losses associated with training or a low dietary intake. This chapter describes the symptoms of this condition and also explains the causes of the related conditions, sports anaemia and latent iron deficiency. The appropriate use of iron supplements is also covered.

Finally, details of specific nutritional considerations for female athletes during pregnancy are given, and the effect a low body fat percentage may have on the chances of conception and successful pregnancy are discussed.

Relative energy deficiency in sport

In 1992 this combination of disorders was given the formal name of the 'female athlete triad' during a consensus conference convened by the American College of Sports Medicine, and documented in a position stand published in 1997 (Otis *et al.*, 1997). In the 2005 IOC Consensus Statement, the Female Athlete Triad was defined as 'the combination of disordered eating (DE) and irregular menstrual cycles eventually leading to a decrease in endogenous oestrogen and other hormones, resulting in low bone mineral density' (BMD) (IOC, 2005). In 2007, the American College of Sports Medicine redefined the Triad as a clinical entity that refers to the 'relationship between three interrelated components: energy availability (EA), menstrual function and bone health' (Nattiv *et al.*, 2007).

Since then, researchers have shown that the clinical phenomenon is not a triad of three components, but rather a syndrome under-pinned by an energy deficiency relative to the balance between energy intake (EI) and energy expenditure required for health and daily living, growth and sporting activities. In 2014, the IOC replaced the term 'Female Athlete Triad' with a broader and more comprehensive term, 'Relative Energy Deficiency in Sport' (RED-S) (Mountjoy *et al.*, 2014).

The underlying problem of RED-S is a low energy availability (EA). This is calculated as energy intake (EI) minus exercise energy expen-diture (EE). It is the amount of energy available to the body to perform all other functions after exercise training expenditure is subtracted. In healthy adults, a value of 45 kcal/kg fat-free mass (FFM)/day equates with energy balance and optimum health. It has been suggested that 30 kcal/kg FFM/day should be the lower threshold of energy availability in females. Fat-free mass includes muscles, organs, fluid and bones.

It may occur when energy intake is too low, energy expenditure is too high or a combination of both. Although it is more common in female athletes, it can also occur in males. A low EA may compromise athletic performance in the short and long term.

Disordered eating

Many athletes are very careful about what they eat and often experiment with different dietary programmes in order to improve their perfor-mance. However, there is a thin line between paying attention to detail and obsessive eating behaviour. The pressure to be thin or attain higher performance makes some athletes develop eating habits that not only put their performance at risk but also endanger their health.

Disordered eating is one of the risk factors for the development of amenorrhoea, a loss of normal menstrual periods. This condition is often the result of a chronic low calorie intake, low body fat and weight, high intensity training and volume, and psychological stress.

Eating disorders represent the extremes in a continuum of eating behaviours. An eating disor-der is defined as: a *distorted pattern of thinking and behaviour about food*. In all cases, preoccupa-tion and obsession with food occurs and eating is out of control. It's as much about attitude and behaviour towards food as it is about consump-tion of food.

What is relative energy deficiency in sport?

Relative Energy Deficiency in Sport (RED-S) refers to the impaired physiological function including metabolic rate, menstrual function, bone health, immunity, protein synthesis and cardiovascular health caused by relative energy deficiency or low EA in male and female athletes. It more accurately describes the clinical syndrome previously known as the Female Athlete Triad.

Clinical eating disorders such as anorexia, bulimia and compulsive eating are defined by official, specific criteria by the American Psychiatric Association (APA). *Anorexia nervosa* is the extreme of restrictive eating behaviour in which the individual continues to restrict food and feel fat despite being 15% or more below an ideal body weight. *Bulimia* refers to a cycle of food restriction followed by bingeing and purging. Compulsive eating is a psychological craving for food that results in uncontrollable eating.

However, many people who don't fall into these clinical categories may still have a subclinical eating disorder. This is often called *disordered eating*. Sufferers have an intense fear of gaining weight or becoming fat even though their weight is normal or below normal. They are preoccupied with food, their weight and body shape. Like anorexics, they have a distorted body image, imagining they are larger than they really are. They attempt to lose weight by restricting their food, usually consuming less than 1200 kcal a day, and may exercise excessively to burn more calories. The result is a chaotic eating pattern and lifestyle.

ARE FEMALE ATHLETES MORE LIKELY TO DEVELOP DISORDERED EATING?

Female athletes are more vulnerable to disordered eating than the general population – disordered eating affects approximately 20% of female elite athletes and 8% of elite male athletes but up to 60% in certain sports (Sundgot-Borgen & Torstveit, 2010); Sundgot-Borgen 1994(a) and (b); Petrie, 1993). Disordered eating appears to be more common in athletes in sports where a low body weight, low body fat level or thin physique is perceived to be advantageous, as well as weight-category sports (*see* Table 11.1) (Sundgot-Borgen & Torstveit, 2010; Beals & Manore, 2002; Sundgot-Borgen & Torstveit, 2004). In a US study, 30% of elite female skaters considered themselves overweight, had a poor body image and indicated a preference for a thinner body shape (Jonnalagadda *et al.*, 2004). A 2004 study of 1620 male and female elite Norwegian athletes found that 42% of women competing in aesthetic sports and 24% of those competing in endurance events met the clinical criteria for an eating disorder (Sundgot-Borgen & Torstveit, 2004). And in a 2007 survey carried out at Coastal Carolina University, US, 19% of female cross-country runners reported having

Table 11.1	EATING DISORDERS – HIGH RISK SPORTS
Lean sports	Distance running and cycling, horse racing
Aesthetic sports	Gymnastics, figure skating, ballet, synchronised swimming
Weight category sports	Lightweight rowing, judo, karate, weightlifting, boxing, wrestling, mixed martial arts
Gym sports	Bodybuilding, competitive aerobics

Source: Beals & Manore, 1994.

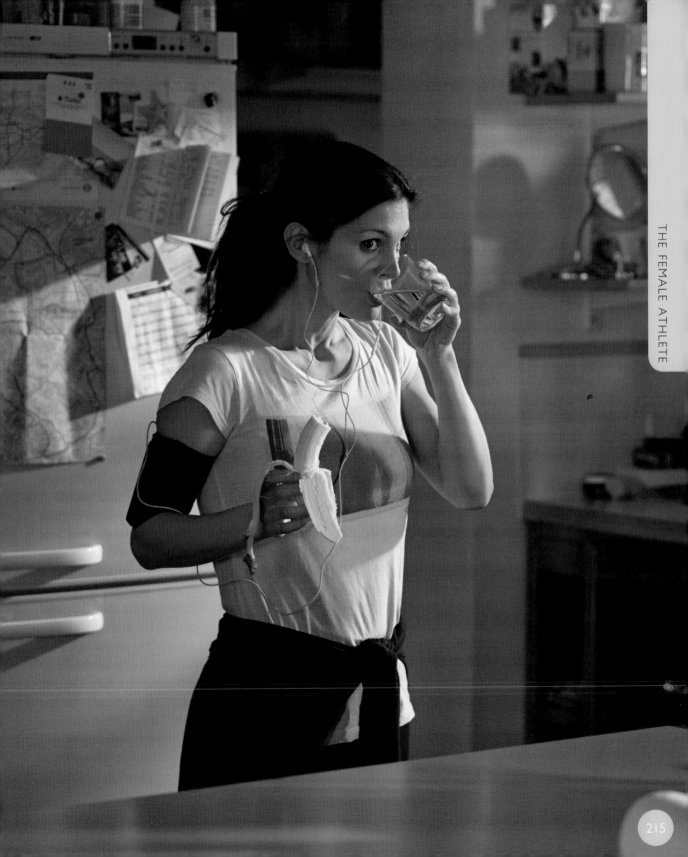

a current or previous eating disorder. Another study suggests that females involved in sports that favour leanness and a high power-to-weight ratio, such as figure skating and gymnastics, are more likely to be at risk of developing disordered eating and be over-concerned about their body weight and dieting (Zucker *et al.*, 1999).

Although most athletes with eating disorders tend to be female, males are also at risk, especially those who compete in sports that place a high emphasis on appearance and leanness (e.g. body-building, crew and distance running) or where there is a culture of 'weight cutting' to achieve a competitive edge (e.g. wrestling, boxing and horse racing).

The causes differ depending on the sport. Distance runners are at greater risk of developing disordered eating because of the close link between low body weight and performance. Those participating in aesthetic sports such as dancing, bodybuilding and gymnastics are at risk because success depends on body shape as well as physical skill. Athletes competing in weigh-category sports such as judo and lightweight rowing are also more likely to develop eating disorders due to the pressures of meeting the weight criteria.

There is no single cause of disordered eating but, typically, it stems from a belief that a lower body weight enhances athletic success. The athlete begins to diet and, for reasons not completely understood, then adopts more restrictive and unhealthy eating behaviour.

It is not the sport itself that creates the risk for the athlete, but rather certain aspects of the sport and/or the sport environment. Put simply, there are particular personality variables that predispose an athlete to developing an eating disorder, and specific sport environments seem to

Health Problems Associated With Eating Disorders

- Amenorrhoea (cessation of periods) and infertility
- Heart problems, such as abnormal beat rhythm, low blood pressure and cardiac failure
- Osteoporosis, weakened bones, risk of fracture
- Erosion of dental enamel
- Gastrointestinal problems, such as peptic ulcers
- Kidney problems
- Low white blood cell count and poor immunity
- Metabolic problems
- Difficulty maintaining body temperature
- Dry, scaly, itchy skin
- Fine layer of hair on body

create additional risk. For example, the demands of certain sports or training programmes or the requests made by coaches to lose weight may trigger an eating disorder in susceptible individuals. It is possible that some people with a pre-disposition to eating disorders are attracted to certain sports. Studies have shown that athletes in sports demanding a high degree of leanness have a more distorted body image, and are more dissatisfied with their body weight and shape compared to the general population. Researchers have found that the personality characteristics of elite athletes are very similar to those with eating disorders: obsession, competitiveness, perfectionism, compulsiveness and self-motivation. Training then becomes a way to lose weight and the positive relationship

Have you got disordered eating?

This questionnaire is not intended as a diagnostic method for disordered eating or as a substitute for a full diagnosis by an eating disorders specialist. If you answer yes to six or more of the following questions, you could be at risk of developing disordered eating and may benefit from further help.

• Do you count the calories of everything you eat?
• Do you think about food most of the time?
• Do you worry about gaining weight?
• Do you worry about or dislike your body shape?
• Do you diet excessively?
• Do you feel guilty during or after eating?
• Do you feel your weight is one aspect of your life you can control?
• Do your friends and family insist that you are slim while you feel fat?
• Do you exercise to compensate for eating extra calories?
• Does your weight fluctuate dramatically?
• Do you ever induce vomiting after eating?
• Have you become isolated from family and friends?
• Do you avoid certain foods even though you want to eat them?
• Do you feel stressed or guilty if your normal diet or exercise routine is interrupted?
• Do you often decline invitations to meals and social occasions involving food in case you might have to eat something fattening?

between leanness and performance further legitimises the athlete's pursuit of thinness.

Evidence is also emerging that sufferers have a disturbed body chemistry as well as a psychological predisposition to disordered eating. For example, studies have found that more than half of those suffering from anorexia have a severe zinc deficiency and that recovery is more successful if zinc supplements are given (Bryce-Smith & Simpson, 1984). There may also be a genetic link. Around 10% of anorexics have siblings similarly affected, and it occurs more commonly than would be expected in identical twins. Researchers have identified certain genes that influence personality traits such as perfectionism and thus predispose an individual to eating disorders (Garfinkel & Garner, 1982; Davis, 1993). Scientists have also proposed that sufferers have a defective gene that results in abnormally high levels of the brain chemical serotonin. This causes a reduction in appetite, lowered mood and anxiety. They suggest that anorexics use starvation as a means of escaping anxiety.

WHICH ATHLETES ARE AT RISK?

A number of factors predispose an athlete to developing an eating disorder. Risk factors include the following (Sundgot-Borgen, 1994b; Williamson *et al.*, 1995):

• pressure from influential people (coaches or parents) to lose weight to improve sports performance
• over-involvement in sports, with limited other social and recreational activities
• training even when sick or injured
• training outside of scheduled practice times or more than other athletes on the team
• a traumatic event

- injury
- poor performance
- a change in coaching personnel.

WHAT ARE THE WARNING SIGNS?

Athletes with disordered eating try to keep their disorder a secret. However, there are physical and behavioural signs you can look out for. These are detailed in Tables 11.2 and 11.3 (*see also* 'Have you got disordered eating?', p. 217).

WHAT ARE THE HEALTH EFFECTS OF DISORDERED EATING?

The chaotic and restricted eating patterns of disordered eating often result in menstrual and fertility problems. Menstrual dysfunction (irregularities in the menstrual cycle – oligomenorrhoea – or a complete loss of menstrual periods – amenorrhoea) is common among anorexics. The combination of low body fat levels, restricted calorie intake, low calcium intake, intense training and stress can result in bone thinning, stress fractures and other injuries and, ultimately, premature osteoporosis. One study found that disordered eating was associated with low bone mineral density in runners who had regular menstrual cycles (Cobb *et al.*, 2003). Another found that 45 out of 53 female competitive track and field runners had suffered stress fractures, and this was correlated with high levels of weight and eating concerns (Bennell *et al.*, 1995). Researchers at the University of British Columbia, Vancouver, found that women runners with a recent stress fracture were more likely to have a high degree of dietary restraint compared with runners without a history of stress fractures (Guest & Barr, 2005).

Table 11.2 CHARACTERISTICS OF ANOREXIA NERVOSA		
Physical signs	**Psychological signs**	**Behavioural signs**
Severe weight loss	Obsessive about food, dieting and thinness	Eating very little
Well below average weight	Claiming to be fat when thin	Relentless exercise
Emaciated appearance	Obsessive fear of weight gain	Great interest in food and calories
Periods stop or become irregular	Low self-esteem	Anxiety and arguments about food
Growth of downy hair on face, arms and legs	Depression and anxiety	Refusing to eat in company
Feeling cold, bluish extremities	Perfectionism	Lying about eating meals
Restless, sleeping very little	High need for approval	Obsessive weighing
Dry/yellow skin	Social withdrawal	Rituals around eating

Table 11.3	CHARACTERISTICS OF BULIMIA NERVOSA	
Physical signs	**Psychological signs**	**Behavioural signs**
Tooth decay, enamel erosion	Low self-esteem and self-control	Out of control bingeing on large amounts of food (up to 5000 kcal)
Puffy face due to swollen salivary glands	Impulsive	Eating to numb feeling/provide comfort
Normal weight or extreme weight fluctuations	Depression, anxiety, anger	Guilt, shame, withdrawal and self-deprecation after bingeing
Abrasions on knuckles from self-induced vomiting	Body dissatisfaction and distortion	Purging – vomiting, laxative abuse
Menstrual irregularities	Preoccupied with food, body image, appearance and weight	Frequent weighing
Muscle cramps/weakness		Disappearing after meals to get rid of food
Frequently dehydrated		Secretive eating May steal food/laxatives

Gastrointestinal problems, electrolyte imbalances, kidney and bowel disorders and depression are also common. Anorexics may develop low blood pressure and chronic low core body temperature. In bulimics, repeated vomiting and use of laxatives can lead to stomach and oesophagus pain, enamel erosion and tooth decay.

HOW CAN ATHLETES WITH DISORDERED EATING CONTINUE TRAINING?

It seems extraordinary that athletes with apparently very low calorie intake continue to exercise and compete, apparently unabated. Undoubtedly, a combination of psychological and physiological factors are involved.

On the psychological side, anorexics are able to motivate and push themselves to exercise, despite feelings of exhaustion. Sufferers are strong willed, highly driven and have a strong desire to succeed. Thus, in the short term they are able to continue training and competing, despite their low calorie intake.

Some scientists believe that some athletes under-report their food intake and, in fact, eat more than they admit. For example, a study at Indiana University on 9 highly trained cross-country runners found that they were eating, on average, 2100 kcal per day but their predicted energy expenditure was 3000 kcal (Edwards, 1993). After analysing the results of a Food Attitude Questionnaire, the researchers suggested that many had a poor body image and had inaccurately reported what they ate during the study.

On the physiological side, it is likely that the body adapts by becoming more energy efficient, reducing its metabolic rate (10–30% is possible).

Improve your body image

This guide is not intended as a treatment for disordered eating. Treatment should always be sought from an eating disorders specialist.

- Learn to accept your body's shape – emphasise your good points.
- Realise that reducing your body fat will not solve deep-rooted problems or an emotional crisis.
- Don't set rigid eating rules for yourself and feel guilty when you break them.
- Don't ban any foods or feel guilty about eating anything.
- Don't count calories.
- Think of foods in terms of taste and health rather than a source of calories.
- Establish a sensible healthy eating pattern rather than a strict diet.
- Listen to your natural appetite cues – learn to eat when you are hungry.
- If you do overeat, don't try to 'pay for it' later by starving yourself or exercising to burn off calories.
- Enjoy your exercise or sport for its own sake; have fun instead of enduring torture to lose body fat.
- Set positive exercise goals not related to losing weight.

This would allow the athlete to train and maintain energy balance on fewer calories than would be expected. Some scientists, however, suggest that excessive exercise during dieting may augment the fall in metabolic rate.

To overcome physical and emotional fatigue, many anorexics and bulimics use caffeine-containing drinks such as strong coffee and 'diet' cola. However, in the long term, performance ultimately falls. As glycogen and nutrient stores become chronically depleted, the athlete's health will suffer and optimal performance cannot be sustained indefinitely. Maximal oxygen consumption decreases, cardiac output decreases and chronic fatigue sets in.

Without enough protein to maintain and repair muscle, there will be a loss of lean body mass, strength and endurance. The athlete quickly becomes more susceptible to injury, illness and infection. If fat intake is too low (less than 10% of calories), the lack of fat-soluble vitamins and essential fatty acids will result in fatigue and poor performance. Deficiencies of vitamins and minerals will eventually develop, and these will affect performance too, increasing the risk of muscle weakness, injuries and infections.

Athletes who use diuretics or laxatives or self-induce vomiting will become dehydrated. This quickly results in fatigue and poor performance. It can also have serious effects on health. The reduced blood volume results in decreased blood flow to the skin, which means the body is not able to sweat properly and maintain a normal temperature during exercise. This, in turn, increases core temperature and increases the risk of heat exhaustion and heatstroke.

In summary, athletes with disordered eating and eating disorders are likely to suffer from nutritional deficiencies, chronic fatigue, dehydration and a dramatic reduction in performance.

HOW SHOULD I APPROACH SOMEONE SUSPECTED OF HAVING DISORDERED EATING?

Approaching someone you suspect has disordered eating requires great tact and sensitivity. Sufferers are likely to deny that they have a problem; they may feel embarrassed and their self-esteem threatened, so it is vital to avoid a direct confrontation about their eating behaviour or physical symptoms. Be tactful, tread very gently – do not suddenly present 'evidence' – and avoid accusations.

If the sufferer admits to having an eating problem (*see* 'Have you got disordered eating?'), suggest that it would be best to consult an eating disorders specialist. Various forms of specialist help are available, such as trained counsellors from a self-help organisation or private eating disorders clinic (*see* pp. 377–8), or with a GP's referral, treatment within a multidisciplinary team of psychologists and dietitians.

Menstrual dysfunction and bone loss

ARE FEMALE ATHLETES AT GREATER RISK OF MENSTRUAL DYSFUNCTION?

Female athletes are more likely to develop menstrual dysfunction. Several studies have found that menstrual dysfunction is more prevalent among female athletes participating in endurance or aesthetic sports (Beals & Hill, 2006; Torstveit & Sundgot-Borgen, 2005; Sundgot-Borgen, 1994; Sundgot-Borgen & Larsen, 1993).

In a study at the University of Utah and the University of Indianapolis, significantly more

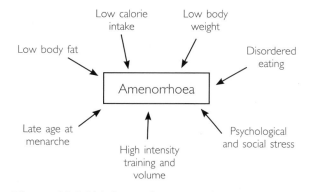

Figure 11.1 Risk factors for amenorrhoea among athletes

lean-build athletes suffered menstrual irregularities than non lean-build athletes (Beals & Hill, 2006). This may be due to the greater volume of training associated with endurance sports. However, a study at San Diego State University indicates that approximately 20% of female high school athletes, regardless of sport, are at risk of disordered eating or menstrual dysfunction and that the two conditions are often inter-related (Nichols *et al.*, 2007). Nearly 27% of lean-build athletes had menstrual dysfunction, compared with 17% non lean-build athletes.

Menstrual dysfunction is unlikely to develop as a result of exercise alone, nor does there seem to be a specific body fat percentage below which regular periods stop. Studies have shown that female athletes who have a low EA are at increased risk of menstrual dysfunction (Loucks, 2003). A combination of factors, such as low EA, disordered eating, intense training before menarche, high intensity training and volume, low body-fat levels and physical and emotional stress are usually involved (*see* Fig. 11.1). The more of these risk factors that you have, the greater the chance of developing menstrual dysfunction.

Girls who begin intense training pre-puberty usually start their periods at a later age than the average. This may be due to a combination of high-volume exercise and low body-fat levels. Some female athletes, particularly runners, may have shorter than average menstrual cycles due to anovulatory cycles, which are cycles during which an egg is not produced. This pattern is linked to low levels of female hormones: oestrogen and progesterone, follicle-stimulating hormone (FSH) and luteinising hormone (LH).

ARE DISORDERED EATING AND MENSTRUAL DYSFUNCTION LINKED?

Studies show that female athletes who consistently have low EA are more likely to have menstrual dysfunction. It has been suggested that this is an energy-conserving adaptation by the body to a very low calorie intake. In other words, the body tries to save energy by economising on the energy costs of menstruation i.e. 'shutting down' the normal menstrual function.

The body mechanism is as follows: the combination of mental or physiological stress and a chronic negative energy balance increases cortisol production by the adrenals, which disrupts the release of gonadotrophin-releasing hormone (GnRH) from the brain. This, in turn, reduces the production of the gonadotrophin-releasing hormone, luteinising hormone (LH) and follicle-stimulating hormone (FSH), oestrogen and progesterone (Loucks et al., 1989; Edwards et al., 1993).

HOW DOES MENSTRUAL DYSFUNCTION CAUSE BONE LOSS?

It's a myth that amenorrhoea is simply a consequence of hard training; it should be regarded as a clinical state of overtraining, because of the adverse effects it has on many systems in the body.

One of the most severe effects is the reduction in bone density and increased risk of early osteoporosis and stress fractures. This is partly due to low levels of oestrogen and progesterone, both of which act directly on bone cells to maintain bone turnover (Drinkwater et al., 1984). When hormone levels drop, the natural breakdown of old bone exceeds the speed of formation of new bone. The result is loss of bone minerals and a loss of bone density. Training, then, no longer has a positive effect on bone density: it cannot compensate for the negative effects of low oestrogen and progesterone. But high levels of cortisol and poor nutritional status – both linked to menstrual dysfunction – are also thought to contribute to bone loss and low bone density (Carbon, 2002). Canadian researchers have found that disordered eating is correlated with menstrual irregularities and increased cortisol levels, all of which are risk factors for stress fractures (Guest & Barr, 2005).

Studies have found that the bone mineral density in the lumbar spine can be as much as 20–30% lower in amenorrhoeic distance runners compared with normally menstruating runners (Cann et al., 1984; Nelson et al., 1986). Whether bone mineral density 'catches up' once menstruation resumes is not known for certain. One long-term study found that bone mass increased initially, but in the long term, it remained lower compared to active and inactive women (Drinkwater, 1986).

DOES MENSTRUAL DYSFUNCTION AFFECT PERFORMANCE?

Menstrual dysfunction results in many performance-hindering effects, all of which are linked to very low oestrogen levels. These include an increased risk of soft tissue injuries, stress fractures, prolonged healing of injuries and reduced ability to recover from hard training sessions (Lloyd *et al.*, 1986). For example, low oestrogen levels result in a loss of suppleness in the ligaments, which then become more susceptible to injury. Low oestrogen levels slow down bone adaptation to exercise and micro-fractures occur more readily and heal more slowly.

The good news is that performance will most likely improve once menstruation resumes. Studies show that when amenorrhoeic athletes improve their diet and restructure their training programme to improve energy balance, normal menstruation resumes within about 3 months and performance improves consistently (Dueck *et al.*, 1996). This is perhaps the most persuasive reason to seek treatment if you have amenorrhoea.

HOW CAN MENSTRUAL DYSFUNCTION BE TREATED?

You should definitely seek advice if you have suffered amenorrhoea (absence of periods) for longer than 6 months. An initial consultation with your GP will rule out medical causes of amenorrhoea. You should then get a referral to a specialist, such as a gynaecologist, sports physician, endocrinologist or bone specialist. As part of your treatment you should consider advice from a sports nutritionist, exercise physiologist or sports psychologist. Treatment will centre on resuming 'normal' body weight and body fat, and reducing or changing your training programme. For example, you may have to reduce your training frequency, volume and intensity or change your current programme to

include more cross-training. You may need to increase your food intake in order to bring your body weight and body fat within the normal range. If you have some degree of disordered eating, you will need help in overcoming this problem (*see* p. 221).

If amenorrhoea persists after this type of treatment, hormone therapy may be prescribed to prevent further loss of bone mineral density. Doses of oestrogen and progesterone, similar to those used for treating postmenopausal women, are usually used. Supplements containing calcium, magnesium and other key minerals may be advised simultaneously.

Iron deficiency

Iron is required for:

- making haemoglobin, the oxygen-carrying protein in red blood cells
- making myoglobin, the protein that carries and stores oxygen in your muscle cells
- aerobic energy production (the 'electron transport system' that controls the release of energy from cells)
- a healthy immune system.

It is estimated that 30% of female athletes, although not anaemic, have iron deficiency. This is termed 'non-anaemic iron deficiency', or 'latent iron deficiency'. Iron deficiency can reduce the amount of oxygen delivered to the muscles during exercise, as well as the amount of energy that can be generated in muscle cells. It reduces your maximal oxygen consumption (VO_2max), your endurance capacity and your performance. The American College of Sports

Medicine states that iron deficiency can have negative effects on exercise performance as well as bone health (Rodriguez *et al.*, 2009).

WHAT ARE THE SYMPTOMS OF IRON DEFICIENCY?

There are 3 stages of iron deficiency:

1. Storage iron depletion – when serum ferritin levels drop below 18 nanograms per millilitre (ng/ml)

2. Early functional deficiency – when red blood cell formation starts to become impaired but not enough to cause anaemia

3. Iron-deficiency anaemia – when haemoglobin levels fall below 13 g/100 ml in men and 12 g/100 ml in women; ferritin levels below 12 ng/ml

The first stage of iron deficiency is characterised by symptoms such as tiredness, chronic fatigue, pallor, headaches, light-headedness, above-normal

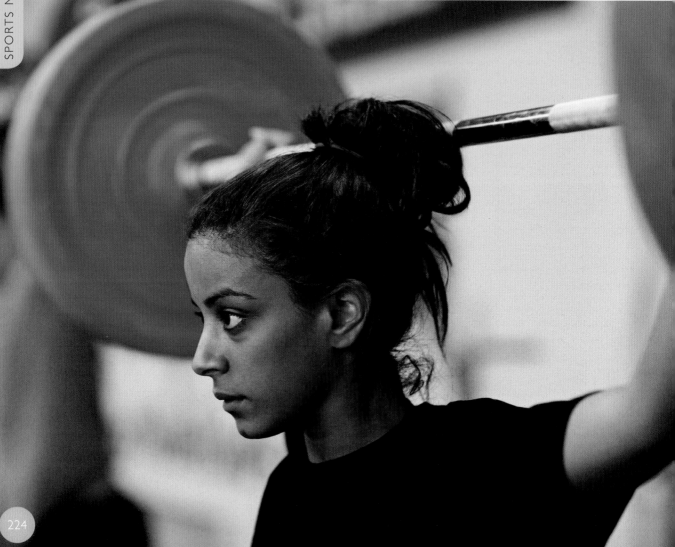

breathlessness during exercise and palpitations, frequent injuries, loss of endurance and power, loss of appetite and loss of interest in training. In stage-2 iron deficiency, the body makes smaller red blood cells with less haemoglobin, which impairs the body's ability to carry oxygen around the body and affects physical performance. Stage 3, iron-deficiency anaemia, occurs when there is insufficient haemoglobin to meet the body's needs. It can be diagnosed by a simple blood test.

WHAT IS SPORTS ANAEMIA?

Sports anaemia, although associated with a low haemoglobin concentration, is not really anaemia. It arises as a consequence of regular aerobic training, which causes an increase in blood plasma volume. It is most likely to occur in the early stages of a training programme or when training load increases. As a result the red blood cells are more diluted, and measures of haemoglobin and ferritin appear lower since they have effectively been 'watered down'.

WHAT ARE THE CAUSES OF IRON-DEFICIENCY ANAEMIA IN FEMALE ATHLETES?

Iron-deficiency anaemia may be the result of increased blood losses associated with training or a deficient dietary intake.

Training effects

Blood losses in the urine, a condition called *haematuria*, may occur in female distance runners. This is due to bruising of the bladder lining caused by repeated pounding by the abdominal contents during running. Another condition, called *haemoglobinuria* (the presence of haemoglobin in the urine), can result from repetitive foot strikes associated with poor running gait or pounding on hard surfaces. This causes some destruction of red blood cells in the soles of the feet. In haematuria, the urine has a cloudy appearance, whereas in haemoglobinuria it is clear, like rosé wine. Another route of blood loss in distance runners may be via the digestive tract and may be visible with diarrhoea. This is caused by the repeated minor trauma as the abdominal contents bounce up and down with each foot strike. However, iron losses via any of these routes are relatively small.

Diet

Studies reveal that many female athletes consume less than the RNI of iron. This may be due to a low food or calorie intake, which is common among weight-conscious athletes and those involved in sports requiring a low body fat level. It is very difficult to consume enough iron on a calorie intake of less than 1500 kcal a day. Many female athletes avoid red meat (a readily absorbed source of iron) or eat very little and perhaps do not compensate by eating other sources of iron.

HOW MUCH IRON DO I NEED?

The UK recommended intake is 8.7 mg/day for men; 14.8 mg/day for women aged 19–50 years; and 8.7 mg for women over 50 years. There is no official recommendation for athletes (Rodriguez *et al.*, 2009). Table 11.4 shows the iron content of various foods.

CAN IRON SUPPLEMENTS IMPROVE PERFORMANCE?

Many studies suggest that iron supplementation may be beneficial for athletes who are iron deficient

Table 11.4	THE IRON CONTENT OF VARIOUS FOODS	
Food	Portion size	mg iron
Calves' liver	Average (100 g)	12.2
Dried apricots (ready to eat)	5 (200 g)	7.0
Red lentils (boiled)	4 tbsp (160 g)	4.0
Prunes (ready to eat)	10 (110 g)	3.0
Baked beans	1 small tin (205 g)	2.9
Chickpeas (boiled)	4 tbsp (140 g)	2.8
Pumpkin seeds	Small handful (25 g)	2.5
Lean beef fillet (grilled)	Average (105 g)	2.4
Spinach	3 tbsp (100 g)	2.1
Wholemeal bread	2 large slices (80 g)	2.0
Wholemeal roll	1 (50 g)	1.8
Cashew nuts	30 (30 g)	1.8
Walnuts	12 halves (40 g)	1.2
Eggs	1 large (61 g)	1.2
Broccoli	2 spears (90 g)	1.0
Dark chicken meat	2 slices (100 g)	0.8

but do not have anaemia (Brownlie *et al.*, 2004). It not only improves haemoglobin, serum ferritin levels and iron status but also increases work capacity as evidenced by increasing oxygen uptake, reducing heart rate, and decreasing lactate concentration during exercise (Lukaski, 2004). A review of 22 studies by researchers at the University of Melbourne found that iron supplementation improved maximal and sub-maximal exercise performance in women with and without anaemia (Pasricha *et al.*, 2014). The usual recommended dose is 200 mg iron sulphate 3 times a day for 1 month. However, you should not take supplements without medical advice. They can cause unpleasant side effects such as reduced bowel motility, constipation and dark faeces.

WHICH FOODS CONTAIN IRON?

Foods rich in iron include red meat, offal, poultry (dark part of the meat), fish, pulses, whole grains, dark green leafy vegetables, eggs, fortified foods and dried fruit (*see* Table 11.4). Meat, offal and fish contain 'haeme iron', which the body can absorb more readily than 'non-haeme iron' from plant foods such as wholegrain cereals, egg yolks, beans, lentils, green leafy vegetables, dried apricots, nuts and seeds. The absorption of non-haeme iron can be increased by:

- Adding a vitamin C-rich food, such as red peppers, broccoli, spinach, tomatoes, oranges, berries (strawberries, raspberries, blueberries, blackberries) or kiwi fruit.
- Including fruit and vegetables with meals – they contain citric acid, which increases iron absorption.
- Avoiding coffee or tea with your meal as they contain tannins that reduce iron absorption.

- Avoiding bran – it contains high levels of phytates, which inhibit the absorption of iron.

Pregnancy

Female athletes share the same nutritional recommendations for pregnancy as non-athletes, but there are additional issues that need to be addressed. These relate to body weight and body composition, which tend to differ markedly from non-athletic women. Many female athletes, particularly those in sports requiring a very lean physique, such as endurance events, aesthetic sports and weight-category sports, tend to have a lower body fat percentage than non-athletic women. In addition, the physical and psychological demands of regular exercise may affect your chances of conception and of a successful pregnancy. This section highlights the sports-specific issues associated with pregnancy.

DOES MY BODY FAT LEVEL AFFECT MY FERTILITY?

A lower than average body fat level is often associated with a drop in oestrogen production which, in turn, affects normal menstrual function and can result in oligomenorrhoea or amenorrhoea (*see* p. 221, 'Are female athletes at greater risk of menstrual dysfunction?'). Research shows that body fat is important for oestrogen production and for converting the hormone from its inactive form into its active form. However, as explained previously, loss of normal menstrual function is not simply a result of attaining a very low body fat percentage. It is often the result of a combination of factors, including a chronic low calorie intake, high training volume and intensity, and emotional and physical stress. Many female athletes are affected by one or more of these factors and, thus, fertility can be low and the chances of pregnancy small. Normal menstrual function and fertility can usually be restored within 6 months by adopting a more appropriate training programme, increasing your food intake so that energy intake matches energy output, and reducing stress.

WHAT ARE THE PROBLEMS WITH HAVING A VERY LOW BODY FAT PERCENTAGE DURING PREGNANCY?

A low body fat level is less likely to be a problem than a small pregnancy weight gain. Provided you are in good health and are gaining weight at the recommended rate (*see* p. 228), low body fat levels should not present a problem. However, a small weight gain suggesting prolonged food restriction can have an adverse effect on the baby. The baby is more likely to be underweight when born, to be shorter in length and to have a smaller head circumference than normal. Dieting or restricting your weight gain during pregnancy is not recommended.

Short-term dietary imbalances (e.g. during the first trimester due to sickness) do not affect the baby. Hormones are produced by the mother and placenta to ensure the baby continues to receive the necessary growth factors and nutrients during occasional times of adversity. During these periods, it is the mother's health that is more likely to suffer.

HOW MUCH WEIGHT SHOULD I GAIN DURING PREGNANCY?

The recommended average weight gain is 10–12.5 kg over 40 weeks. Although there are no specific recommendations for weight gain during pregnancy in the UK, the American College of Obstetricians and Gynaecologists encourages thinner women to gain a little more weight, around 12.8–18 kg (28–40 lb).

The majority of the weight will be spread fairly evenly over the last two trimesters, about ½ kg (1 lb) per week, with a little more at the end. About one quarter of your weight gain (3–4 kg/6–9 lb) will be the weight of your baby; about half (6 kg/13 lb) will be pregnancy-related weight (placenta, amniotic fluid, uterus, extra blood, breast tissue); and about one quarter (3–4 kg/6–9 lb) will be extra body fat. Table 11.5 shows the body component changes during pregnancy.

Most of the extra fat gain occurs in the second trimester, when an increased level of progesterone favours body fat deposition, mainly subcutaneously in the thighs, hips and abdomen. This extra fat deposit acts as a buffer of energy for late pregnancy when the developing baby's energy needs are highest. The hormone lactogen is produced during late pregnancy and post-pregnancy to mobilise these fat stores to provide energy for the developing baby and breast milk production, should your calorie intake drop. In practice, this extra fat is not necessary because there is little danger of a drop in food supply (i.e. famine). Most women already have enough body fat to buffer against a food shortage.

Gaining extra body fat is unlikely to be advantageous for female athletes because it represents surplus weight that can potentially reduce your performance once you resume training. Thus, the 3.35 kg fat allowance in the recommended 12.5 kg pregnancy weight gain may be regarded as optional for female athletes. Provided you consume a well-balanced diet during pregnancy,

Table 11.5	BODY COMPONENT CHANGES DURING PREGNANCY
Body component	**Average increase in weight (kg)**
Baby	3.4
Placenta	0.65
Amniotic fluid	0.8
Uterus	0.97
Breasts	0.41
Blood	1.25
Extra-cellular fluid	1.68
Fat	3.35
Total	**12.5**

Source: Hytten & Leitch, 1971.

you can aim to gain 9–10 kg. However, do not try to stay below this level.

HOW MANY CALORIES SHOULD I EAT?

The Department of Health recommends no change in calorie intake during the first two trimesters of pregnancy for the general population. However, as an athlete, you may need to adjust your food intake if you reduce your training substantially during pregnancy. It is fine to continue exercising during pregnancy, but you will almost certainly need to reduce the intensity and/or frequency of your training, particularly during the third trimester (due to your increased weight and the physiological changes associated with pregnancy). Prolonged high-impact activities such as running, jumping, plyometrics and high-impact aerobics, and heavy-weight training are not recommended during the second and third trimesters as they cause undue stress on the joints. During pregnancy, the ligaments, which support the joints, become softer and more lax owing to the effects of the hormone relaxin. Therefore, if you omit these activities from your routine your energy expenditure may be considerably lower than normal and you risk unnecessary fat gain unless you eat less or substitute an alternative exercise programme.

During the third trimester, there is a greater increase in your energy needs as the baby grows larger and additional pregnancy-related tissues are laid down. The DoH recommends an extra 200 kcal daily during this time. However, you may not need to eat more food because the discomfort of the growing bump may curtail your normal physical activity level. Your training may be further reduced or even stopped during the last few weeks of pregnancy, so there may be no change in your net calorie intake.

GENERAL NUTRITIONAL GUIDELINES FOR PREGNANCY

- Include foods rich in omega-3 and omega-6 fatty acids in your diet. These are needed for the normal development of brain tissue, and for brain, central nervous system and eye function. (*See* Chapter 8, p. 180: 'What are the best food sources of essential fatty acids?')
- A daily multivitamin and mineral supplement may be useful to help meet your increased needs. *See* Chapter 5 p. 100.
- The DoH recommends taking a daily folic acid supplement containing 400 µg (0.4 mg) prior to pregnancy and during the first 12 weeks to reduce the risk of neural tube defects. (*See* Appendix 2, 'Glossary of Vitamins and Minerals', for food sources of folic acid.)
- Avoid alcohol altogether, especially during the first trimester.
- You should avoid vitamin A supplements (*see* Appendix 2, 'Glossary of Vitamins and Minerals'), fish liver oil supplements, liver, and liver paté since very high doses (more than 10 times the RNI) may lead to birth defects.
- Avoid raw or lightly cooked eggs and products made with them to reduce the risks of salmonella poisoning.
- Avoid mould-ripened soft cheeses such as Camembert and Brie, and also blue-veined cheeses, to reduce the risk of listeria poisoning.
- Avoid unpasteurised milk.
- Avoid undercooked meat as well as all types of paté to avoid the risk of food poisoning.
- Avoid shark, swordfish and marlin as they may contain high levels of mercury. You should also avoid raw shellfish.
- Do not eat more than two tuna steaks (weighing 140 g each) or 4 cans (140 g when drained) of tuna a week as they may contain high levels of mercury.
- Do not eat more than two portions of oily fish a week because it contains pollutants such as dioxins and polychlorinated biphenyls.

Summary of key points

- Relative Energy Deficiency in Sport (RED-S) is relatively common among female athletes participating in sports where emphasis is placed on being lean or attaining a very low body weight.

- RED-S is characterised by impaired menstrual function, metabolic rate, bone health, immunity, protein synthesis and cardiovascular health.
- The underlying problem of RED-S is a low energy availability (EA), calculated as energy intake (EI) minus exercise energy expenditure (EE).
- 30 kcal/kg FFM/day should be the lower threshold of EA in females.
- Intense and excessive training programmes combined with restrictive diets may lead to an obsessive preoccupation with body weight and calorie intake and eventually disordered eating.
- Eating disorders are much more common in athletes in sports where a low body weight, low body fat level or thin physique is perceived to be advantageous.
- It is possible that some people with a predisposition to eating disorders are attracted to certain sports.
- Female athletes who have a low EA are at increased risk of menstrual dysfunction.
- Amenorrhoea develops due to a combination of factors, such as EA, disordered eating, the commencement of intense training before menarche, high training intensity and volume, low body fat levels and physical and emotional stress.

- Amenorrhoea has an adverse effect on many systems in the body, including a reduction in bone density, putting you at risk of early osteoporosis and stress fractures; soft tissue injuries; prolonged healing of injuries and reduced ability to recover from hard training sessions.
- Iron-deficiency anaemia is characterised by a concentration of haemoglobin in the blood below 12 g/dl and/or a level of ferritin below 12 ng/ml, but occurs no more frequently among athletes than in non-athletes.
- Iron-deficiency anaemia may be the result of increased blood losses associated with training or a deficient dietary intake.
- Sports anaemia, although associated with a low haemoglobin concentration, arises as a consequence of regular aerobic training, which causes an increase in blood plasma volume.
- The physical and psychological demands of regular exercise, together with a very low body fat, may reduce your chances of conception.
- A low body fat level is less likely to be a problem than a small pregnancy weight gain, which may result in reduced growth of the developing baby. Dieting or restricting your weight gain during pregnancy is not recommended.
- You may need to reduce your food intake if you reduce your training substantially during pregnancy.

The young
//athlete

Like adults, young athletes need to eat a balanced diet to maintain good health and achieve peak performance. While there has been relatively limited research performed with active children, it is possible to adapt nutritional guidelines for children and adolescents to the specific demands of exercise and sport as well as use some of the research on adult athletes. This chapter covers the energy, protein and fluid needs for young athletes as well as meal timing, travelling and competing. Weight is also an important issue for some young athletes. Being overweight not only affects their health but also reduces their athletic performance and their self-esteem. Similarly, some young athletes struggle to keep up their weight or put on weight because of the high energy demands of their sport. This chapter details some key strategies to help parents and coaches manage these issues.

HOW MUCH ENERGY DO YOUNG ATHLETES REQUIRE?

There are no specific data on energy requirements for children who train regularly, but you can get a rough estimate using the values in Tables 12.1 and 12.2. Table 12.1 shows the estimated average requirements for children for standard ages

published by the Department of Health. These figures do not take account of regular exercise or sport, so you will need to make an allowance for this.

More relevant to young athletes are the figures shown in Table 12.2, which shows energy requirements according to body weight and physical activity level (PAL). PAL is the ratio of overall daily energy expenditure to BMR based on the intensity and time spent being active. You can work out the PAL from Table 12.3. Sedentary children (and adults) would have a PAL of 1.4, while active children are likely to have a PAL between 1.6 and 2.0.

Table 12.4 lists the estimated calorie expenditure for various activities for a 10-year-old child weighing 33 kg. These values are based on measurements made on adults, scaled down to the body weight of a child, with an added margin of 25% (Astrand, 1952). (There are no published values relating to children.) This margin takes account of the relative 'wastefulness' of energy in children compared with adults performing the same activity, due mainly to their lack of coordination between agonist and antagonist muscle groups. This makes children metabolically less economical than adolescents and adults. Also they are biomechanically less efficient (e.g. they tend to have a faster stride frequency when running) – again, raising the energy cost of any given activity. However, the energy cost decreases as children become more proficient at performing the activity. Exactly how much active children should eat is difficult to predict, but for children who are not overweight or underweight, you can use their appetite as a guide to portion sizes. Be guided, too, by their energy levels. If children are not eating enough, then their energy levels will be persistently low, they will feel lethargic and under-perform at sports. On the other hand, if they appear to have plenty of energy and get-up-and-go, then they are probably eating enough.

Table 12.1	ESTIMATED AVERAGE REQUIREMENTS FOR ENERGY OF CHILDREN	
Age	Boys (kcal)	Girls (kcal)
4–6 years	1715	1545
7–10 years	1970	1740
11–14 years	2220	1845
15–18 years	2755	2110

Department of Health Dietary reference values for food energy and nutrients for the United Kingdom (1991). London: HMSO.

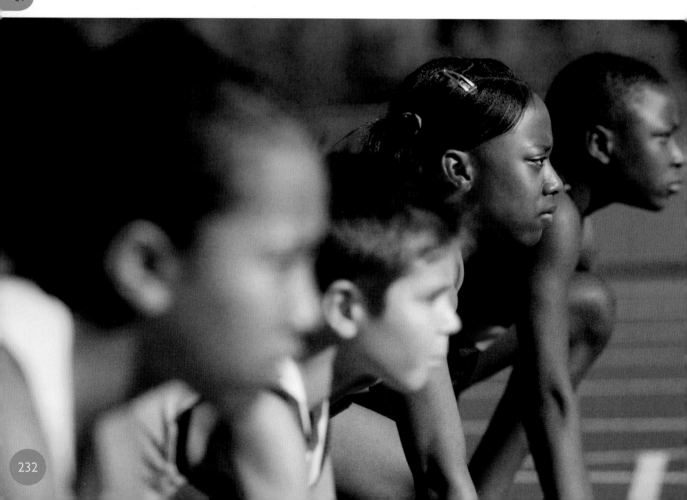

Table 12.2	ESTIMATED AVERAGE REQUIREMENTS OF CHILDREN AND ADOLESCENTS ACCORDING TO BODY WEIGHT AND PHYSICAL ACTIVITY LEVEL						
	Weight (kg)	BMR kcal/d	PAL				
			1.4	1.5	1.6	1.8	2.0
Boys	30	1189	1675	1794	1914	2153	2368
	35	1278	1794	1914	2057	2297	2559
	40	1366	1914	2057	2177	2464	2727
	45	1455	2033	2177	2320	2632	2919
	50	1543	2153	2321	2464	2775	3086
	55	1632	2297	2440	2608	2943	3253
	60	1720	2416	2584	2751	3086	3445
Girls	30	1095	1531	1651	1746	1962	2201
	35	1163	1627	1715	1866	2081	2321
	40	1229	1722	1842	1962	2201	2464
	45	1297	1818	1938	2081	2344	2584
	50	1364	1913	2033	2177	2464	2727
	55	1430	2009	2153	2297	2584	2871
	60	1498	2105	2249	2392	2703	2990

Department of Health Dietary reference values for food energy and nutrients for the United Kingdom (1991). London: HMSO.

DO YOUNG ATHLETES BURN FUEL DIFFERENTLY FROM ADULTS?

Studies suggest that during exercise children use relatively more fat and less carbohydrate than do adolescents or adults (Martinez & Haymes, 1992; Berg & Keul, 1988). This applies to both endurance and short, higher intensity activities, where they tend to rely more on aerobic metabolism (in which fat is a major fuel). The nutritional implications are not clear, but there is no reason to recommend they should consume more than the recommended maximum for fat for the general population (35% of energy).

Table 12.3	PHYSICAL ACTIVITY LEVEL (PAL)
1.4	Mostly sitting, little physical activity
1.5	Mostly sitting, some walking, low levels of exercise
1.6	Daily moderate exercise
1.8	Daily moderate–high exercise level
2.0	Daily high exercise level

Table 12.4	CALORIES EXPENDED IN VARIOUS ACTIVITIES	
Activity		**Calories in 30 minutes**
Cycling (11.2 km/h)		88
Running (12 km/h)		248
Sitting		24
Standing		26
Swimming (crawl, 4.8 km/h)		353
Tennis		125
Walking		88

Values are based on measurements made on adults, scaled down to the body weight of 33 kg, with an added margin of 25%. Heavier children will burn slightly more calories; lighter children will burn less.

HOW MUCH PROTEIN SHOULD YOUNG ATHLETES CONSUME?

Because children are growing and developing, they need more protein relative to their weight than adults. The reference nutrient intakes for protein published by the Department of Health give a general guideline for boys and girls of different ages. These are given in Table 12.5. Most children need about 1 g per kg body weight (adults need 0.75 g/kg BW). For example, a child who weighs 40 kg should eat about 40 g of protein daily. However, the published values do not take account of exercise, so active children may need a little more protein, around 1.1–1.2 g/kg body weight/day (Ziegler *et al.*, 1998).

Young athletes can meet their protein needs by including 2–4 portions of protein-rich foods in their daily diet (lean meat, fish, poultry, eggs,

Table 12.5	DAILY PROTEIN REQUIREMENTS OF CHILDREN	
Age	**Boys**	**Girls**
4–6 years	19.7 g	19.7 g
7–10 years	28.3 g	28.3 g
11–14 years	42.1 g	41.2 g
15–18 years	55.2 g	45.0 g

Department of Health Dietary reference values for food energy and nutrients for the United Kingdom (1991). London: HMSO.

beans, lentils, nuts, tofu and Quorn) as well as balanced amounts of grains (bread, pasta, cereals) and dairy foods (milk, yoghurt, cheese), all of which also supply smaller amounts of protein.

Vegetarian children should eat a wide variety of plant proteins: beans, lentils, grains, nuts, seeds, soya and Quorn (*see* Chapter 13, 'The Vegetarian Athlete').

SHOULD YOUNG ATHLETES USE PROTEIN SUPPLEMENTS?

Protein supplements, such as protein shakes and bars, are unnecessary for children. Even the very active should be able to get enough protein from their diet. While such supplements may have a role to play in the diets of some adult athletes, there is no justification for giving them to children. It is more important that children learn how to plan a balanced diet from ordinary foods and how to get protein from the right food combinations.

HOW MUCH CARBOHYDRATE SHOULD YOUNG ATHLETES CONSUME?

There are no specific recommendations for young athletes. However, those previously detailed for adults would be appropriate for this age group since they are expressed in terms of body weight (Burke *et al.*, 2011). Thus, young athletes training between 1 and 2 hours a day would need around 5–7 g carbohydrate for each 1 kg body weight. For example, a 60 kg athlete training 1–2 hours each day would need 360–420 g carbohydrate daily. As a rule of thumb, young athletes should be able to meet their carbohydrate requirements by eating the following:

- 4–6 portions of carbohydrate-rich foods (grains, potatoes)
- 5+ portions of fruit and vegetables
- 2–4 portions of dairy products

See Table 1.3 (p. 14) for guidance on food portion sizes.

The exact portion size depends on their energy need. Generally, older, heavier and more active children need bigger portions. Be guided by their appetite but don't get too prescriptive about the exact amount they should eat. Check the carbohydrate content of foods in the table in Appendix 1: Glycaemic Index and Glycaemic Load (pp. 338–41).

WHAT SHOULD YOUNG ATHLETES EAT BEFORE TRAINING OR COMPETITION?

Most of the energy needed for exercise is provided by whatever the athlete has eaten several hours or even days before. Carbohydrate in their food will have been converted into glycogen and stored in their muscles and liver. If they have eaten the right amount of carbohydrate, they will have high levels of glycogen in their muscles,

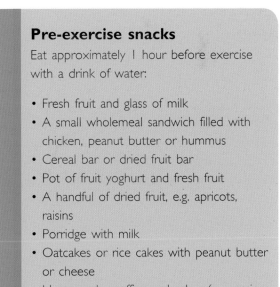

Pre-exercise snacks

Eat approximately 1 hour before exercise with a drink of water:

- Fresh fruit and glass of milk
- A small wholemeal sandwich filled with chicken, peanut butter or hummus
- Cereal bar or dried fruit bar
- Pot of fruit yoghurt and fresh fruit
- A handful of dried fruit, e.g. apricots, raisins
- Porridge with milk
- Oatcakes or rice cakes with peanut butter or cheese
- Homemade muffins and cakes (see recipes on pages 333–37).

ready to fuel their activity. If they have not eaten enough carbohydrate, they will have low stocks of glycogen, putting them at risk of early fatigue during exercise.

Food eaten before exercise needs to stop children feeling hungry during training, be easily digested and have a moderate to low GI. Such a snack or meal provides sustained energy and will help the athlete keep going longer during exercise. But don't let them eat lots of sugary foods such as sweets and soft drinks just before exercising. This may cause a surge of blood glucose and insulin followed by a rapid fall, resulting in hypoglycaemia, early fatigue and reduced performance.

The boxes above and overleaf give some ideas for suitable pre-exercise meals and snacks. It takes a certain amount of trial and error to find out which foods and what amounts suit an individual best. Adjust the quantities according to their appetite, how they feel and what they like. It's important that they feel comfortable with the types and amounts of foods. Don't offer anything new before a competition, as it may not agree with them.

TIMING THE PRE-EXERCISE MEAL

The exact timing of the pre-exercise meal will probably depend on practical constraints – for example, the training session may be straight after school, leaving very little time to eat. If there is less than 1 hour between eating and training, give them a light snack (see box 'Pre-exercise snacks').

If they have more than 2 hours between eating and training, their normal balanced meal will be suitable. This should be based around a carbohydrate food such as bread or potatoes together with a little protein such as chicken or beans, as well as a portion of vegetables and a drink.

Pre-exercise meals

Eat 2–3 hours before exercise with a drink of water:

- Sandwich/roll/bagel/wrap filled with chicken, fish, cheese, egg or peanut butter and salad
- Jacket potato with beans, cheese, tuna, coleslaw or chicken
- Pasta with tomato-based pasta sauce and cheese and vegetables
- Chicken with rice and salad
- Vegetable and prawn or tofu stir fry with noodles or rice
- Pilaff or rice/fish/vegetable dish
- Mixed bean hot pot with potatoes
- Chicken and vegetable casserole with potatoes
- Porridge made with milk
- Wholegrain cereal (e.g. bran or wheat flakes, muesli or Weetabix) with milk or yoghurt
- Fish and potato pie

WHAT SHOULD YOUNG ATHLETES EAT BEFORE AN EVENT?

If they are competing, you need to make sure that the young athletes have access to the right kinds of food. It's definitely a good idea to pack a supply of food because suitable foods and drinks may not be available at the event venue. Young athletes should have their normal meal about 2–3 hours before the event – enough time to digest the food and for the stomach to empty. For example, if the event is in the morning, schedule breakfast 2–3 hours before the event start time. Similarly, if the event is in the afternoon, adjust the timing of lunch to 2–3 hours before the event.

Like adults, children may feel too nervous or excited to eat on the day of the event. So, offer nutritious drinks (such as diluted fruit juice, sports drinks, milk-based drinks or yoghurt drinks) or light snacks. If they skip meals, children may become light-headed or nauseous during the event and will not perform at their best. Here are some simple rules to follow on the day of the event:

- Do not eat or drink anything new
- Stick to familiar foods and drinks
- Take your own foods and drinks wherever possible
- Drink plenty of water or diluted juice before and after the event
- Have high carbohydrate snacks (*see* 'Pre-exercise snacks')
- Avoid high fat foods before the event
- Avoid eating sweets and chocolate during the hour before the event
- Avoid soft drinks (containing more than 6 g sugar/100 ml) an hour before the event
- Encourage children to go to the toilet just before the event.

WHAT SHOULD YOUNG ATHLETES EAT DURING EXERCISE?

If young athletes will be exercising continually for less than 90 minutes, they won't need to eat anything during exercise. They should, however, be encouraged to take regular drink breaks, ideally every 15–20 minutes or whenever there is a suitable break in training or play. Make sure they take a water bottle and keep it within easy reach – for example, at the poolside, at the side of the football pitch or by the track.

During an all-day training session or competition, have food and drink available during the short breaks. For example, make opportunities to refuel between swimming heats, tennis games and gymnastic events. During matches or tournaments lasting more than an hour (e.g. football, cricket or hockey), offer them food and drink during the half-time interval. High carbohydrate, low fat foods and drinks are the obvious choice because these will help to keep energy levels high, maintain their blood glucose level, delay the onset of fatigue and prevent hypoglycaemia. As you will almost certainly need to take them with you, they should also be non-perishable, portable and quick and easy to eat. Sometimes food is provided at events, but you will need to check exactly what will be available beforehand – it may be crisps, chocolate bars, biscuits and soft drinks, all of which are unhelpful for good performance! Check the box below for suitable snacks.

Snacks for short breaks during training or competition
- Water, diluted fruit juice or sports drinks
- Bananas
- Fresh fruit – grapes, apples, satsumas, pears
- Dried fruit – raisins, apricots, mango
- Oatcakes and rice cakes with bananas or honey
- Rolls, sandwiches, English muffins, mini-bagels, mini-pancakes
- Fruit, cereal and energy bars

WHAT SHOULD YOUNG ATHLETES EAT AFTER EXERCISE?

After exercise, the priority is to replenish fluid losses. So give young athletes a drink straight away – water or diluted fruit juice are the best drinks.

They also need to replace the energy they have just used. The post-exercise snack or meal is perhaps the most important meal, as it determines how fast athletes will recover before the next training session. Unless they will be eating a meal within half an hour, give them a snack to stave off hunger and promote recovery. The exact amounts you should provide will depend on their appetite and body size. As a guide, give just enough to alleviate their hunger and keep them going until their mealtime. Studies with adult athletes have shown that 1 g of carbohydrate per kg body weight eaten within 2 hours of exercise speeds recovery.

Suitable recovery snacks

Accompany all snacks with a drink of water or diluted fruit juice.

• Milk or milk-based drink
• Fresh fruit e.g. bananas, grapes, and apples
• Dried fruit
• Nuts and raisins
• Yoghurt
• Yoghurt drink
• Smoothie
• Roll or bagel with jam or honey
• Mini-pancakes
• Homemade muffins, bar, biscuits (see recipes on pp. 333–37)
• Homemade apple, carrot or fruit cake

Suitable recovery meals

Accompany all meals with a drink of water or diluted fruit juice, and 1–2 portions of vegetables or salad.

• Jacket potatoes with beans, tuna or cheese
• Pasta with tomato sauce and cheese
• Rice with chicken and stir-fried vegetables
• Fish pie
• Baked beans on toast
• Fish cakes or bean burgers or falafel with jacket potatoes.

Opt for foods with a moderate or high GI, which will raise blood glucose levels fairly rapidly and then be converted into glycogen in the muscles. Studies with adult athletes have found that including a little protein (in a ratio of about 3:1) enhances recovery further. Check the box below for suitable recovery snacks and meals. In practice, many of the snacks on offer in the canteen or vending machines at leisure clubs and sports centres are unsuitable. Foods like crisps, chocolate bars, sweets and fizzy drinks will not promote good recovery after exercise. They are little more than concentrated forms of sugar, fat or salt, and actually slow down rehydration. Because they provide a lot of calories too, these foods can take away the young athlete's appetite for healthier foods at the next meal.

So what can you do? Let your leisure centre know that you are unhappy with the choice of snacks on offer to children, ask other parents and coaches to do the same and suggest that they replace these 'junk' snacks with healthier foods. Any of the suggestions in the box ('Suitable recovery snacks') would be appropriate. Encourage children to take their own drinks and snacks.

WHAT SHOULD YOUNG ATHLETES EAT WHEN TRAVELLING OR COMPETING AWAY?

When young athletes are travelling to compete away from home, organise their food and drink in advance and take these with you. They may need snacks for the journey so take a supply of suitable foods – use any of the suggestions in the box 'Snacks for eating on the move'. Do not rely on roadside cafés, fast food restaurants, railway or airport catering outlets – healthy choices are often limited at these places. Make sure you take plenty of drinks, in case of delays. Air-conditioned travel in cars, coaches and planes can quickly make children dehydrated.

Try to find out what catering arrangements have been made at the venue. Check the local restaurants and takeaways. Encourage children to choose dishes that are high in carbohydrate, such as pasta, pizza or rice dishes. And warn them against trying anything unfamiliar or unusual

Snacks for eating on the move
- Sandwiches filled with chicken or tuna or cheese with salad; banana and peanut butter; Marmite
- Rice cakes, oatcakes and wholemeal crackers
- Granola or cereal bars
- Flapjacks
- Yoghurt drinks
- Individual cheese portions
- Small bags of nuts – peanuts, cashews, almonds
- Fresh fruit – apples, bananas, grapes
- Dried fruit
- Fruit bar or liquorice bar
- Boiled eggs
- Vegetable crudités e.g. carrots, peppers, cucumber and celery with hummus

Suitable restaurant meals and fast foods when travelling to an event
- Simple pasta dishes
- Simple stir-fried dishes
- Thin pizza with tomato and vegetable toppings
- Simple noodle or rice dishes
- Jacket potatoes with tuna, chicken, beans or cheese
- Pancakes with fruit

– the last thing they need is an upset stomach before the event! When travelling abroad, it's best to avoid common food-poisoning culprits – chicken, seafood and meat dishes – unless you are sure they have been properly cooked and heated to a high temperature. Be wary of such foods served lukewarm. Check the box below for suitable meals when travelling away.

Remember, too, that young athletes will probably be feeling nervous or apprehensive when travelling away. They may not feel like eating much food. In this case, encourage them to have plenty of nutritious drinks instead, such as fruit juice, smoothies, yoghurt drinks and milkshakes. Pack their favourite foods – of the non-perishable variety – to tempt their appetite. Sometimes it's a case of simply getting them to eat something

Restaurant meals and fast foods to avoid

- Burgers and chips
- Chicken nuggets
- Pasta with creamy or oily sauces
- Hot curries
- Kebabs
- Battered fish and chips
- Lukewarm chicken, turkey, meat, fish or seafood dishes
- Hot dogs
- Fried chicken meals.

rather than nothing. If they stop eating they will run down their energy reserves, putting them at a disadvantage for competition.

ARE YOUNG ATHLETES MORE SUSCEPTIBLE TO DEHYDRATION THAN ADULTS?

Young athletes are much more susceptible to dehydration and overheating than adults for the following reasons:

- they sweat less than adults (sweat helps to keep the body's temperature stable)
- they cannot cope with very hot conditions as well as adults
- they get hotter during exercise
- they have a greater surface area for their body weight
- they often fail to recognise or respond to feelings of thirst.

The increase in core temperature at any given level of dehydration is quite a bit greater in young athletes than in adults. Encourage young athletes to check their hydration status with a 'pee test' (*see* p. 144).

On average, young athletes lose between 350 and 700 ml of body fluid per hour's exercise. If it's hot and humid or they are wearing lots of layers of clothing, they will sweat more and lose even more fluid. Encourage them to drink plenty of fluid before, during and after exercise. As for adults, fluid losses depend on:

- The temperature and humidity of the surroundings – the warmer and higher the humidity, the greater their sweat losses, so they will need to drink more.
- How hard they are exercising – the harder they exercise, the more they sweat, so they will need to drink more.
- How long they are exercising – the longer they exercise, the greater the sweat losses, so they will need to drink accordingly.
- Their size – the bigger they are, the greater the sweat loss, so the more they need to drink.
- Their fitness – the fitter they are, the earlier and more profusely they sweat (it's a sign of good body temperature control), so they will need to drink more than their less fit friends.

In some sports where body weight is a factor in performance (e.g. gymnastics), coaches (hopefully a minority) restrict fluids during training, in the misguided belief that the human body will eventually adapt to low fluid intakes, or perhaps this is simply to remove the hassle and distraction of drinking itself! However, even if children manage to exercise, they will be performing below par. They will also be at risk of developing heat cramps and heat exhaustion.

Warning signs of dehydration

Children can become dehydrated more easily than adults. Here are some of the signs to look out for.

Early symptoms

- Unusually lacking in energy
- Fatiguing early during exercise
- Complaining of feeling too hot
- Skin appears flushed and feels clammy
- Passing only small volumes of dark-coloured urine
- Nausea

Action: Drink 100–200 ml water or sports drink every 10–15 minutes.

Advanced symptoms

- A bad headache
- Becomes dizzy or light-headed
- Appears disorientated
- Short of breath

Action: Drink 100–200 ml sports drink every 10–15 minutes. Seek professional help.

The risks of dehydration in young athletes are similar to those in adults. Here's a reminder:

- Exercise feels much harder
- Heart rate increases more than usual
- May develop cramps, headaches and nausea
- Concentration is reduced
- Ability to perform sports skills drops
- Fatigues sooner and loses stamina

HOW MUCH SHOULD YOUNG ATHLETES DRINK BEFORE EXERCISE?

Like adults, young athletes should aim to be well hydrated before exercise. If they are slightly dehydrated at this stage, there is a bigger risk of overheating once they start exercising. Encourage them to drink 6–8 cups (1–1.5 litres) of fluid during the day and, as a final measure, top up with 150–200 ml (a large glass) of water 45 minutes before exercise.

HOW MUCH SHOULD YOUNG ATHLETES DRINK DURING EXERCISE?

While adult athletes are encouraged to drink to thirst during exercise (*see* p. 147), children may need more encouragement to drink since their thirst mechanism is a less reliable indicator of their fluid status. Use the following guidelines, in conjunction with the considerations below, to plan a drinking strategy:

Before exercise
150–200 ml 45 mins before activity

During exercise
75–100 ml every 15–20 mins

After exercise
Drink freely until no longer thirsty, plus an extra glass, or drink 300 ml for every 0.2 kg weight loss.

You can estimate how much fluid young athletes have lost during exercise by weighing them before and after training. For each 1 kg lost, they should drink 1.5 litres of fluid. This accounts for the fact that they continue to sweat after exercise and lose more fluid through urine during this time. For example, if the young athlete weighs 0.3 kg less after exercise, he has lost 0.3 litres (300 ml) of fluid. To replace 300 ml of fluid, he needs to drink 450 ml of fluid during and after training. But don't expect young athletes to drink large volumes after exercising. Divide their drinks into manageable amounts to be taken during and after exercise. A good strategy would be to drink, say, 100 ml at three regular intervals during exercise, then 150 ml afterwards.

How can young athletes be encouraged to drink enough while exercising?

- Make drinking more fun with a squeezy bottle or a novelty water bottle.
- Make sure they place the bottle within easy access, e.g. at one end of the pool or by the side of the track, court, gym or pitch.
- Allow drinking time during training/play – encourage them to take regular sips, ideally every 10–20 mins. This may take practice.
- Tell them not to wait until they are thirsty – plan a drink during the first 20 minutes of exercise, then at regular intervals during the session, even if they are not thirsty.
- If they are playing in a team, work out suitable drink breaks, e.g. half-time during a match, or while listening to the coach during practice sessions.
- If they don't like water, offer a flavoured drink such as diluted fruit juice, dilute squash or a sports drink (see 'What should young athletes drink?').
- Slightly chilling the drink (to around 8–10°C) usually encourages children to drink more.

WHAT SHOULD YOUNG ATHLETES DRINK?

As with adults, plain water is best for most activities lasting less than 90 minutes. It replaces lost fluids rapidly and so makes a perfectly good drink for sport. But there are two potential problems with drinking water. Firstly, many young athletes are not very keen on drinking water, so they may not drink enough. Secondly, water tends to quench one's thirst even if the body is still dehydrated. Encourage water whenever possible, but if young athletes find it difficult to drink enough water, give them a flavoured drink. Diluted pure fruit juice (diluted one or two parts water to one part juice), sugar-free squash or ordinary diluted squash are less expensive alternatives. But bear in mind that most brands are laden with additives, including artificial sweeteners, colours and flavourings, which you may prefer to avoid. Organic squashes are better options, although they are more expensive.

Although commercial sports drinks may not benefit young athletes' performance for activities lasting less than 90 mins (compared with water or flavoured drinks), they will encourage them to drink larger volumes of fluid (Wilk & Bar-Or, 1996; Rivera-Brown *et al.*, 1999). But a word of caution with commercial sports drinks: in practice, many children find that sports drinks sit 'heavily' in their stomachs. So, you may either dilute the sports drink down with water (if making up from powder, add a little extra water) or alternate sports drinks with water.

If children will be exercising hard and continuously for more than 90 minutes, sports drinks containing around 4–6 g of sugars per 100 ml may benefit their performance. This is because the sugars in these drinks help fuel the exercising muscles and postpone fatigue. The electrolytes (sodium and potassium) in the drinks are designed to stimulate thirst and make them drink more (*see* Chapter 7: Hydration). On the downside, sports drinks are relatively expensive. It's cheaper to make your own version by diluting fruit juice (one part juice to one or two parts water) or organic squash (diluted one part squash to six parts water). Both would also help maintain energy (blood glucose) levels during prolonged exercise. The most important thing is that children drink enough. Therefore, the taste is important. If they don't like it, they

Choosing the best drink for exercise

Exercise lasting less than 90 minutes

- Water
- Fruit juice diluted 2 parts water to 1 part juice
- Sports drink alternated with water

Exercise lasting more than 90 minutes

- Sports drink (4–6 g sugars/100 ml)
- Fruit juice diluted 1–2 parts water to 1 part juice
- Squash (ideally organic), diluted 6 parts water to 1 part squash

What young athletes shouldn't drink!

- Fizzy drinks – the bubbles in fizzy drinks may cause a burning sensation in the mouth, especially if drunk quickly, and will certainly stop children from drinking enough fluid. Fizzy drinks can also upset the stomach and make them feel bloated and uncomfortable during exercise.
- Ready-to-drink soft drinks – these are too concentrated in sugar and will tend to sit in the stomach too long during exercise. They may make children feel nauseous and uncomfortable.
- Drinks containing caffeine – caffeinated soft drinks, cola, coffee and tea increase the heart rate and may cause trembling and restlessness at night – children are more sensitive to caffeine than adults.

Six ways to keep cool

1. Provide extra water during hot and humid weather.
2. Schedule exercise for the cooler times of the day during hot weather.
3. Schedule regular drink breaks during sessions, ideally in the shade during hot weather.
4. Encourage young athletes to wear loose fitting, natural fibre clothing during exercise, which allows them to sweat freely and permits moisture to evaporate.
5. Let them acclimatise gradually to hot or humid weather conditions – allow 2 weeks.
6. Make sure they drink extra water 24 hours before a competition.

How to choose a supplement

1. Choose a comprehensive formula designed for your children's age range; ideally the following nutrients should be there: vitamin A, vitamin C, vitamin D, vitamin E, thiamin, riboflavin, niacin, vitamin B_6, folic acid, vitamin B_{12}, biotin, pantothenic acid, beta carotene, calcium, phosphorus, iron, magnesium, zinc, iodine.
2. Check that the quantities of each nutrient are no more than 100% of the NRV stated on the label.
3. Avoid supplements with added colours.
4. Try to choose brands that have been produced by established manufacturers with a good reputation for quality control and clinical research.

won't drink it! So, experiment with different flavours until you find the ones they like. A little trial and error may be needed to find the best strength drink, too. If it's too concentrated, it will sit in their stomachs and make them feel uncomfortable.

SHOULD YOUNG ATHLETES TAKE VITAMIN SUPPLEMENTS?

In theory, young athletes should not need supplements if they are eating a well-balanced diet and a wide variety of foods. But, in practice, not many children manage to do this. Reliance on fast foods, ready-meals and processed snacks, as well as peer pressure and time pressure, make this very difficult to achieve. The National Diet and Nutrition Survey of British Schoolchildren revealed that the most commonly eaten foods among 4–18 year olds, eaten by 80% of children, are white bread, crisps, biscuits, potatoes and chocolate bars (Gregory *et al.*, 2000). On average, they ate only 2 portions of fruit and vegetables a day and less than half ever ate green leafy vegetables. Intakes of zinc, magnesium, calcium and iron were below the RNI among 15–18 year olds.

A well-formulated children's multivitamin and mineral supplement can help ensure they get enough vitamins and minerals so that their growth, physical and mental development and physical performance will not be impaired. Low intakes of certain vitamins and minerals have been linked with lower IQ, reasoning ability, physical performance, poor attention and behavioural problems.

It is possible that supplementation can help correct deficiencies and produce a significant improvement in these aspects in children. However, extra vitamins and minerals won't make children more brainy or sporty if they are already well nourished.

SHOULD YOUNG ATHLETES TAKE CREATINE?

There is no research to support the use of sports supplements in young athletes and the long-term risks are unknown (Unnithan *et al.*, 2001). One of the most popular supplements is creatine. No sports organisation has recommended its use in people under 18. The American College of Sports Medicine and American Academy of Paediatrics position statements advise against the use of creatine for athletes under 18 years of age. Because dietary supplements are not regulated, there is a possibility that creatine supplements may contain impurities that would cause a positive drug test.

Creatine would in any case have little benefit in young athletes. Firstly, they rely more on aerobic than anaerobic metabolism, so any attempt to enhance anaerobic energy production through creatine supplementation would be of limited effect. Secondly, the biggest improvement to performance comes from training at this stage of development. Hard training and a balanced diet, not supplements, are the keys to optimal performance.

WHEN SHOULD YOUNG ATHLETES LOSE WEIGHT FOR THEIR SPORT?

Some young athletes may feel pressurised to lose weight to improve their performance in sport. Low body weights or fat percentages are often correlated with improved running speed, jumping ability, endurance and performance in many sports. Whether they are overweight or not, unfortunately young athletes are often influenced to lose weight by the successes of thinner teammates or by the remarks of a well-meaning coach.

So what should you do? Young athletes who are a healthy weight or body fat percentage (*see* Figures 12.1 and 12.2) should not be encouraged to lose weight. If they are unhappy about their weight, the problem may be one of poor self-esteem or being ill matched to their sport. For example, children with a naturally large build would not be well matched to sports requiring a naturally slim physique such as long-distance running, ballet or gymnastics.

If you feel that a young athlete has a genuine weight problem and that reducing body fat would benefit their performance, health and self-esteem, follow the advice on p. 247 ('The healthy way to tackle weight'), or consult a registered nutritionist or dietitian (*see* www. senr.org.uk). Usually, a strategy that increases their daily activity level and training intensity, together with a healthier diet, is all that is needed. Allow plenty of time – months rather than weeks – for fat loss. Under professional guidance, young athletes should lose no more than 1–2 kg per month, depending on their age and weight. Weight loss goals must be realistic and achievable for their build and degree of maturity. They should reach this goal at least 3 or 4 weeks before competition. This will allow them to compete at their best. You should discourage strict dieting, diuretics, excessive exercise and use of saunas as weight loss methods, as they can be very dangerous for growing athletes. In the short term, these methods could result in an excessive loss of water, low muscle glycogen stores, fatigue and poor

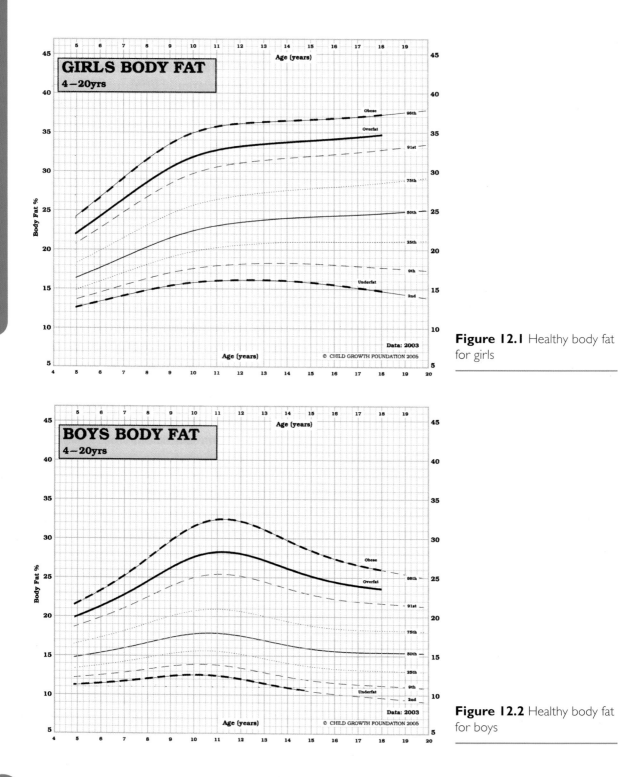

Figure 12.1 Healthy body fat for girls

Figure 12.2 Healthy body fat for boys

performance. Long term, they could lead to yo-yo dieting, eating disorders, poor health and impaired development.

How to assess overweight and body fatness in children and adolescents

Body mass index (BMI = weight (kg)/height $(m)^2$) (*see* Table 12.6) is commonly used in adults to define overweight. There are also international standards, which define cut-off points related to age to define overweight and obesity in children (Figures 12.1 and 12.2). A BMI higher than the normal limit for their age means they are overweight; a BMI higher than the obese value suggests their health is at risk. However, as with adults, using BMIs with athletic children can be misleading and lead to a misclassification of overweight, as they do not distinguish between weight in the form of fat or lean tissue.

Body fat centile charts provide more accurate information for assessing children and young athletes. The simplest way to measure body fat percentage is with a body composition scale based on bioelectrical impedance and calibrated for children.

THE HEALTHY WAY TO TACKLE WEIGHT

The best thing you can do is to encourage a balanced diet and regular physical activity. Talk to young athletes about healthy eating and exercise, teach by example and let them make their own decisions about food.

- **Don't** tell a young athlete that they are 'greedy' or 'lazy'.
- **Do** tell them that you recognise how hard it is to make healthy choices at times.
- **Don't** make a young athlete feel guilty about their eating habits.
- **Do** praise them lavishly when you see them eating healthily.

Build self-esteem

If you can build young athletes' self-esteem and help them feel more positive about themselves, they are more likely to make healthier food choices. Make a point of praising their accomplishments, emphasising their strengths, and encouraging them to try new skills to foster success. Never call them fat or tell them to lose weight. Let them know that its what's inside that matters and play down your concerns about their weight – or even your own weight.

Table 12.6	BMIs FOR OVERWEIGHT OR OBESITY IN CHILDREN			
Age	Overweight		Obese	
	Boys	Girls	Boys	Girls
5	17.4	17.1	19.3	19.2
6	17.6	17.3	19.8	19.7
7	17.9	17.8	20.6	20.5
8	18.4	18.3	21.6	21.6
9	19.1	19.1	22.8	22.8
10	19.8	19.9	24.0	24.1
11	20.6	20.7	25.1	25.4
12	21.2	21.7	26.0	26.7
13	21.9	22.6	26.8	27.8

Source: Cole et al., 2000.

Don't say 'diet'

You shouldn't restrict a young athlete's calorie intake without the advice of a nutritionist dietitian. Nutritional needs during childhood are high and important nutrients essential to a child's health could be missed out. Instead, make healthy changes to what they eat.

Table 12.7	DIETARY REFERENCE VALUES FOR BOYS 4–18 YEARS				
	Dietary Reference Value (DRV)	**4–6**	**7–10**	**11–14**	**15–18**
Energy	EAR	1715 kcal	1979 kcal	2220 kcal	2755 kcal
Fat	Max 35% energy	67 g	77 g	86 g	107 g
Saturated fat	Max 11% energy	21 g	24 g	27 g	34 g
Carbohydrate	Min 50% energy	229 g	263 g	296 g	367 g
Added sugars*	Max 11% energy	50 g	58 g	65 g	81 g
Fibre **	8 g per 1000 kcal	14 g	16 g	18 g	22 g
Protein		19.7 g	28 g	42 g	55 g
Iron		6.1 mg	8.7 mg	11.3 mg	11.3 mg
Zinc		6.5 mg	7.0 mg	9.0 mg	9.5 mg
Calcium		450 mg	550 mg	1000 mg	1000 mg
Vitamin A		500 ug	500 ug	600 ug	700 ug
Vitamin C		30 mg	30 mg	35 mg	40 mg
Folate		100 ug	150 ug	200 ug	200 ug
Salt***		3 g	5 g	6 g	6 g

Department of Health Dietary reference values for food energy and nutrients for the United Kingdom (1991). London: HMSO.

EAR = Estimated Average Requirement

* Non-milk extrinsic sugars

** Proportion of adult DRV (18 g) i.e. 8 g/1000 kcal

*** Scientific Advisory Committee on Nutrition (2003): Salt and Health. London: HMSO.

Source: S. Jebb et al., 2004.

Set a good example

Young athletes are more likely to copy what you do than what you say. They learn a lot about food and activity by watching their parents. They should see that you exercise and eat a balanced diet. Share mealtimes as often as possible and eat the same meals.

Table 12.8	DIETARY REFERENCE VALUES FOR GIRLS 4–18 YEARS				
	Dietary Reference Value (DRV)	**4–6**	**7–10**	**11–14**	**15–18**
Energy	EAR	1545 kcal	1740 kcal	1845 kcal	2110 kcal
Fat	Max 35% energy	60 g	68 g	72 g	82 g
Saturated fat	Max 11% energy	19 g	21 g	23 g	26 g
Carbohydrate	Min 50% energy	206 g	232 g	246 g	281 g
Added sugars*	Max 11% energy	45 g	51 g	54 g	62 g
Fibre **	8 g per 1000 kcal	12 g	14 g	15 g	17 g
Protein		19.7 g	28 g	41 g	45 g
Iron		6.1 mg	8.7 mg	14.8 mg	14.8 mg
Zinc		6.5 mg	7.0 mg	9.0 mg	7.0 mg
Calcium		450 mg	550 mg	800 mg	800 mg
Vitamin A		500 ug	500 ug	600 ug	600 ug
Vitamin C		30 mg	30 mg	35 mg	40 mg
Folate		100 ug	150 ug	200 ug	200 ug
Salt***		3 g	5 g	6 g	6 g

Department of Health Dietary reference values for food energy and nutrients for the United Kingdom (1991). London: HMSO.

EAR = Estimated Average Requirement

* Non-milk extrinsic sugars

** Proportion of adult DRV (18 g) i.e. 8 g/ 1000 kcal

*** Scientific Advisory Committee on Nutrition (2003) Salt and Health. London: HMSO.

Source: S. Jebb et al., 2004.

Don't use food as a reward

Rewarding good behaviour with sweet treats only reinforces the idea that they are a special treat and makes children crave them more. Allow them in moderation, say, on one day of the week and at the end of a meal.

Don't ban any foods

Allow all foods, but explain that certain ones should be eaten only occasionally or kept as occasional treats. Banning a food increases children's desire for it and makes it more likely that they will eat it in secret.

Provide healthy snacks

Instead of biscuits, crisps and chocolate, make sure there are healthier alternatives to hand. Fresh fruit, vegetables, salad and plain yoghurt are good choices. Keep them in a place where your child can easily get them – for example, a fruit bowl on the table, yoghurts at the front of the fridge.

Get them moving more

Although a young athlete trains and plays sport, they may be very inactive the rest of the time. Look for opportunities to increase their daily activity. For example, encourage them to walk or cycle to and from school. Try to increase the amount of exercise you do together as a family – swimming, playing football, a family walk or bike ride.

Limit screen time

Plan and agree exactly what they will watch on television and agree on a defined time period. Once the programmes have finished, switch off the television, no matter how much they protest. Don't place a television in your children's bedrooms.

Let them eat fruit... and other healthy snacks

- Fresh fruit e.g. apple slices, satsumas, clementines, grapes, strawberries
- Wholemeal toast with Marmite
- Grilled tomatoes on wholemeal toast
- Low fat yoghurt
- Low fat milk
- Nuts e.g. cashews, peanuts, almonds, brazils
- Wholegrain breakfast cereal with milk
- Plain popcorn
- Vegetable crudités (carrot, pepper and cucumber sticks)
- Rice cake with sliced bananas or cottage cheese.

How much exercise should children get?

According to current advice (Department of Health, 2011), to maintain a basic level of health, children and young people aged 5–18 need to do:

- At least 60 minutes (1 hour) of moderate to vigorous activity every day, which should be a mix of moderate intensity aerobic activity, such as fast walking, and vigorous intensity aerobic activity, such as running.
- On 3 days a week, these activities should involve muscle-strengthening activities, such as push-ups, and bone-strengthening activities, such as running.

Balance activity and viewing time

Let the number of hours they have exercised equal the number of hours they are allowed to watch television. If they have done an hour's physical activity during the day, you could allocate an hour's television watching.

Don't snack and view

Discourage eating meals or unhealthy snacks while watching television. Because their mind will be on the television and not on the food, they won't notice when they are full up.

TOP TIPS TO MAINTAIN A HEALTHY WEIGHT

- Aim for five portions of fruit and vegetables a day.
- Follow the one-third rule – vegetables should fill at least one-third of the plate. This will help satisfy hunger as well as providing protective nutrients.
- Always eat food sitting at a table – eating in front of the TV or eating on the run makes you eat more because you don't concentrate fully.

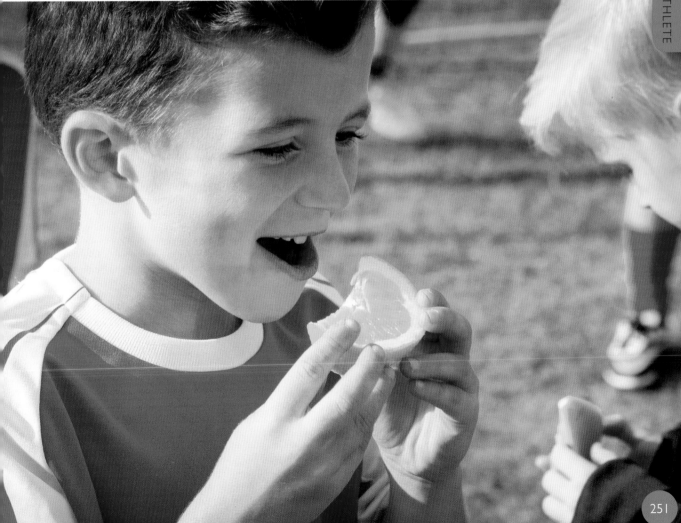

- Give them fruit to take to school for break times – apples, satsumas and grapes are all suitable.
- Don't ditch dairy products in a bid to save calories: switch to low fat or skimmed versions. They contain just as much calcium.
- Give brown rather than white – wholegrain bread, bran cereals and wholewheat pasta are rich in fibre, which makes your child feel fuller. Switch gradually, though, to avoid stomach upsets.
- Don't ban chocolate – for treats, offer a fun-sized chocolate bar.
- Have soup made with lots of veggies more often – it's filling, low in calories, and nutritious. Your child can help make it, or you can buy ready-made fresh versions.
- Make healthier chips by thickly slicing potatoes, tossing in a little olive oil and baking in the oven.
- Include fruit for desserts – fresh fruit, stewed apples or pears with custard, baked apples and fruit crumble.
- Encourage them to eat slowly and enjoy every mouthful. Teach by example.
- Start the day with porridge – oats keep your child fuller for longer and keep cravings at bay.
- Include baked beans and lentils in meals – they are filling, nutritious and don't cause a rapid rise in blood sugar.
- Encourage them to drink at least 6 glasses of fluid a day. Thirst is sometimes mistaken for hunger.

HOW CAN YOUNG ATHLETES PUT ON WEIGHT?

Many young athletes struggle to keep up their weight or put on any weight, because they burn

High energy snacks for weight gain

- Nuts – peanuts, almonds, cashews, brazils, pistachios
- Dried fruit – raisins, sultanas, apricots, dates
- Wholemeal sandwiches with cheese, chicken, ham, tuna, peanut butter or banana
- Yoghurt and fromage frais
- Milk, milkshakes, flavoured milk and yoghurt drinks
- Breakfast cereal or porridge with milk and dried fruit
- Cheese – slices, cubes or novelty cheese snacks
- Cheese on toast
- Scones, fruit buns, malt loaf
- Small pancakes
- English muffins, rolls or bagels
- Cereal or breakfast bars (check they contain no hydrogenated fat)
- Bread or toast spread with jam or honey

a lot of energy in sport. Encourage them to eat more frequent meals and snacks – six or seven times a day. They may not be able to meet their daily energy demands for growth and activity from three meals.

Aim to add in three or four snacks or mini meals a day. To gain weight, children need to consume more calories than they use for growth and exercise. Make the energy and nutrient content of the food more concentrated. Here are some suggestions:

- Serve bigger portions, particularly of pasta, potatoes, rice, cereals, dairy products and protein-rich foods.
- Provide three to four nutritious energy-giving snacks between meals (*see* box for suggestions).
- Include nutritious drinks, e.g. milk, homemade milkshakes, yoghurt drinks, fruit smoothies and fruit juice.
- Scatter grated cheese on vegetables, soups, potatoes, pasta dishes and hotpots.
- Add dried fruit to breakfast cereals, porridge and yoghurt.
- Spread bread, toast or crackers with peanut butter or nut butter.
- Serve vegetables and main courses with a sauce, such as cheese sauce.
- Avoid filling up on stodgy puddings, biscuits and cakes as they supply calories but few essential nutrients.
- Try milk-based or yoghurt-based puddings, e.g. rice pudding, banana custard, fruit crumble with yoghurt, fruit salad with yoghurt, custard, bread pudding, fruit pancakes.

IS STRENGTH TRAINING APPROPRIATE FOR YOUNG ATHLETES?

A well-designed strength training or weight training programme will improve a young athlete's strength, reduce their risk of sports injuries and improve their sports performance. Contrary to the belief that strength training can damage the growth cartilage or stunt their growth, recent studies suggest that it can actually make bones stronger. In fact, there are no reported cases of bone damage in relation to strength training. Children who strength train tend to feel better about themselves as they get stronger, and have higher self-esteem. But strength training is not the same as power lifting, weightlifting or bodybuilding, none of which are recommended for children under 18 years old.

Bulking up should not be the goal of a strength training programme. Children and teenagers should tone their muscles using a light weight (or body weight) and a high number of repetitions, rather than lifting heavy weights. Only after they have passed puberty should children consider adding muscle bulk. Younger children should begin with body weight exercises such as push-ups and sit-ups. More experienced trainees may use free weights and machines.

Sports scientists say that a well-designed strength training programme can bring many fitness benefits for children and can complement an existing training programme. Indeed, the American Academy of Paediatrics Committee on Sports Medicine endorses it. Here are some guidelines:

- Children should be properly supervised during training sessions.
- They should use an age-appropriate routine (adult routines are not suitable) – typically 30 second intervals with breaks in between, with a thorough warm-up and cool-down period.
- Ensure the exercises are performed using proper form and technique.
- Children should start with a relatively light weight and a high number of repetitions.
- No heavy lifts should be included.
- The programme should form part of a total fitness programme.
- The sessions should be varied and fun.

Note: children should complete a medical examination before beginning a strength training programme.

Summary of key points

- Young athletes expend approximately 25% more calories for any given activity compared with adults.
- Young athletes need more protein relative to their weight than adults – about 1 g per kg body weight (adults need 0.75 g/kg). Protein supplements are not necessary.
- If young athletes will be exercising continually for less than 90 minutes, they won't need to eat anything during exercise but should be encouraged to take regular drink breaks, ideally every 15–20 minutes.
- After exercise, give young athletes a drink straight away – water or diluted fruit juice are the best drinks – followed by a high carbohydrate, high GI snack to stave off hunger and promote recovery.
- Young athletes are more susceptible to dehydration and overheating than adults.
- Encourage them to drink 6–8 cups (1–1.5 litres) of fluid during the day, then top up with 150–200 ml (a large glass) of water 45 minutes before exercise.
- During exercise, they should aim to drink 75–100 ml every 15–20 minutes.
- After exercise, they should drink freely until no longer thirsty, plus an extra glass, or drink 300 ml for every 0.2 kg weight loss.
- As with adults, plain water is best for most activities lasting less than 90 minutes, otherwise a flavoured drink will encourage them to drink enough fluid (examples above).
- Young athletes should not need supplements if they are eating a well-balanced diet and a wide variety of foods, but a children's multivitamin and mineral supplement may provide assurance.
- There is no research to support the use of sports supplements in young athletes and the long-term risks are unknown. The ACSM specifically warn against the use of creatine in athletes under 18.
- If an athlete has a genuine weight problem, seek professional advice. Talk to young athletes about healthy eating and exercise, teach by example and let them make their own decisions about food.
- Young athletes who struggle to keep up their weight or put on any weight should be encouraged to eat more frequent meals and snacks and focus on energy and nutrient-rich foods (examples above).

The vegetarian athlete

13

Many athletes choose to follow a vegetarian diet or avoid red meat either for ethical reasons or in the belief that such a diet is healthier. Indeed, large-scale prospective dietary surveys have found that vegetarians have higher intakes of fruit and vegetables, fibre, antioxidant nutrients and phytonutrients, and lower intakes of saturated fat and cholesterol than do meat-eaters (Davey *et al.*, 2003; Key *et al.*, 1996). It is estimated that 3% of people in the UK are vegetarian and one in three claim to eat less meat. The question is whether the benefits of a vegetarian diet extend to enhanced physical fitness and performance. This chapter considers the research in this area and covers the key nutritional considerations for vegetarian athletes. It also provides practical advice to help vegetarian athletes meet their requirements.

Is a vegetarian diet suitable for athletes?

Many people imagine that a plant-based diet cannot fulfil an athlete's nutritional requirements, that meat is necessary for building strength and endurance, and that vegetarian athletes are smaller, weaker, less muscular and less powerful than their meat-eating counterparts. There is no truth to support these misconceptions. On the contrary, the American Dietetic Association and Dietitians of Canada's 1997 position paper on vegetarian diets states that the needs of competitive athletes can be met through a vegetarian diet (ADA, 1997). This view is echoed in the 2000 ADA and American College of Sports Medicine joint position paper on physical fitness and athletic performance, which states 'foods of animal origin

What is the definition of a vegetarian?

A vegetarian diet is defined as one that does not include meat, poultry, game, fish, seafood, or slaughter by-products such as gelatine or animal fats. It includes grains, pulses, nuts, seeds, vegetables and fruits with or without the use of dairy products and eggs. A lacto-ovo-vegetarian eats both dairy products and eggs. This is the most common type of vegetarian diet. A lacto-vegetarian eats dairy products but not eggs.

A vegan does not eat dairy products, eggs, or any other animal product.

are not essential to ensure optimal athletic performance' (ADA/DC/ACSM, 2000).

WHAT ARE THE HEALTH BENEFITS OF A VEGETARIAN DIET?

The British Dietetic Association states that 'well planned vegetarian diets can be nutritious and healthy' (BDA, 2014). This is in agreement with the position paper on vegetarian diets from the Academy of Nutrition and Dietetics (formerly the American Dietetic Association), which states that 'appropriately planned vegetarian diets, including total vegetarian or vegan diets, are healthful, nutritionally adequate, and may provide health benefits in the prevention and treatment of certain diseases' (Craig *et al.*, 2009).

Large-scale studies have shown that vegetarians are less likely to suffer from chronic diseases such as heart disease, certain cancers, type 2 diabetes, obesity and high blood pressure (Appleby *et al.*, 1999). Researchers at Loma Linda University, US, found that people following vegetarian diets had a 12% lower risk of death from any cause in a 6-year follow-up, compared with non-vegetarians (Orlich *et al.*, 2013).

The EPIC-Oxford study of 45,000 people found that vegetarians were 32% less likely to develop heart disease compared with meat and fish-eaters (Crowe *et al.*, 2013). They were also significantly less likely to be overweight or have type 2 diabetes, and had lower blood pressure and LDL-cholesterol levels. Bowel cancer is less common among vegetarians. A report by the World Cancer Research Fund (WCRF) and the American Institute of Cancer Research (AICR) found that eating red meat and processed meats increases the risk of bowel cancer (WCRF/AICR, 2007). Both the WCRF and the National Health Service (NHS) recommend eating no more than 500 g of meat a week (or 70 g a day), and as little processed meat as possible. The World Health Organization's International Agency for Research on Cancer (WHO/IARC) states that processed meat 'definitely' causes cancer and that red meat 'probably' causes cancer (Bouvard *et al.*, 2015).

Generally, vegetarians have a lower Body Mass Index (BMI) than meat eaters (Spencer *et al.*, 2003). This is partly due to healthier lifestyles but also due to the fact that plant-based foods contain significantly fewer calories than meat. High intakes of fibre and polyphenols found in plant foods also influence the diversity and balance of gut microbes – they encourage healthy gut bacteria to grow and crowd out the unhealthy gut bacteria. Researchers suggest that having a healthy balance of gut bacteria reduces the amount of energy absorbed from food (Spector, 2015).

CAN A VEGETARIAN DIET BENEFIT ATHLETIC PERFORMANCE?

The position statement on nutrition athletic performance by the American Dietetic Association (ADA), American College of Sports Medicine (ACSM) and Dietitians of Canada (DC) states that 'well-planned vegetarian diets appear to effectively support parameters that influence athletic performance' (ADA, 2009). This view is backed by the Australian Institute for Sport (AIS) who state that 'vegetarian eating can support optimal sports performance'.

An analysis by Australian researchers of eight previous studies compared the performance of athletes eating a vegetarian diet with those whose diets included meat and concluded that well-planned and varied vegetarian diets neither hinder nor improve athletic performance (Craddock *et al.*, 2015). Researchers at the University of British Columbia, Vancouver, Canada, also carried out a review of studies on vegetarian athletes and reached the same conclusion. (Barr & Rideout, 2004). However, a vegetarian diet *per se* is not associated with improved aerobic performance (Nieman, 1999).

Several studies have found no significant differences in performance, physical fitness (aerobic or anaerobic capacities), limb circumference, and strength between vegetarian and non-vegetarian athletes (Williams, 1985; Hanne *et al.*, 1986). Even among female athletes consuming a semi-vegetarian diet (less than 100 g red meat per week), there was no difference in their maximum aerobic capacity – or aerobic fitness – compared with meat-eaters (Snyder, 1989). And long-term vegetarian women (average duration of vegetarianism 46 years) had equal health status to non-vegetarian women, according to another study (Nieman, 1989).

Danish researchers tested athletes after they had consumed either a vegetarian or non-vegetarian diet for 6 weeks alternately (Richter *et al.*, 1991). The carbohydrate content of each diet was kept the same (57% energy). Whichever diet they ate, the athletes experienced no change in aerobic capacity, endurance, muscle glycogen concentration or strength.

In a German study, runners completed a 1000 km race after consuming either a vegetarian or non-vegetarian diet containing similar amounts of carbohydrate (60% energy) (Eisinger, 1994). The finishing times were not influenced by the diet; the running times of the vegetarians were not significantly different from those of the non-vegetarians.

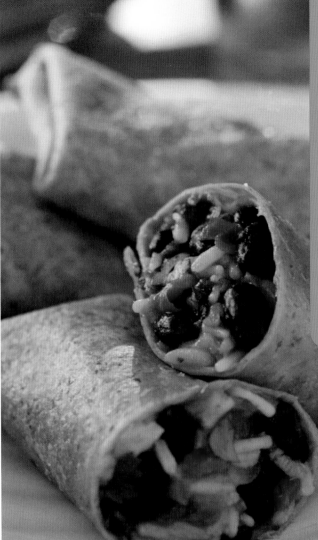

Together, these studies suggest that a vegetarian diet, even when followed for several decades, is compatible with successful athletic performance. However, no studies have examined whether a vegetarian diet will *improve* athletic performance, so we don't know with certainty the true benefits of a vegetarian diet on exercise performance.

CAN A VEGETARIAN DIET PROVIDE ENOUGH PROTEIN FOR ATHLETES?

In general, vegetarian diets are lower in protein than non-vegetarian diets but, nevertheless, they tend to meet or exceed the RNI for protein (Janelle & Barr, 1995). But since athletes need more protein than the RNI for the general population (1.2–2.0 g vs. 0.75 g/kg body weight/day), the question is whether vegetarians can consume enough protein without taking supplements.

Researchers have concluded that most athletes are able to meet these extra demands from a vegetarian diet as long as a variety of protein-rich foods are consumed and energy intakes are adequate (Nielson, 1999; Lemon, 1995; Barr & Rideout, 2004). Good sources of vegetarian proteins are detailed below. The American College of Sports Medicine advises vegetarian athletes to eat around 10% more protein than the recommendations for non-vegetarians to account for the lower levels of essential amino acids in plant foods (Rodriguez *et al.*, 2009). You can achieve this by eating a wide variety of nuts, seeds, beans, lentils, dairy foods, soya products (tofu, tempeh), cereals (oats, pasta, rice, millet and other grains), bread and quinoa, as well as eggs. Aim for around 20 g per meal, including post-training. Studies by researchers at McMaster University have shown this to be the optimal amount to trigger muscle growth and recovery (Moore *et al.*, 2009; Moore *et al.*, 2012).

Contrary to popular belief, even strength athletes can obtain enough protein from a vege-

Table 13.1	THE PROTEIN CONTENT OF VARIOUS FOODS INCLUDED IN A VEGETARIAN DIET		
Good sources	**(g)**	**Fair sources**	**(g)**
Chickpeas, lentils or beans (cooked) (4 heaped tbsp, 200 g)	18 g	Pasta, wholemeal or white (230 g boiled)	7 g
Milk (1 glass/200 ml)	7 g	Rice, brown or white (180 g boiled)	5 g
Egg (1, size 2)	8 g	Bread, wholemeal or white (1 slice)	3 g
Plain yoghurt (125 g)	6 g	Porridge made with water (200 g)	3 g
Strained low fat Greek yoghurt (150 g)	15 g		
Tofu (100 g)	13 g	Potatoes, boiled (200 g)	4 g
Quorn mince (100 g)	12 g	Broccoli (100 g)	3 g
Peanuts (50 g)	12 g		
Pumpkin seeds (50 g)	12 g		

tarian diet – the limiting factor for muscle mass gains appears to be total calorific intake, not protein intake.

WHICH FOODS ARE THE BEST PROTEIN SOURCES FOR VEGETARIANS?

Good protein sources for vegetarians include beans, lentils, nuts, seeds, dairy products, eggs, soya products (tofu, soya milk, soya 'yoghurt' and soya mince), and Quorn. The protein content of various foods is shown in Table 13.1.

Single plant foods do not contain all the essential amino acids you need in the right proportions, but when you combine plant foods, any deficiency in one is cancelled out by higher amounts in the other. This is known as protein complementing. Many plant proteins are low in one of the essential amino acids (the 'limiting amino acid'). For example, grains are short of lysine while pulses are short of methionine. Combining grains and pulses leads to a high quality protein that is just as good, if not better, than protein from animal foods. A few examples are beans on toast, peanut butter on toast, or rice and lentils. Adding dairy products or eggs also adds the missing amino acids, e.g. macaroni cheese or porridge.

Other examples of protein combinations include:

- Tortilla with refried beans
- Bean and vegetable hotpot with rice or pasta
- Dahl with rice
- Falafel wrap
- Lentil soup with a roll
- Quorn korma with chapatti
- Stir-fried tofu and vegetables with rice

Do vegetarians need protein supplements?

If you already get enough protein from food then there is no need to take supplements. However, if you find it difficult to meet your protein requirement from food alone, or if you follow a vegan diet, then protein supplements are a good alternative. They are convenient and can make it easier to obtain your daily protein. Studies show that consuming 20 g protein post-exercise promotes muscle recovery. However, you can also get this amount from 500 ml milk.

Vegetarians may benefit more from creatine supplements

Meat is a major source of creatine in the diet – it typically supplies around 1 g per day for non-vegetarians – so vegetarians tend to have lower muscle creatine concentrations than do non-vegetarians (Maughan, 1995). Because initial muscle creatine levels are lower, vegetarians have an increased capacity to load creatine into muscle following supplementation and are likely to gain greater performance benefits in activities that rely on the ATP–PC system (see pp. 21–22), i.e. sports involving repeated bouts of anaerobic activity (Watt et al., 2004).

In essence, you can achieve protein complementation by combining plant foods from two or more of the following categories:

1. pulses: beans, lentils and peas
2. grains: bread, pasta, rice, oats, breakfast cereals, corn and rye
3. nuts and seeds: peanuts, cashews, almonds, sunflower seeds, sesame seeds and pumpkin seeds
4. Quorn and soya products: soya milk, tofu, tempeh (fermented soya curd similar to tofu but with a stronger flavour), soya mince, soya burgers, Quorn mince, Quorn fillets and Quorn sausages.

It is now known that the body has a pool of amino acids, so that if one meal is deficient, it can be made up from the body's own stores. Because of this, you don't have to worry about complementing amino acids all the time, as long as your diet is generally varied and well balanced. Even those foods not considered high in protein are adding some amino acids to this pool.

WHAT ARE THE PITFALLS OF A VEGETARIAN DIET FOR ATHLETES?

As with any dietary change, it is important to plan your diet well and gain as much knowledge about vegetarian diets as possible. Some athletes adopt a vegetarian or vegan diet in order to lose body fat in the belief that such diets are automatically lower in calories. Many do not substitute suitable foods in place of meat and fail to consume enough protein and other nutrients to support their training. Athletes with disordered eating may omit meat – as well as other food groups – from their diet but disordered eating is certainly not a consequence of vegetarianism!

A very bulky vegetarian diet that includes lots of high fibre foods (e.g. beans, whole grains) may be too filling if you have high energy needs. To ensure you eat enough calories, you may need to include more compact sources of carbohydrate (e.g. dried fruit, fruit juice) or include a mixture of both wholegrain and refined grain products (e.g. wholemeal and white bread) in your diet.

The most common shortfalls are protein, iron, omega-3 fats and vitamin D. Vegans may also fall short on vitamin B_{12} and calcium. Deficiencies of these nutrients will affect your performance and health, and increase your risk of illness, fatigue and injury. The good news is that by eating alternative foods, you can easily avoid these nutritional pitfalls and obtain all nutrients you need for peak health and performance.

SPECIAL CONSIDERATIONS ON A VEGETARIAN DIET
Iron and zinc
Omitting meat may result in lower intakes of iron and zinc and, theoretically, an increased risk of iron-deficiency anaemia. However, there is evidence that the body adapts over time by increasing the percentage of minerals it absorbs from food. Lowered levels of iron and zinc in the diet result in increased absorption.

Despite iron from plants being less readily absorbed, research has shown that iron-deficiency anaemia is no more common in vegetarians than in meat eaters (Alexander *et al.*, 1994; Janelle & Barr, 1995). Even among female endurance athletes, vegetarians are not at greater risk of iron deficiency. Researchers have found that blood levels of haemoglobin and running performance are very similar between non-vegetarian and vegetarian female runners (Snyder, 1989; Seiler, 1989).

Eating vitamin C-rich food (e.g. fruit and vegetables) at the same time as iron-rich foods greatly improves iron absorption. Citric acid (found naturally in fruit and vegetables) and amino acids also promote iron absorption. Good sources of iron for vegetarians include wholegrain cereals, wholemeal bread, nuts, pulses, green vegetables (broccoli, watercress and spinach), fortified cereals, seeds and dried fruit. Table 13.2 shows the iron content of various vegetarian foods.

The absorption of zinc and other trace minerals, such as copper, manganese and selenium, can be reduced by bran and other plant compounds (phytates, oxalic acid), but most studies have failed to show that vegetarians have lower blood levels of these minerals (Fogelholm, 1995). However, it is advisable to avoid eating too many bran-enriched foods. Whole grains, pulses, nuts, seeds and eggs are good sources of zinc. Table 13.3 shows the zinc content of various vegetarian foods.

Omega-3s

Oily fish are rich in long chain omega-3 fatty acids, so vegetarians who don't eat fish will need to obtain them from other foods. One of the main omega-3 fatty acids, alpha-linolenic acid (ALA), is found in certain plant foods such as

Table 13.2	THE IRON CONTENT OF VARIOUS FOODS INCLUDED IN A VEGETARIAN DIET		
Good sources	**Iron, mg**	**Fair sources**	**Iron, mg**
5 heaped tbsp (250 g) cooked quinoa (75 g dry weight)	5.9 mg	Boiled egg (1)	1.3 mg
4 heaped tbsp (200 g) cooked beans	5.0 mg	Cashews (25 g or 4 oz)	1.5 mg
4 heaped tbsp (200 g) cooked lentils (75 g dry weight)	4.8 mg	Avocado (75 g or 3 oz)	1.1 mg
Bran flakes (45 g or 1½ oz)	5.3 mg	Asparagus (125 g or 4 oz)	1.1 mg
Spinach, boiled (100 g or 3½ oz)	4.0 mg	1 slice wholemeal bread (40 g)	1.0 mg
100 g tofu	3.5 mg		
Baked beans (225 g or 8 oz)	3.2 mg	Broccoli, boiled (100 g or 3½ oz)	1.0 mg
Muesli (60 g or 2¼ oz)	2.76 mg	Brown rice (200 g or 7 oz)	0.9 mg
4 dried figs (60 g or 2¼ oz)	2.1 mg	Peanut butter (20 g or ⅔ oz)	0.5 mg
8 dried apricots (50 g or 2 oz)	2.1 mg		

Table 13.3	THE ZINC CONTENT OF VARIOUS FOODS INCLUDED IN A VEGETARIAN DIET			
Good sources	**Zinc, mg**	**Fair sources**	**Zinc, mg**
Chickpeas (200 g or 7 oz)	2.8 mg	Peanut butter (20 g or ⅔ oz)	0.6 mg
Baked beans (225 g or 8 oz)	1.6 mg	Peas, frozen/canned (80 g or 3⅓ oz)	0.6 mg
1 Vegeburger (100 g or 3½ oz)	1.6 mg	3 dried figs (60 g or 2¼ oz)	0.5 mg
Pumpkin seeds (20 g or ⅔ oz)	1.3 mg	3 Brazil nuts (10 g or ⅓ oz)	0.4 mg
Muesli (60 g or 2¼ oz)	1.3 mg	Potatoes, boiled (200 g or 7 oz)	0.4 mg
Cheddar cheese (30 g or 1 oz)	1.2 mg	1 orange (140 g or 5 oz)	0.3 mg
Tahini paste (20 g or ⅔ oz)	1.1 mg	6 almonds (10 g or ⅓ oz)	0.3 mg
1 fruit yoghurt (150 g or 5 oz)	0.9 mg	Peanut butter (20 g or ⅔ oz)	0.6 mg

Table 13.4	THE OMEGA-3 CONTENT OF VARIOUS FOODS INCLUDED IN A VEGETARIAN DIET			
Good sources	**g per 100 g**	**Portion**	**g per portion**
Flaxseed oil	57 g	1 tbsp (14 g)	8.0 g
Flaxseeds (ground)	16 g	1 tbsp (24 g)	3.8 g
Rapeseed oil	9.6 g	1 tbsp (14 g)	1.3 g
Walnuts	7.5 g	1 tbsp (28 g)	2.6 g
Walnut oil	11.5 g	1 tbsp (14 g)	1.6 g
Sweet potatoes	0.03 g	Medium (130 g)	1.3 g
Peanuts	0.4 g	Handful (50 g)	0.2 g
Broccoli	0.1 g	3 tbsp (125 g)	1.3 g
Pumpkin seeds	8.5 g	2 tbsp (25 g)	2.1 g
Omega-3 eggs	0.8 g	1 egg	0.4 g

pumpkin seeds and flaxseed oil (*see* Table 13.4, which gives the omega-3 fatty acid content of various foods). In the body it is converted to eicosapentanoic acid (EPA) and docosapentanoic acid (DPA) – the two fatty acids that are found in plentiful amounts in oily fish but not other foods and which offer greater cardio protective benefits than the parent ALA.

The Vegetarian Society recommends an ALA intake of 1.5% of energy, or roughly 4 g a day. This should provide enough of the parent omega-3 fatty acid to ensure enough EPA and DHA are formed by the body (conversion rates are around 5–10% for EPA and 2–5% for DHA). Include some of the foods listed in Table 13.4 in your daily diet.

You should also aim to achieve an LA to ALA ratio of around 4:1 or slightly lower since a high intake of LA interferes with the conversion process of ALA to EPA and DHA. Replace fat high in omega-6 oils (such as sunflower or corn oil) with fats higher in monounsaturated oils (such as olive oil and nuts), which do not disrupt the formation of EPA and DHA.

It's a good idea to take vegetarian omega-3 supplements if you don't get food sources of omega-3s regularly. Opt for supplements made from algae oil – these are better options than those made from flaxseed oil as they contain high levels of both the omega-3 fatty acids DHA and EPA instead of ALA. The high concentration of omega-3s found in oily fish is due to the algae they consume, which produces the oils.

EASY MENU PLANNER

Plan your vegetarian diet around the following five food groups to ensure you get the right balance of amino acids and other nutrients.

Fruit and vegetables
5 or more servings a day

Serving size = approx 80 g, equivalent to 1 medium fruit e.g. apple; 2 small fruit e.g. kiwi fruit; 1 cupful berries e.g. strawberries; 3 heaped tbsp of cooked vegetables.

Pulses and other protein-rich foods
2–4 servings a day (4–5 if dairy products are excluded)

This group includes beans, lentils, eggs, nuts, seeds, soya milk, soya mince, Quorn, tofu, and tempeh.

Serving size = 125 g (4 oz) cooked pulses, tofu, soya mince; 2 eggs; 25 g (1 oz) nuts or seeds.

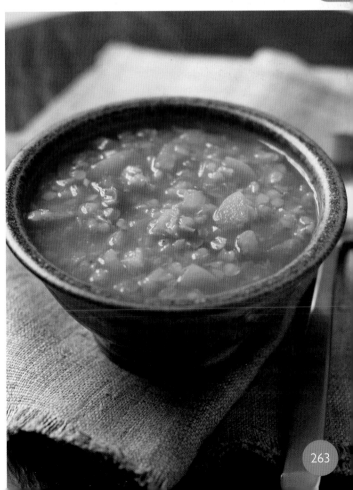

Cereals and starchy vegetables

4–6 servings a day depending on activity level

This group includes bread, rice, pasta, breakfast cereals and potatoes. At least half of your servings should be whole grains.

Serving size = 2 slices of bread; 60 g (uncooked weight) grains or breakfast cereal; 175 g potato.

Milk and dairy products

2–4 servings a day

This group includes milk, yoghurt and cheese. Choose the low fat versions wherever possible.

Serving size = 200 ml (⅓ pint) milk; 1 carton (150 ml) yoghurt/fromage frais; 40 g hard cheese; 125 g cottage cheese.

Healthy fats and oils

2–4 portions a day.

This group includes all vegetable oils (try to include at least one source of omega-3 rich oil daily), nuts, seeds and avocados.

Serving size = 2 tsp (10 ml) oil; 25 g nuts or seeds; ½ avocado.

Summary of key points

- Overall, vegetarians have higher intakes of fruit and vegetables, fibre, antioxidant nutrients and phytonutrients, and lower intakes of saturated fat compared with meat-eaters.
- Vegetarians suffer less heart disease, hypertension, obesity, type 2 diabetes and certain cancers than meat-eaters.
- The nutritional needs of athletes can be fully met through a vegetarian diet.
- Studies have shown that well-planned and varied vegetarian diets don't hinder athletic potential and do indeed support athletic performance.
- There are no significant differences in performance, physical fitness (aerobic or anaerobic capacities), limb circumference, and strength between vegetarian and non-vegetarian athletes.
- Vegetarian diets are lower in protein than non-vegetarian diets but, nevertheless, most athletes are able to meet these extra demands from a vegetarian diet as long as a variety of protein-rich foods are consumed and energy intakes are adequate.
- Vegetarian athletes are likely to gain greater performance benefits from creatine supplementation than meat-eaters, due to their initially lower muscle creatine levels.
- A poorly planned vegetarian diet may result in low intakes of iron, zinc and omega-3 fatty acids but studies show that iron-deficiency anaemia is no more common in vegetarians than meat eaters.
- Vegetarians can obtain omega-3 fatty acids from foods rich in alpha-linolenic acid (ALA) and should aim for an ALA intake of 1.5% of energy, or roughly 4 g a day.

The older
athlete

14

Now, more than ever, many people in their 50s, 60s and beyond want to improve their health, retain a high level of fitness, and remain competitive and at the top of their game. However, the aging process is accompanied by many physiological changes that affect your exercise capacity, muscle mass and strength. Typically, most athletes start to see a drop in their peak performance some time in their 30s.

Fortunately, a combination of regular exercise and good nutrition, especially protein intake, can help prevent or reduce age-related declines in muscle mass, strength and physiological functioning. This chapter explains how you can adjust your diet so you will still be able to perform to your potential in sport as you get older.

HOW DOES AGING AFFECT FITNESS?

For most athletes, peak performance begins to drop some time in our 20s or 30s, depending on the sport and activity. The rate of decline gradually increases to about 0.7% per year throughout our 40s, 50s and 60s, with progressively steeper increases thereafter (Tanaka & Seals, 2008). The major age-related changes that may affect nutritional requirements are summarised in Table 14.1.

The physiological reasons for this decline are varied and not very well understood. What is known is that the natural aging process is associated with a gradual reduction in cardiovascular and respiratory functioning, and muscle mass. Resting stroke volume, maximum heart rate and aerobic capacity (VO_2max) decline at a rate of approximately 10% per decade from the mid 20s (Downes, 2002). From middle age onwards, the drop in endurance performance is due mainly to a reduction in VO_2max, whereas from young adulthood to middle age it is mainly due to a reduction in lactate threshold (Tanaka & Seals, 2008).

Flexibility tends to decrease due to accumulated wear and tear. Recovery from hard workouts and healing after injury take longer, and chronic overuse injuries become more common, accounting for as many as 70% of injuries in athletes over 60 years of age. To reduce your injury risk, you may need to reduce the amount of repetitive impact exercise you do and focus instead on low impact activities, as well as building extra recovery and sleep into your programme.

Power and strength, however, decline much more quickly unless you include resistance exercise in your training programme. Muscle mass

Table 14.1	THE MAIN AGE-RELATED CHANGES THAT MAY INFLUENCE NUTRITIONAL REQUIREMENTS
Age-related change	**Nutritional implication**
Reduced aerobic capacity	Reduced energy requirements
Reduced muscle mass	Reduced energy requirements
Reduced bone mass	Increased requirement for calcium and vitamin D
Reduced skin capacity for vitamin D synthesis	Increased requirement for vitamin D
Reduced gastric acid	Increased requirement for B_{12}, folic acid, calcium, iron and zinc
Reduced absorption of calcium	Increased requirement for calcium and vitamin D
Reduced thirst perception	Increased requirement for fluid
Reduced kidney function	Increased requirement for fluid

loss typically begins in your 30s (Janssen *et al.*, 2000) and then declines by 8% per decade until the age of 70, increasing to about 15% per decade thereafter (Mitchell *et al.*, 2012).

Bone mass also declines from the mid 30s and one in three women over 50 will experience fractures as a result of osteopososis (thinning of the bones), as will one in five men. All of these physiological changes inevitably result in a drop in endurance, strength and physical performance.

The good news is that regular exercise can offset many of the detrimental effects of aging. A study at the Mayo Clinic College of Medicine, US, found that older people (59–76 years of age) who did at least 1 hour of endurance exercise a day had a higher aerobic capacity, less body fat and greater insulin sensitivity (and therefore less risk of developing metabolic syndrome) than those who were sedentary (Lanza *et al.*, 2008).

There was little difference in mitochondria function between older and younger active people in the group, which suggests that regular endurance exercise largely prevented the decline in aerobic capacity that normally occurs with age. According to the researchers at the University of Missouri, US, maintaining a life-long habit of regular aerobic exercise delays the onset of decline in aerobic capacity by 30 years (Booth & Zwetsloot, 2010). An active 80-year-old may have a higher level of fitness than a sedentary 50-year-old, especially when it comes to measures of VO_2max, muscle strength and endurance.

Studies show that resistance training can prevent the muscle loss that occurs with age and even result in muscle gain. A study by researchers at Top Institute Food and Nutrition, The Netherlands, of 24 women and 29 men aged 70–71 years showed that 6 months of resistance training resulted in a 10% increase in leg muscle mass and a 42% increase in leg strength (Leenders *et al.*, 2013).

It is well established that regular physical activity along with a healthy diet (in particular getting adequate calcium and vitamin D) help maintain bone mass, preventing or delaying the onset of osteoporosis (Warburton *et al.*, 2006). Also, exercise has the added benefit of increasing psychological well-being, decreasing the risk of chronic disease and reducing overall mortality rates relative to age.

Energy

Our daily energy needs tend to decrease gradually as we get older. This is partly due to the age-related decrease in lean body mass, resulting in an overall drop in resting metabolic rate (RMR), and partly due to a reduction in physical activity levels. However, this muscle loss can be prevented by incorporating resistance training in your training programme and maintaining your training volume. This is explained more fully in the following section.

Your RMR is an estimate of how many calories you would burn if you were to do nothing but rest for 24 hours. It represents the minimum amount of energy needed to keep your body functioning, including breathing and keeping your heart beating. It can be estimated using the Mifflin-St Jeor equation, which utilises age as well as weight and height to take account of age-related muscle loss (*see* p. 268). However, it does not account for exercise or make any adjustment for body composition.

For example, the RMR for a 60-year-old male athlete who measures 1.78m and weighs 70 kg

Fitness measurements explained

Maximal oxygen consumption (VO$_2$max) is the maximal volume of oxygen that the body can deliver to the working muscles per minute. It is an excellent measure of an athlete's cardiovascular fitness and aerobic endurance. Those who are fit have higher VO$_2$max values than those who are less well conditioned.

Lactate threshold (LT) is the exercise intensity at which blood lactate concentrations increase significantly above baseline. Lactate is the by-product of glucose breakdown by muscle cells. Having a high LT means you can work at a higher intensity for longer.

is 1518 kcal, whereas the RMR for a 30-year-old of the same height and weight is 1668 kcal. In other words, an average 60-year-old man expends 150 fewer calories per day at rest compared with an average 30-year-old. However, this is based on the assumption that the 60-year-old has less muscle mass than the 30-year-old.

The daily energy expenditure will also be correspondingly less. This can be calculated by multiplying RMR by the Physical Activity Level (PAL) and then adding estimated exercise energy expenditure (*see* page 291). For example, for a 60-year-old who is mostly sedentary (PAL 1.4) and expends an average 500 calories per day during exercise:

- Daily energy expenditure = $1518 \times 1.4 + 500$ = 2625 kcal

By comparison, a 30-year-old would expend 2835 kcal per day, a difference of 210 calories. This equates to two chocolate biscuits or a pint of beer! Clearly, you can compensate for the age-related drop in calorie expenditure by consuming fewer calories, increasing energy exercise expenditure or avoiding muscle loss in the first place by including resistance training in your programme.

Calorie intake should come from nutrient-dense foods that promote maximum performance, enhance recovery from workouts and reduce the risk of chronic diseases such as cardiovascular disease, type 2 diabetes, cancer and osteoporosis and other debilitating diseases of aging.

Protein

Both protein ingestion and resistance training are powerful anabolic stimuli, triggering muscle protein synthesis (MPS). However, as you get older, the muscles become less able to respond to the anabolic effects of dietary protein and exercise on muscle protein synthesis (MPS), and develop an 'anabolic resistance' (Burd *et al.*, 2013; Rennie, 2009). The exact mechanisms are unclear but it is thought that the absorption of amino acids from the gut is reduced as well as the uptake of amino acids by the muscles. In essence, this means that, without regular resistance exercise, MPS declines and many people experience an age-related loss of muscle.

After the age of 50, most people tend to lose 0.5–1.2% of their muscle mass and 3% of their strength per year (Bell *et al.*, 2016). In inactive people, this age-related loss of muscle and strength, called sarcopenia, can dramatically reduce your mobility, quality of life and abil-

The Mifflin-St Jeor equation for estimating RMR

Men
$10 \times$ weight (kg) $+ 6.25 \times$ height (cm) $- 5 \times$ age (y) $+ 5$

Women
$10 \times$ weight (kg) $+ 6.25 \times$ height (cm) $- 5 \times$ age (y) $- 161$

Mifflin et al., 1990.

What is sarcopenia?

Sarcopenia is the gradual loss of muscle mass, strength and mobility that occurs with age. It can begin in your 30s but usually accelerates in your 60s onwards unless specific measures are taken to prevent it. Losses are typically 0.5–1.2% per year; most people in their 70s have only 60–80% of the muscle mass they had in their 30s. This age-related muscle loss is the result of a chronic disruption in the balance between protein synthesis and breakdown (Koopman, 2011) and is caused by lack of exercise as well as poor nutrition (particularly insufficient protein intake), a drop in hormone (growth hormone and testosterone) levels, chronic inflammation and DNA damage.

ity to perform everyday activities (*see* 'What is sarcopenia?' above). It also increases the risk of falls and fractures, and contributes to the development of chronic metabolic diseases such as type 2 diabetes.

But sarcopenia isn't inevitable. With adequate protein intake in conjunction with regular weight-bearing exercise and resistance training performed at least twice a week, you can prevent and reverse sarcopenia and even gain lean body mass (Booth & Zwetsloot, 2010; Peterson *et al.* 2011).

HOW MUCH PROTEIN SHOULD I CONSUME?

New findings suggest that older people (both inactive and active) may require a higher protein intake than previously thought to offset protein loss and maintain muscle mass, strength and physiological functioning (Moore *et al.*, 2015; Gray-Donald *et al.*, 2014; Deutz *et al.*, 2014; Bauer *et al.*, 2013).

For healthy non-active adults aged over 65, the European Society for Clinical Nutrition and Metabolism recommend 1.0–1.2 g/kg BW/day to prevent sarcopenia and maintain muscle mass (Deutz *et al.*, 2014), which is more than the amount recommended for younger adults (0.75 g/kg BW/day). For healthy active older adults, researchers recommend a daily protein intake of 1.2–1.5 g/kg BW/day to help preserve muscle mass and strength (Witard *et al.*, 2016). This equates to 84 g–105 g per day for a 70 kg person.

It is more practical, however, to express protein intake recommendations per meal, rather than per day. The optimal protein dose for stimulating maximal muscle protein synthesis (MPS) is believed to be in the region of 0.4 g/kg BW per meal, which is considerably higher than the recommendation for younger athletes (0.25 g/kg BW/day) (Moore *et al.*, 2015; Witard *et al.*, 2016). This equates to 28 g for an athlete weighing 70 kg.

In one study of older men (average age 73), those who consumed 35 g whey protein showed significantly greater amino acid absorption and subsequent MPS than those who consumed 10 or 20 g (Pennings *et al.*, 2012).

The following amounts of foods provide 30 g protein, which equates to the optimal protein needs of a 70 kg older athlete.

- 2 slices (100 g) red meat
- 1 average (125 g) chicken or turkey breast
- 1 fillet (150 g) fish
- 1 small tin (120 g) tuna
- 6 tbsp (300 g) strained Greek yoghurt
- 4 glasses (900 ml) milk (any type)
- 4 large eggs
- 1 tin (400 g) beans and 2 slices wholemeal toast
- 2 bowls (600 g) porridge made with milk
- 400 ml protein shake (20 g whey protein plus 400 ml milk)

IS PROTEIN TIMING IMPORTANT FOR MUSCLE BUILDING?

As well as quantity, the timing of protein intake is also important when it comes to stimulating maximal MPS in older athletes. Studies have found that consuming protein either during or immediately after exercise improves the anabolic response and allows more of the dietary protein to be used to build new muscle proteins (Pennings *et al.*, 2011). This not only helps to prevent protein breakdown during exercise but also helps to compensate for the anabolic resistance that occurs with age, and builds new muscle.

Since the anabolic effect of exercise is now known to extend at least 24 hours after exercise, there are further muscle-building benefits to be gained by consuming protein through-out the day, not only in the post-workout meal (Wall *et al.*, 2014). A study at the University of Texas Medical Branch, US, found that 24-hour MPS was significantly greater when volunteers consumed 90 g protein as 3 × 30 g meals evenly spaced, compared with a skewed meal pattern that biased protein intake towards the evening meal (Mamerow *et al.*, 2014). In practice, this means including similar quantities of foods such as milk, eggs, meat, fish, poultry, tofu, beans and lentils at every meal, including breakfast. Suitable high protein snack options include yoghurt, nuts and nut butter.

WHICH TYPE OF PROTEIN IS BEST?

Ideally, you should include high quality proteins that provide all 8 essential amino acids, including the amino acid leucine, such as milk and dairy products, whey protein supplements, eggs and meat. Leucine not only provides a substrate for building new muscle proteins but also acts as an important anabolic signal for MPS by activating enzymes within the mTOR signalling pathway (*see* p. 85). Vegans should include a mixture of plant proteins (such as beans and grains) in order to get the full complement of EAAs.

SHOULD I CONSUME PROTEIN BEFORE SLEEP?

Studies have also shown that consuming protein before sleep can result in greater MPS in younger athletes (*see* p. 83). However, this is also advantageous for older athletes. In a study involving 16 healthy older men (average age 74) at the Maastricht Medical Centre in The Netherlands, those who were given an infusion of 40 g casein protein overnight had significantly greater MPS

and whole body protein synthesis compared with those who received a placebo (Groen *et al.*, 2012). While consuming protein overnight is not a practical strategy for most people, having a high protein snack or drink before bed could help maximise the effects of resistance exercise and help you gain more muscle. Suitable options include:

- 300 ml milk or hot chocolate (10 g protein)
- 300 ml milk blended with 20 g casein protein, a banana or a handful of berries (30 g protein)
- 250 g strained Greek yoghurt mixed with berries, honey or granola (20 g protein)

Carbohydrate

As we get older, we retain the abilities to store carbohydrate as glycogen in the liver and muscles; to use glycogen as a source of fuel during exercise; and to recover muscle glycogen levels following exercise. So, the carbohydrate needs of older athletes are no different from those of younger athletes. However, as mentioned previously, since daily energy expenditure typically drops then your daily carbohydrate requirement may become smaller too.

HOW MUCH CARBOHYDRATE?

Your carbohydrate intake should match the fuel needs of your training programme. Thus, the guidelines for carbohydrate requirements in Table 3.1 (Guidelines for daily carbohydrate intake, p. 34) apply equally to older athletes. These are based on body weight and exercise load, so the greater your body weight (a proxy for muscle mass) and exercise volume, the higher your carbohydrate requirement. For example,

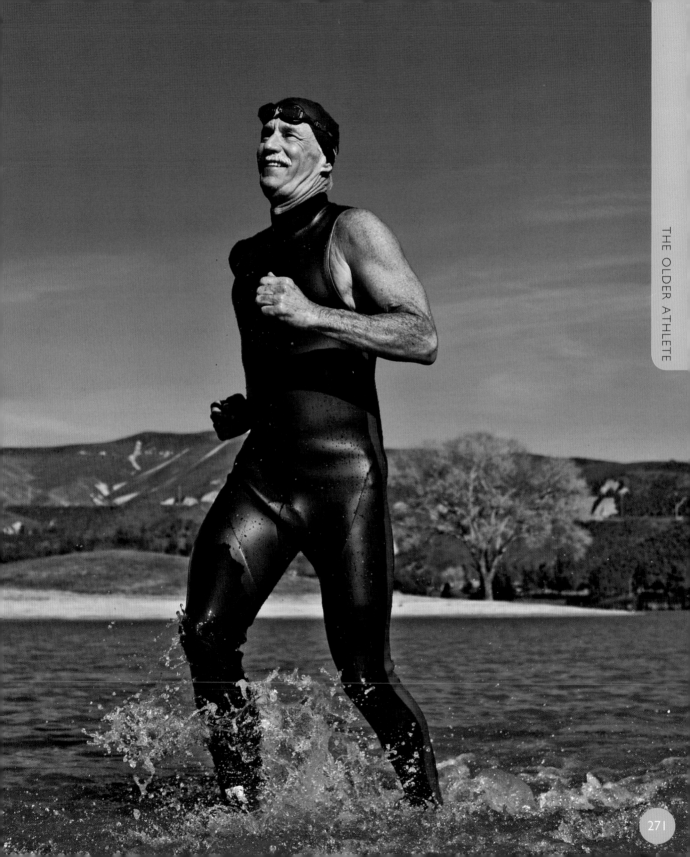

you will require 5–7 g carbohydrate/kg BW/ day when performing moderate intensity exercise for approximately 1 hour per day; or 3–5 g/kg BW/day if you do several hours of low intensity exercise. For athletes with a higher training load, 6–10 g/kg/day would be appropriate.

HOW SHOULD I TIME MY CARBOHYDRATE AROUND EXERCISE?

As detailed in Chapter 2, the timing of your carbohydrate intake before, during and after exercise is important. For your pre-exercise meal, it is recommended you should consume 1–4 g carbohydrate/kg BW 1–4 hours before exercise (ASCM/AND/DC, 2016). Essentially you need to leave enough time to digest the food but not too long, otherwise this energy will be used up by the time you begin exercising and you may feel hungry and lacking in energy. The closer your pre-workout meal is to your workout, the smaller the amount of carbohydrate it should contain. And the longer and harder your workout, the more carbohydrate you will need beforehand. As a rule of thumb, consume 1 g carbohydrate/kg BW 1 hour before exercise, 2 g carbohydrate/ kg BW 2 hours before, and so on.

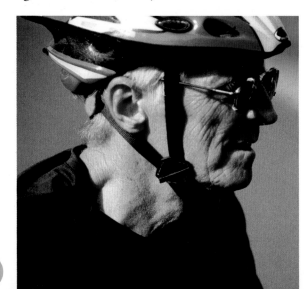

For exercise lasting less than 45–60 minutes, there is no benefit to be gained by consuming carbohydrate during exercise. For exercise lasting longer than 60 minutes, consuming between 30 and 60 g carbohydrate/hour helps maintain blood glucose concentration, spare muscle glycogen, delay the point of exhaustion and improve endurance. However, for high intensity exercise lasting 45–75 minutes, 'mouth-rinsing' – whereby a carbohydrate-containing drink is simply swilled around the mouth but not swallowed – may improve performance. The carbohydrates stimulate sensors in the mouth that signal to the brain that carbohydrates are on their way, thus stimulating the brain's pleasure and reward centres, masking fatigue and reducing perceived exertion.

Muscles become more susceptible to the damage caused by eccentric exercise (where the muscle lengthens as it contracts, such as during the lowering phase of resistance training exercises, plyometric training or downhill running) and are not able to repair this damage as quickly between workouts. You can reduce muscle damage and protein breakdown during prolonged intense exercise by consuming carbohydrate and protein (*see* p. 81).

To promote rapid recovery after exercise, especially if you plan to train within 8 hours, you should consume 1.0–1.2 g carbohydrate/kg BW/hour for the first 4 hours. Adding protein to your post-exercise meal or snack will enhance muscle repair, glycogen storage and MPS. High or moderate GI carbohydrates will facilitate fastest glycogen refuelling but for recovery periods of 24 hours or longer, the type and timing of carbohydrate intake is less critical. Opt for nutrient-dense sources, such as oats, wholegrain pasta or bread, fruit, potatoes, brown rice or quinoa wherever possible, rather than sugars.

ARE THERE BENEFITS OF CONSUMING A LOW CARBOHYDRATE DIET?

The concept of training with 'low carbohydrate availability' (restricting carbohydrate intake and training in a glycogen-depleted state) has become popular with elite endurance athletes (*see* p.36–46). The idea is to stimulate greater training adaptations, encourage the muscles to burn fat more readily and improve your performance in endurance events. However, 'training low' can also hamper the muscles' ability to use carbohydrate at high exercise intensities (above 65% VO_2max), reducing power output and making exercise at any given intensity feel significantly harder. In other words, you can't train as hard. There is no clear evidence that following a low carbohydrate diet long term provides any performance advantage for those exercising above 65% VO_2max or participating in races that involve sprints or high intensity efforts.

On the other hand, low carbohydrate diets may suit certain older athletes, particularly those who do mostly low to moderate intensity exercise, those with type 2 diabetes or those with insulin resistance (when your cells are less sensitive to insulin so cannot process carbohydrate into fuel efficiently). It may also appeal to those wishing to prevent weight gain or lose body fat, but, as mentioned previously, the consensus of evidence suggests that low carbohydrate diets are no more effective in reducing body weight and insulin resistance than other types of diets (Pagoto & Appelhans, 2013; Hu *et al.*, 2012, Johnston *et al.*, 2006). What matters most when it comes to weight loss is achieving a calorie deficit and then being able to sustain the diet long term.

Carbohydrate periodisation, whereby you do certain (low intensity) workouts with low carbohydrate availability and high intensity sessions with high carbohydrate availability, may be a better option if you are competing at elite level. The idea is to match your carbohydrate intake to the demands of your training sessions so you get the dual benefits of 'training low' (fat adaptation) as well as the performance benefits of high intensity training.

Fat

HOW MUCH FAT SHOULD I CONSUME?

Because fat is very calorie-dense (9 calories per gram), it can be an excellent source of fuel. However, your main focus should be on meeting your carbohydrate and protein goals, with fat making up the calorie balance. Stick to the recommended distribution range of 20–35% of total energy (*see* p. 176). Lower fat intakes are not recommended as you risk deficient intakes of fat-soluble vitamins and essential fatty acids.

WHICH TYPES OF FAT ARE HEALTHIEST?

When it comes to minimising cardiovascular risk, the type of fat you eat is more important than the amount. Artificial trans fatty acids (found in hydrogenated fats) appear to raise cardiovascular risk the most and should be avoided. Saturated fats are now thought to be less harmful for the heart than previously. Some types of saturated fatty acids increase LDL cholesterol while other types decrease it, making it difficult for scientists to come to an overall conclusion, but the overall effect is likely to be neutral.

Follow the UK public health guidelines to limit daily saturated fat intake to less than 11% of total energy. Most studies also recommend replacing some of the saturated fat in your diet with unsaturated fats (found in vegetable oils, nuts, seeds and oily fish). Unsaturated fats lower LDL cholesterol and raise HDL cholesterol and therefore lower the risk of cardiovascular disease.

DO I NEED TO CONSUME MORE OMEGA-3S?

You should try to include essential fatty acids in your daily diet. Omega-3s may help reduce cardiovascular risk, lower cholesterol, protect against abnormal heart rhythms and build-up of plaque in the arteries, as well as helping brain function and preventing loss of memory. However, omega-3s have also been shown to have anti-inflammatory effects. Chronic inflammation is believed to be a key factor in the development of many chronic diseases, including heart disease, certain cancers, type 2 diabetes, osteoarthritis and dementia. For athletes, omega-3s may enhance aerobic metabolism, improve oxygen delivery to cells, minimise post-exercise soreness and reduce post-exercise inflammation.

The DoH recommends a minimum of 450–900 mg omega-3 fatty acids per day, and advises people to eat at least 2 portions of fish a week, one of which should be oily fish. The best sources of omega-3s include oily fish, such as mackerel and salmon, flaxseeds, pumpkin seeds, walnuts, chia seeds and their oils.

Fluid

As we get older, our perception of thirst decreases and sweat rate decreases. You may notice that you sweat less and begin sweating later during exercise compared with younger athletes. Kidney function is also reduced, which means the ability of your kidneys to concentrate urine is reduced. Kenney & Chiu, 2001; Miescher et al., 1989; Phillips et al., 1984).

All of this means that as you age you are more susceptible to dehydration, so make sure you begin training sessions well hydrated. Achieve this by drinking plenty of fluid in the 24 hours prior to training and approximately 5–10 ml/kg BW in the 2 to 4 hours before exercise. This promotes hydration and allows enough time for the excretion of excess water (ACSM/AND/DC, 2016). During exercise, you may prefer to drink to a planned schedule rather than relying totally on thirst, since thirst becomes less pronounced as we get older and is therefore a less reliable indicator of the body's fluid needs.

As a rule of thumb, an intake of 400–800 ml/hour prevents dehydration as well as over-hydration (Sawka et al., 2007; ACSM/AND/DC, 2016). You can work out how much fluid you lose through sweating by weighing yourself before and after a typical workout, then aim to drink sufficient to ensure a weight loss of no more than about 2% (see p. 146). After each session, you should drink an additional 1.2–1.5 litres of fluid for each 1 kg lost during exercise (IAAF, 2007; Shirreffs et al., 2004; Shirreffs et al., 1996).

Vitamin D

Low blood levels of vitamin D are common across all age groups but this is particularly problematic as we get older as the skin's capacity to produce vitamin D from UV light diminishes. Data from the UK National Diet and Nutrition

Survey (NDNS) showed that 17% of men aged 65 or older and 24% of women had vitamin D deficiency (Bates *et al.*, 2014).

Vitamin D plays an important role in healthy bones and teeth, muscle function, supporting our immune system, lung function, cardiovascular health, and the brain and nervous system. Low levels may reduce muscle function and strength and impair performance (Hamilton, 2011; Larson-Meyer, 2010; Halliday *et al.*, 2011). Getting adequate levels of vitamin D – whether from sun exposure or diet – is, therefore, important for optimal performance.

There are only three categories of foods that contain significant amounts of vitamin D: eggs, liver and oily fish. Each of the following provides the recommended daily intake of 10 mcg (400 IU):

- 5 eggs
- 1 tsp (5 ml) cod liver oil
- 200 g tinned sardines
- 120 g mackerel
- 140 g salmon
- 340 g tinned tuna (in oil).

Summary of key points

- Aerobic capacity, muscle mass and bone density gradually decline with age.
- Energy needs may decrease due to loss of muscle mass (and the resultant drop in RMR), and reduced physical activity levels.
- Muscles are less responsive to the anabolic effects of dietary protein and exercise.
- An increased daily protein intake (1.2–1.5 g/kg BW/day) can help offset protein loss and maintain muscle mass and strength.

- To maximise MPS, an intake of 0.4 g protein/kg BW per meal is recommended.
- Including proteins rich in leucine as well as consuming protein post-exercise may also help increase MPS.
- Adjust your carbohydrate intake to the fuel needs of your training programme.
- Omega-3s are particularly important for older athletes, and may help reduce cardiovascular risk and chronic inflammation and enhance aerobic metabolism.
- Thirst becomes less pronounced with age and is therefore a less reliable indicator of your body's fluid needs.
- The skin's capacity to produce vitamin D from UV light diminishes so dietary sources become more important.

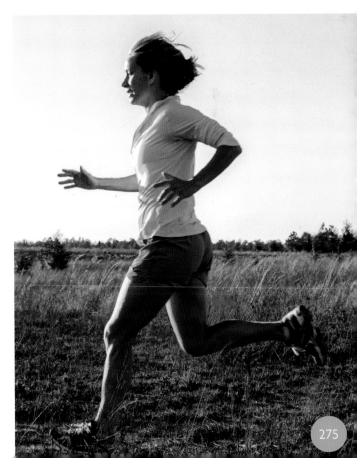

Competition //nutrition

Your diet before a competition will have a big impact on your performance, and could provide you with that winning edge. In addition, what you eat and drink on the day of the event can affect your ability to recover between heats and your performance in subsequent heats. This chapter covers the whole of the competition period, including the week before the event, during, and after the event. It consolidates much of the information presented in preceding chapters, in particular Chapter 3 on carbohydrate intake and Chapter 7 on fluid intake, and provides specific guidelines for arriving at your competition well hydrated and with full glycogen stores. It gives pre-competition sample eating plans, which you can use as a basis for developing your personal programme, suitable pre-competition meals and snacks that can be eaten between heats and events. For those athletes who need to make weight for their competition, this chapter gives a simple step-by-step nutrition strategy that will help you lose body fat safely and effectively.

The week before

During the week before a competition, your two main aims are:

1. to fill your muscle and liver glycogen stores so that you compete with a 'full' fuel supply;
2. to keep well hydrated.

Your preparation will be dictated by the kind of event that you are competing in, the importance of the event and how frequently you compete.

Short duration events lasting less than 4 minutes

Short duration, all-out events lasting less than 4 minutes are fuelled by ATP, PC and muscle glycogen. If you are competing in a sprint event, it is important to allow enough recovery time after your last training session, and to make sure your muscle glycogen stores are replenished. The presence of muscle damage will delay the recovery process. Training that may cause muscle fibre damage should either be scheduled earlier in the week to allow for recovery or avoided altogether. Such training includes plyometrics, heavy-weight training and hard running. Reduce your training over the pre-competition week and rest for the last 1–3 days prior to the competition. There is no advantage to be gained by carbohydrate loading so continue eating your usual diet, adjusting your carbohydrate intake according to your daily activity. Use Table 15.1 as a guide to the amount of carbohydrate you should be eating during the final 3 days.

Endurance events lasting more than 90 minutes

If you are competing in an endurance event lasting longer than 90 minutes, you may benefit from carbohydrate loading. This is detailed in Chapter 3, 'Carbohydrate loading', pp. 71–2. In summary, you should consume a moderate carbohydrate diet (5–7 g/kg body weight/day) for the first 3 days, followed by a high carbohydrate intake (10–12 g/kg body weight/day) for the final 36–48 hours. Use Table 15.1 as a guide to the amount of carbohydrate you should be eating during the pre-competition week. Your last hard training session should be completed one week before your competition. Then taper your training during the final week so that you perform only very light exercise and rest the day prior to your competition.

Endurance events lasting less than 90 minutes; or multiple heats

If your event lasts less than 90 minutes, or if your competition schedule includes several short heats in one day, your muscle glycogen stores can become depleted. Examples of events with multiple heats include swimming, track cycling and track and field athletics. You can fill your muscle glycogen stores by tapering your training during the final week and maintaining or increasing your carbohydrate intake to about 7–8 g/kg body weight/day during the 3 days prior to your competition. Use Table 15.1 as a guide to the amount of carbohydrate you should be eating during the final 3 days.

Weekly events

If you compete weekly or even more frequently (e.g. in seasonal competitions such as football, netball and cycling), it may not be possible to rest for 3 days prior to each match or race. You would end up with virtually no training time.

Table 15.1	RECOMMENDED CARBOHYDRATE INTAKE FOR ATHLETES OF DIFFERENT BODY WEIGHTS	
Body weight (kg)	Daily carbohydrate intake equivalent to 7–8 g/kg body weight	Daily carbohydrate intake equivalent to 8–10 g/kg body weight
55	385–440 g	440–550 g
60	420–480 g	480–600 g
65	455–520 g	520–650 g
70	490–560 g	560–700 g
75	525–600 g	600–750 g
80	560–640 g	640–800 g

Perform lower intensity training or technical training during the 2 days before the match and taper only for the most important matches or races. Increase your carbohydrate intake during the final 2 days to 8–10 g/kg body weight/day. Use Table 15.1 as a guide to the amount of carbohydrate you should be eating during the final 3 days.

For all events, your total calorie intake should remain about the same as usual during the pre-competition week, but the proportions of carbohydrate, fat and protein will change. Eat larger amounts of carbohydrate-rich foods (e.g. potatoes, bread, rice, dried fruit) and carbohydrate drinks, and smaller amounts of fats and proteins. However, if you are performing a week-long taper, you may need to reduce your calories slightly to match your reduced training needs. You can do this by reducing your fat intake; otherwise you may experience fat gain.

In practice, divide your carbohydrate evenly between meals, avoid gaps longer than 3 hours, and include some protein and fat in your meals to achieve a sustained glycaemic response and maximum glycogen replenishment. Use the sample eating plans in Table 15.2 as a basis for developing your own plan during the pre-competition week. While they provide the requirements for carbohydrate prior to competition, they are low in fat and protein and are not ideal for the rest of the season.

Check:

- Make sure that you rehydrate fully after training. *See* pp. 146–154 to calculate how much fluid you should consume before and after training. Check your hydration status by monitoring the frequency, volume and colour of your urine during the pre-competition week.

- Avoid any new or untried foods or food combinations during the pre-competition week.
- If you will be travelling or staying away from home, be prepared to take food with you. Try to find out beforehand what type of food will be available at the event venue and predict any nutritional shortfalls.

WHAT IS THE BEST WAY TO MAKE WEIGHT FOR MY COMPETITION?

For weight-class sports such as boxing, judo, mixed martial arts, lightweight rowing and bodybuilding, it is an advantage to be as close as possible to the upper limit of your weight category. However, this should not be achieved at the expense of losing lean tissue (by rapid and severe dieting), depleting your glycogen stores (by starving) or dehydration (by fluid restriction, saunas, sweatsuits, diuretics). The principles for making weight for competition are similar to those for weight loss. In summary:

- Set a realistic and achievable goal.
- Allow enough time – aim to lose 0.5 kg body fat per week. This is crucial to your strategy and *cannot be overemphasised*. You must plan to begin 'making weight' many weeks before your event and *not* at the last minute, as is often the case.
- Monitor your weight and body composition by skinfold thickness measurements and girth measurements (*see* Chapter 8, p. 168–70).
- Reduce your calorie intake by 15% and never eat less than your resting metabolic rate (*see* Chapter 16, pp. 289–93).
- Increase the amount and frequency of aerobic training.
- Adjust your carbohydrate intake according to your training load, eating less on days

Table 15.2	PRE-COMPETITION SAMPLE EATING PLANS	
	Providing 500 g carbohydrate	**Providing 700 g carbohydrate**
Breakfast	1 large bowl (85 g) breakfast cereal	4 thick slices toast with honey
	200 ml skimmed milk	1 glass (200 ml) fruit juice
	2 tbsp (60 g) raisins	1 banana
	1 glass (200 ml) fruit juice	
Morning snack	1 banana sandwich (2 slices bread and 1 banana)	2 scotch pancakes
		2 apples
Lunch	1 large jacket potato (300 g)	1 large bowl (125 g uncooked weight) rice salad with 60 g turkey or 125 g beans and vegetables
	3 tbsp (90 g) sweetcorn and 1 tbsp (50 g) tuna or cottage cheese	2 slices bread
	2 pieces fresh fruit	
	1 carton low fat fromage frais	2 pieces fruit
Pre-workout snack	1 energy bar	2 bananas
Workout	1 litre sports drink	1litre sports drink
Post-workout snack	500 ml milk	2 cereal bars
		1 carton (500 ml) flavoured milk
Dinner	1 bowl (85 g uncooked weight) pasta	2 large (2 × 300 g) jacket potatoes
	125 g stir-fried vegetables	100g chicken or fish
	60 g stir-fried chicken or tofu	Broccoli or other vegetable
	2 slices bread and butter	1 piece fresh fruit
	1 large bowl (200 g) fruit salad	
Snack	2 slices toast with honey	1 carton (200 g) low fat rice pudding
	1 carton low fat yoghurt	

when you perform lower intensity or shorter workouts.

- Adjust fat intake to achieve a 15% calorie deficit.
- Minimise muscle loss by consuming approximately 1.8–2.7 g protein/kg BW/day and at least 0.25 g protein/kg BW/meal.

Avoid rapid weight loss by starvation or dehydration just before your competition, as this can be dangerous. Rapid weight loss leads to depleted glycogen stores, so you will be unable to perform at your best. Dehydration leads to electrolyte disturbances, cramp and heartbeat irregularities. It is doubtful whether you can refuel and rehydrate sufficiently between the weigh-in and your competition, so aim to be at or within your weight category at least a day before the weigh-in. If you find it very difficult to make weight without resorting to these dangerous methods, consider competing in the next weight category.

A major problem with increasing the carbohydrate content of your diet in the pre-competition week is that the extra carbohydrate, stored with an amount of water equivalent to 3 times its weight, can result in weight gain. While this extra glycogen is advantageous in most sports, it can be a disadvantage in weight-class sports where the cut-off weight is often reached by a whisker. Ideally, you should allow for an extra weight gain of up to 1 kg during the final week.

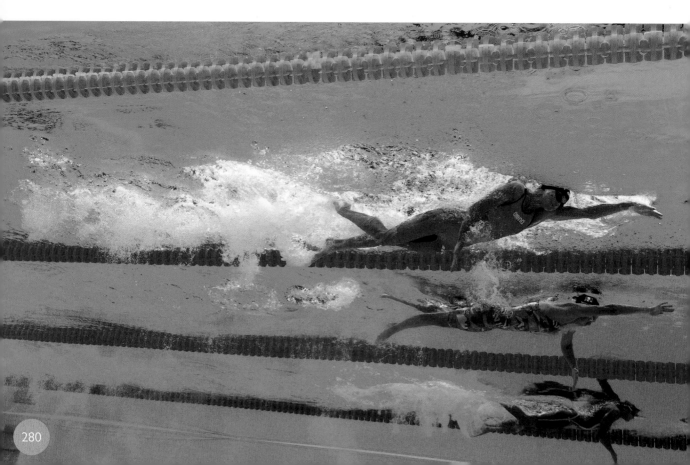

In other words, make weight in advance – aim to attain a weight at least 1 kg below your competing weight.

The day before

The day before your competition your main aims are:

1. to top up muscle glycogen levels
2. to ensure you are well hydrated.

Continue eating meals high in carbohydrate throughout the day and drinking plenty of fluids. To maximise muscle glycogen replenishment, perform only very light exercise or rest completely. Do not skip your evening meal, even if you experience pre-competition 'nerves', as this is an important time for topping up muscle glycogen. However, stick to familiar and simple foods, avoid fatty or oily foods and avoid alcohol, as it is a diuretic.

WHAT SHOULD I EAT WHEN I AM NERVOUS BEFORE COMPETITION?

Most athletes get pre-competition 'nerves' and this can reduce your appetite and result in problems such as nausea, diarrhoea and stomach cramps. If you find it difficult to eat solid food during this time, consume liquid meals such as meal replacement products (protein-carbohydrate sports supplements), sports drinks, milkshakes, yoghurt drinks and fruit smoothies. Try smooth, semi-liquid foods such as puréed fruit (e.g. apple purée, mashed banana, apple and apricot purée), yoghurt, porridge, custard and rice pudding. Bland foods such as semolina, mashed potato, or a porridge made from cornmeal or ground

rice may agree with your digestive system better. To reduce gastrointestinal problems, avoid high fibre foods such as bran cereals, dried fruit and pulses. You may wish to avoid vegetables that cause flatulence such as the brassica vegetables (cabbage, cauliflower, Brussels sprouts, broccoli). When you're nervous, caffeine can cause anxiety and problems such as diarrhoea so you may wish to avoid it the day before your competition. In essence, avoid anything that is new or unfamiliar. The golden rule with pre-competition eating is stick with tried and tested foods, which you know agree with you!

On the day

On the day of your competition, your aims are to:

1. top up liver glycogen stores following the overnight fast
2. maintain blood sugar levels
3. keep hunger at bay
4. keep well hydrated.

Plan to have your main pre-competition meal 2–4 hours before the event. This will allow enough time for your stomach to empty sufficiently and for blood sugar and insulin levels to normalise. It will also top up liver glycogen levels. Nervousness can slow down your digestion rate, so if you have pre-competition nerves you may need to leave a little longer than usual between eating and competing.

The actual timing of your pre-competition meal and the quantity of food eaten depends on the individual, despite the fact that studies recommend consuming 200–300 g carbohydrate during the 4 hours prior to exercise. The key is to find out what works for you and stick with it.

So, for example, if you are competing in the morning, you may need to get up a little earlier to eat your pre-competition breakfast. If your event is at 10.00 a.m., have your breakfast at 7.00 a.m. Some athletes skip breakfast, preferring to feel 'light' when they compete. However, it is not a good strategy to compete on an empty stomach, particularly if your event lasts longer than 1 hour or you will be competing in a number of heats. Low liver glycogen and blood sugar levels may reduce your endurance and result in early fatigue. As explained in Chapter 3, liver glycogen is important for maintaining blood sugar levels and supplying fuel to the exercising muscles when muscle glycogen is depleted.

If you are competing in the afternoon, have a substantial breakfast and schedule lunch approximately 2–4 hours before the competition. If you are competing in the evening, eat your meals at 3-hourly intervals during the day, again scheduling your last meal approximately 2–4 hours before competition.

WHAT SHOULD I EAT ON THE DAY OF MY COMPETITION?

Your pre-competition meal should be:

- based on low GI carbohydrates
- low in fat
- low or moderate in protein
- low or moderate in fibre
- not too bulky or filling
- not salty or spicy
- enjoyable and familiar
- easy to digest
- include a drink – approx. 500 ml 2 hours before the event.

Suitable types of meals are given in the box, 'Pre-competition meals'. Remember, you can reduce the GI of a meal by adding protein. If you really do not feel like eating, have a liquid meal or semi-liquid foods (*see* 'What should I eat when I am nervous before competition?' on p. 281).

Pre-competition meals

Pre-competition breakfasts
(2–4 hrs before event)
- Porridge with bananas
- Cereal with milk and dried fruit
- Toast or bread with jam/honey; low fat yoghurt
- Eggs on toast
- Meal replacement shake

Pre-competition lunches
(2–4 hrs before event)
- Sandwiches or rolls with tuna, cottage cheese or chicken; fresh fruit
- Pasta or rice with tomato-based sauce; fresh fruit
- Baked potato with low fat filling; fresh fruit

Pre-competition snacks
(1 hr before event)
- Smoothie
- Fruit and nut bar or granola bar
- Fresh or dried fruit
- Energy bar
- Low fat fruit yoghurt
- Rice cakes with peanut butter
- Mini (Scotch) pancakes

SHOULD I EAT OR DRINK JUST BEFORE MY COMPETITION?

Consume your pre-event meal 2–4 hours before the start of the event. This will provide a sustained supply of energy, maintain blood sugar levels during the event (particularly during the latter stages), and delay fatigue. Aim to consume about 2.5 g carbohydrate/kg body weight. Most athletes find that low GI foods avoid any risk of hypoglycaemia at the start of the competition. However, make sure that you have rehearsed your eating strategy plenty of times during training before the event. Do not try anything new on the day of competition. The timing is fairly individual, so experiment in training first!

You should also make sure that you are well hydrated before the competition (check the colour of your urine!) and aim to drink a further 125–250 ml fluid about 15–30 minutes before the event. Carry a drink bottle with you at all times.

SHOULD I EAT OR DRINK DURING MY COMPETITION?

If you are competing for more than about 60 minutes, you may find that extra carbohydrate will help delay fatigue and maintain your performance, particularly in the latter stages.

Depending on your exercise intensity and duration, aim to take in 30–60 g carbohydrate per hour. Start consuming the food or drink after about 30 minutes and continue at regular intervals, as it takes approximately 30 minutes for digestion and absorption.

If your glycogen stores are low at the start of the event (which hopefully they are not!), then consuming additional carbohydrate during the event will have a fairly immediate effect on your performance.

Any carbohydrate with a high or moderate GI would be suitable, but you may find liquids easier to consume than solids. Isotonic sports drinks or carbohydrate (maltodextrin) drinks are popular because they serve to replenish fluid losses and prevent dehydration as well as supplying carbohydrate. Avoid high fructose drinks because they are not absorbed as fast as sucrose, glucose and glucose polymers. They may also cause stomach cramps or diarrhoea. Recommended quantities of isotonic drinks for different types of events are given in Table 15.3.

In events lasting more than 2.5 hours, it may be beneficial to increase carbohydrate intake to up to 90 g per hour. This may be in the form of dual energy source drinks or gels, containing a mixture of glucose/maltodextrin and fructose to achieve faster carbohydrate absorption.

Table 15.3	RECOMMENDED QUANTITY OF A 6% ISOTONIC DRINK DURING EXERCISE (60 G GLUCOSE/SUCROSE/GLUCOSE POLYMER DISSOLVED IN 1 LITRE WATER)		
Moderate intensity (30 g carbohydrate/h)		**Moderate–high intensity (45 g carbohydrate/h)**	**High intensity (60 g carbohydrate/h)**
500 ml/h		750 ml/h	1000 ml/h

Table 15.4	FOODS SUITABLE TO EAT BETWEEN HEATS OR IMMEDIATELY AFTER EVENTS	
Sports drink	Milk-based drink or meal replacement shake
Bananas	Breakfast cereal
Dried fruit bar or energy bar	Granola bars or flapjack
Sandwiches or rolls	Oatcakes or rice cakes
Fresh or dried fruit	Home-made muffins and bars – *see* recipes on pp. 333–37
Smoothie	Yoghurt drink

(Accompany solid foods with sufficient water to replace fluid losses)

Drink to thirst or follow the drinking strategy you used in training, although you should be prepared to adjust this according to the temperature and humidity.

If you are competing in certain events such as cycling, sailing, distance canoeing or running, you may be able to take solid foods with you or arrange pick-up points. Suitable foods include energy bars, dried-fruit bars, cereal bars, bananas, gels, granola bars or raisins. If you are competing in matches and tournaments (e.g. football, tennis), take suitable snacks and drinks for the intervals and position them close by.

WHAT TO EAT BETWEEN HEATS OR EVENTS?

If you compete in several heats or matches during the day, it's important to refuel and rehydrate as fast as possible so that you have a good chance of performing well in your next competition. Consume 1–1.2 g carbohydrate/kg body weight during the 2-hour post-exercise period (muscle glycogen replenishment is faster during this time). If you've only a few hours between heats, you may prefer liquid meals such as meal replacement products, sports drinks and milk-based drinks. These will help replace both glycogen and fluid. If you are able to eat solid food, choose carbohydrates with a high GI that you find easy to digest and that are not too filling. Suitable foods are listed in Table 15.4. Take these with you in your kit bag. Drink fluid immediately after competing and continue drinking at regular intervals to replace fluid losses.

WHAT TO EAT AFTER COMPETITION?

After your competition, your immediate aims are to replenish glycogen stores and fluid losses. If you are competing the following day or within the next few days, your post-event food intake is crucial. Again, choose foods with a moderate or high GI to ensure rapid refuelling, and aim for 1–1.2 g carbohydrate per kg body weight during the 2–6-hour post-exercise period. Consuming protein (in 15–25 g servings) in the recovery period also promotes glycogen recovery and

Gastrointestinal problems in athletes

Gastrointestinal (GI) problems and transit troubles are common among athletes, especially when competing. It is estimated that 30 to 50% of endurance athletes experience exercise-related GI problems, such as abdominal pain and cramping, belching, bloating, nausea, heartburn, flatulence, urge to defecate, bowel movements, diarrhoea and vomiting (de Oliveira et al., 2014). In cases of extreme frequency or discomfort, this is known as runners' diarrhoea or 'runners' trots'. In a study at Maastricht University, The Netherlands, 91% of triathletes had at least one GI symptom, of which 29% were serious enough to affect performance (Jeukendrup et al., 2000).

GI problems are more common in running-type sports, possibly due to the physical 'jostling' of the intestines during running. All the food inside your GI tract gets shaken and loosened. The reduced blood flow in the intestines and increased levels of stress hormones (due to anxiety before competitions) affect gut motility and can further exacerbate the condition. And some people's guts are simply more sensitive than others.

Certain foods may irritate the gut, for example high intakes of fibre, fat, protein or fructose. Dehydration, or consuming a drink that is too concentrated in carbohydrate, can also add to the stress on the GI tract.

Exercise – specifically more exercise than your body is used to doing – increases intestinal activity.

Solutions

1. To help alleviate the problem, try doing a short run before the race or doing a warm-up loop around your house before a training run. Alternatively, having a little food before a morning run can help get things moving to enable you to empty your bowels before you head off. Experiment with training at different times of the day.

2. Reduce your intake of high fibre and gas-producing foods the day before as well as the day of the race. Common culprit foods include bran cereals, cruciferous vegetables (such as cabbage, cauliflower and broccoli), beans, lentils and caffeine. For some people, energy gels and bars can cause problems, as can high fructose foods and drinks. Fructose is absorbed relatively slowly from the gut and in high concentrations (especially in the form of a drink) can cause GI symptoms.

3. Start your workout or race fully hydrated. Some athletes avoid drinking in the misguided belief that it causes GI symptoms whereas, in fact, dehydration may be the culprit.

4. Make your sports drink more dilute. Some people find anything above 5 g/100 g sits in their stomach and causes discomfort.

5. Train your gut by regularly consuming carbohydrate foods or drinks during training. Start with very small amounts then gradually increase the amount and frequency. It is possible to increase the number of carbohydrate transporters in your gut so that you become better able to digest and absorb carbohydrate during exercise.

6. Find what works for you. It may take quite a bit of 'trial and error' but by practising your race fuelling and hydration strategy during training there will be less risk of problems on race day.

enhances muscle protein resynthesis. Any of the foods listed in Table 15.4 would be suitable. Drink fluid immediately after competing and continue drinking at regular intervals to replace fluid losses.

Your immediate post-event food should be followed by a carbohydrate-rich meal approximately 2 hours later. Suitable post-event meals include pasta, noodle, potato and rice dishes. Avoid rich or fatty meals (e.g. oily curries, chips, burgers), as these will delay refuelling and can make you feel bloated after competing. Don't forget to drink plenty of rehydrating fluid before embarking on that celebratory alcoholic drink! Rehydrate with 25–50% more fluid than that lost in sweat.

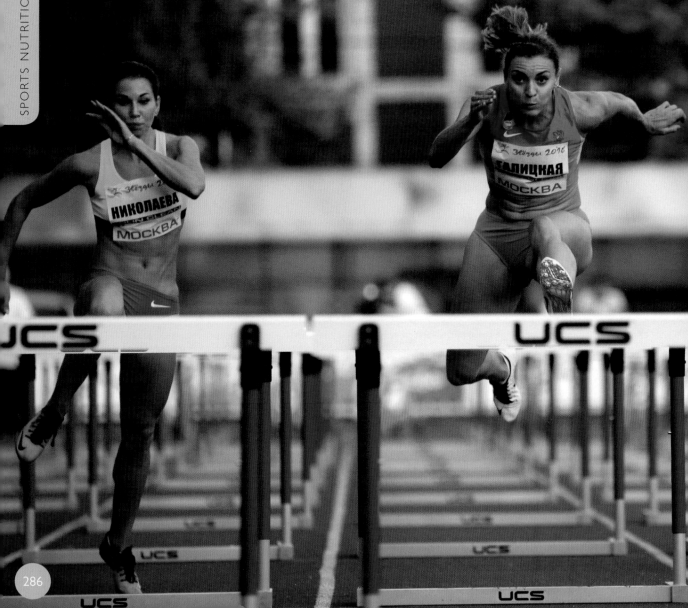

Summary of key points

Timing	Aims	Food and drink recommendations	Examples
The week before	1 Fill muscle glycogen stores	Taper training	• Pasta with fish or beans • Rice with chicken or tofu • Jacket potatoes with tuna or cottage cheese
	2 Maintain hydration	If carbohydrate loading, 10–12 g carbohydrate/kg BW/day for 36–48h pre-event	
		Low GI meals	
		Monitor fluid intake and urine	
The night before	1 Top up muscle glycogen 2 Maintain hydration	• High carbohydrate meal (low GI) • Plenty of fluid • Moderate–low fibre • Low fat • Familiar foods	• Pasta dish with tomato-based sauce • Rice or noodle dishes
2–4 hours before	1 Top up liver glycogen 2 Maintain hydration 3 Prevent hunger	• Low GI meal • High carbohydrate, low fat and low protein • Easily digestible • 400–600 ml fluid	• Porridge or cereal and low fat milk • Bread, toast, sandwiches, rolls • Potato with tuna or cottage cheese
1 hour before	1 Maintain blood sugar	1 g carbohydrate/kg body weight	Sports drink
	2 Maintain hydration	Easy to digest	• Banana • Smoothie • Energy or dried fruit bar • Dried fruit
15–30 min before	1 Maintain hydration	Up to 150 ml fluid	• Water • Sports drink
During events lasting < 75 min	Offset fluid losses	• None • Carbohydrate mouth rinse	• Water • Sports drink

Timing	Aims	Food and drink recommendations	Examples
During events lasting 1–2.5 h	1 Maintain blood sugar 2 Offset fluid losses	• 30–60 g carbohydrate/ hour • High or moderate GI	• Sports drinks • Energy bars or gels with water • Dried fruit, bananas
During events lasting > 2.5 h		• Up to 90 g carbohydrate/h • High or moderate GI • 150–350 ml fluid every 15–20 min	• Dual energy source drinks
Between heats or events	1 Replenish muscle and liver glycogen 2 Replace fluid	• 1–1.2 g/kg body weight within 2 hours • High GI carbohydrate	• Sports drink • Milk-based drink
		500 ml fluid immediately after	• Fresh or dried fruit • Rice cakes, energy bars,
		Continue fluids	Bananas
Post-competition	1 Replenish muscle and liver glycogen	1–1.2g/kg body weight within 2 hours	• Water • Sports drinks
	2 Replace fluid	High GI carbohydrate	Energy bars
		25–50% more fluid than that lost in sweat	Pasta, rice, potato or noodle dishes

Your personal
//nutrition plan

16

Nutrition scientists have provided general guidelines for the amounts of nutrients athletes should consume to optimise their performance. Tailoring this information to suit your specific goals is the next critical step. Your nutritional requirements depend on many factors, including your body weight, your body composition, the energy demands of your training programme, your daily activity levels, your health status and your individual metabolism.

This chapter provides a summary of the macronutrient recommendations for athletes and gives a step-by-step guide to calculating your individual calorie, carbohydrate, protein and fat needs. Some of the calculations have been detailed previously in other chapters but are amalgamated here to help you devise your personal nutrition plan.

To help guide you through, sample calculations are shown for a 30-year-old male athlete, who measures 1.78 m, weighs 70 kg, leads a moderately active lifestyle and does 1 hour high intensity training (cycling 14–16 km/hour) per day.

1: ESTIMATE YOUR CALORIE NEEDS

Your daily calorie needs will depend on your genetic make-up, age, weight, body composition, your daily activity and your training programme.

Table 16.1	SUMMARY OF SPORTS NUTRITION MACRONUTRIENT GUIDELINES
Macronutrient	**Daily guideline**
Carbohydrate	3–5 g/kg BW for low intensity training days 5–7 g/kg BW for moderate intensity training days (approx. 1 h) 6–10 g/kg BW for moderate to high endurance training (1–3 h) 8–12 g/kg BW for high intensity training (> 4 h) or fuelling up for an endurance event
Protein	1.2–2.0 g/kg BW 0.25 g/kg BW/meal 0.25 g/kg BW post-training
Fat	20–35% of daily energy

Equations for estimating RMR

Several equations have been developed to estimate RMR from body weight. The classic equations of Harris and Benedict, developed in the early 1900s, have been frequently used, but have been superseded by newer equations, such as the Mifflin-St Jeor equation, which uses an individual's weight, height and age (Mifflin et al., 1990). Studies comparing various predictive equations for RMR have found the Mifflin-St Jeor to be the most accurate (Frankenfield et al., 2005). However, the Mifflin-St Jeor equation does not account for exercise or make any adjustment for body composition, so applies to people with average body composition.

Step 1: Estimate your resting metabolic rate (RMR)

Your RMR is an estimate of how many calories you would burn if you were to do nothing but rest for 24 hours. It represents the minimum amount of energy needed to keep your body functioning, including breathing and keeping your heart beating. It can be estimated using the Mifflin-St. Jeor equation.

Men

$10 \times$ weight (kg) $+ 6.25 \times$ height (cm) $- 5 \times$ age (y) $+ 5$

Women

$10 \times$ weight (kg) $+ 6.25 \times$ height (cm) $- 5 \times$ age (y) $- 161$.

Table 16.2	SUMMARY OF FLUID INTAKE GUIDELINES
Before exercise	• Ensure you are fully hydrated. • Drink 5–10 ml/kg BW of fluid slowly in the 2 to 4 hours before exercise to promote hydration and allow enough time for excretion of excess water. That's equivalent to 300–600 ml for a 60 kg person, or 350–700 ml for a 70 kg person.
During exercise	• Drink according to thirst. • For most athletes and events, an intake of 400–800 ml/hour prevents dehydration as well as overhydration. • For most exercise lasting 1 hour or less, water is fine for replacing fluid losses. • For high intensity exercise lasting more than 1 hour, a hypotonic or isotonic sports drink containing 40–80 g carbohydrate/litre may reduce fatigue and improve performance. • For high intensity exercise lasting 1–3 hours, consuming between 30 and 60 g carbohydrate/hour will help increase endurance. • For high intensity exercise lasting more than 3 hours, an intake of 90 g carbohydrate/hour is recommended. This should be provided by a mixture of glucose and fructose, e.g. dual source energy drinks.
After exercise	• Drink 1.2–1.5 litres for every 1 kg body weight lost as sweat during exercise.

Example for male athlete (70 kg, 178 cm):
RMR = (10 × 70) + (6.25 × 178) − (5 × 30) + 5 = 1668 kcal

Step 2: Calculate your daily energy expenditure

Estimate your physical activity level (PAL). This is the ratio of your overall daily energy expenditure to your RMR – a rough measure of your lifestyle activity.

- Mostly inactive or sedentary: 1.2
- Fairly active: 1.3
- Moderately active: 1.4
- Active: 1.5
- Very active: 1.7

Example for male athlete (moderately active):
Daily energy expenditure = 1668 × 1.4 = 2335 kcal

Step 3: Estimate the number of calories expended during exercise (see Table 16.3)

Example for male athlete (1 hour cycling, 14–16 km/hour):
Calories expended during exercise = 715 kcal

Step 4: Add figures from steps 2 and 3

This is the number of calories you need to maintain your body weight.

Example:
Maintenance calorie intake = 2335 + 715 = 3050 kcal

Then, if your aim is to:

- lose body fat/weight: reduce your calorie

Table 16.3	CALORIES EXPENDED DURING EXERCISE	
Sport		**kcal/ hour**
Aerobics (high impact)		500
Aerobics (low impact)		357
Badminton		250
Boxing (sparring)		643
Cycling (14–16 km/hour)		715
Cycling (10–12mph km/hour)		429
Judo, karate, kickboxing		715
Rowing machine, 100W (moderate)		500
Rowing machine, 200W (vigorous)		751
Running, 6mph (10min/mile)		715
Running, 8mph (7.5min/mile)		965
Rugby		715
Soccer		715
Swimming, crawl (fast)		786
Swimming, crawl (slow)		572
Tennis (singles)		572
Weight training		429

Source: Ainsworth et al., 2011.

intake by 15% – i.e. multiply your maintenance calories by 0.85 (85%).
Example: 3050 × 0.85 = 2593 kcal

- increase lean body weight/muscle: increase your calorie intake by 20% – i.e. multiply your maintenance calories by 1.2 (120%).
  Example: 3050 × 1.2 = 3660 kcal

2: CALCULATE YOUR CARBOHYDRATE REQUIREMENT

Calculate your carbohydrate requirement according to your activity level and body weight, using Table 16.1: Summary of Sports Nutrition Macronutrient Guidelines.

- For weight loss: as your calorie needs decrease by 15%, so should your usual carbohydrate intake.

- For weight gain: as your calorie needs increase by 20%, so should your usual carbohydrate intake.

Table 16.4 shows sample calculations for weight maintenance, fat loss and muscle gain for a 70 kg male athlete.

3: CALCULATE YOUR PROTEIN INTAKE

Your protein requirement is based on the following recommendations:

- Endurance training: 1.2–1.4 g/kg body weight/day

Table 16.4	CALORIE AND CARBOHYDRATE REQUIREMENTS FOR WEIGHT MAINTENANCE, FAT LOSS AND MUSCLE GAIN		
	Weight maintenance	Weight loss	Weight gain
Calorie requirement	3050	2593	3660
Carbohydrate requirement, g/kg BW	5–7 g	(5–7 g) × 0.85	(5–7 g) × 1.2
Example: 70 kg athlete Carbohydrate requirement, g/day	350–490 g	298–417 g	420–588 g

Table 16.5	PROTEIN REQUIREMENTS FOR WEIGHT MAINTENANCE, WEIGHT LOSS AND WEIGHT GAIN			
	Endurance training	Power & strength training	Weight loss	Weight gain
Protein, g/kg BW/day	1.2–1.4 g/kg BW	1.4–2.0 g/kg BW	1.8–2.7 g/kg BW	20% increase
Example: 70 kg athlete, g/day	84–98 g	98–140 g	126–189 g	101–118 g (endurance) 118–168 g (power & strength)

- Power and strength training: 1.4–2.0 g/kg body weight/day
- Weight loss: 1.8–2.7 g/kg body weight/ day
- Weight gain: 20% increase

Table 16.5 shows the calculations for estimating the protein requirements for different training and body composition goals.

4: CALCULATE YOUR FAT INTAKE

This is the balance left once you have calculated your carbohydrate and protein requirements. Use the following calculation:

- Carbohydrate calories = grams carbohydrate × 4
- Protein calories = grams protein × 4
- Fat calories = total daily calories – carbohydrate calories – protein calories
- Grams fat = fat calories ÷ 9

Table 16.6 shows the calculations for estimating the fat requirements for different training and body composition goals.

Meal plans

To help you plan your personal diet, here are 2 sets of daily meal plans, providing 2000 kcal, 2500 kcal, 3000 kcal, 3500 kcal, 4000 kcal, 4500 kcal and 5000 kcal for meat-eaters and vegetarians. Each meal plan is in line with the nutritional recommendations outlined in this chapter. Opt for the meal plan that most closely matches your calorie requirement and use it as a blueprint for devising your individual diet. Adapt the types and foods to suit your particular food preferences, and adjust portion sizes to suit your day-to-day training goals. For example, on low intensity training or recovery days you will need

Table 16.6	FAT REQUIREMENTS FOR WEIGHT MAINTENANCE, WEIGHT LOSS AND WEIGHT GAIN		
		Weight maintenance	Weight loss	Weight gain
A	Total daily calories	3050	2593	3660
B	Carbohydrate intake	420 g (350–490 g)	358 g (298–417 g)	504 g (420–588 g)
C	Average carbohydrate calories (B × 4)	1680	1432	2016
D	Average protein intake (endurance)	91 g (84–98 g)	158 g (126–189g)	110 g (101–118 g)
E	Protein calories (D × 4)	364	632	440
F	Fat calories (A – C – E)	1006	529	1204
	Fat intake (F × 9)	112 g	59 g	134 g

fewer calories and less carbohydrate than on high intensity training days, so adjust portion sizes accordingly. Similarly, when performing higher intensity or longer workouts you will need to eat larger portions. For meal ideas, *see* Chapter 17, which includes more than 50 recipes for all types of diets.

The macronutrient composition of each food has been listed to show its relative contribution of calories, protein, carbohydrate and fat to your daily totals. If you wish to carry out similar calculations for other foods and construct new meal plans, you may use a reputable set of food composition tables, an online nutrition calculator or a nutritional analysis software program (*see* Further Reading, p. 376)

Notes:

- For cooking and dressings, use oils rich in monounsaturated fats e.g. olive, rapeseed, flax, soya, walnut.
- Use spreads high in monounsaturates or poly-unsaturates, containing no hydrogenated or trans fatty acids.

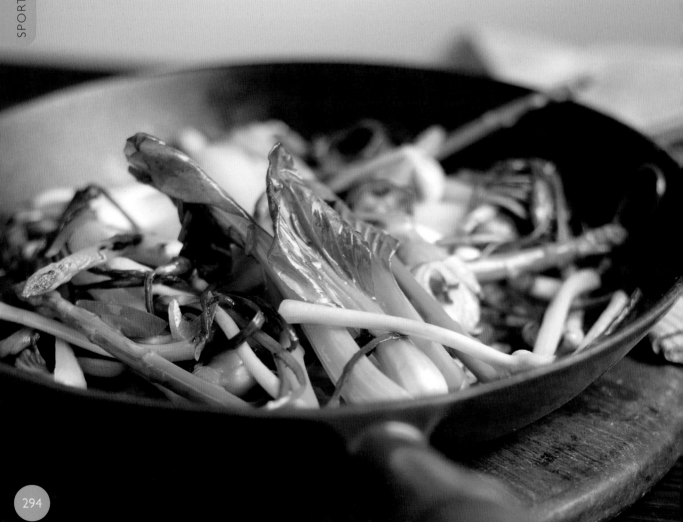

2000 KCAL MEAL PLAN

		Kcal	Protein (g)	Carbohydrate (g)	Fat (g)
Breakfast	2 clementines	65	1	13	0
	1 slice (40 g) wholegrain toast	95	4	16	1
	2 tsp (10 g) olive oil spread	57	0	0	6
	2 scrambled or poached eggs	148	12	0	11
Mid-morning	100 g 0% fat Greek yoghurt	57	10	4	0
	100 g strawberries	30	1	6	0
Lunch	50 g pasta	179	7	35	1
	75 g tuna in brine	75	18	0	1
	100 g chopped peppers	36	1	6	0
	100 g tomatoes	20	1	2	0
	1 tbsp (11 g) oil dressing	69	0	0	7
	1 pear	69	1	14	0
Mid-afternoon	25 g mixed nuts	149	7	3	12
Workout	Water	0	0	0	0
Post-workout	25 g whey protein	174	18	26	0
Dinner	100 g grilled turkey breast	155	35	0	2
	75 g rice noodles	249	4	58	0
	100 g kale	42	3	1	2
	100 g cauliflower	39	4	3	1
	150 g mango	98	1	20	0
Total		2037	122	256	51

2500 KCAL MEAL PLAN

		Kcal	Protein (g)	Carbohydrate (g)	Fat (g)
Breakfast	75 g oats	320	10	52	7
	300 ml skimmed milk	104	10	14	1
	100 g blueberries	68	1	15	0
Mid-morning	25 g almonds	158	6	2	14
	100 g low fat plain Greek yoghurt	98	8	9	4
Lunch	200 g baked potato	158	4	33	0
	10 g olive oil spread	57	0	0	6
	100 g tuna in brine	99	24	0	1
	Rocket salad	16	1	2	0
	15 g oil/vinegar dressing	69	0	0	7
	2 kiwi fruit	65	1	12	1
Mid-afternoon	1 Flapjack	265	5	24	16
Workout	Water	0	0	0	0
Post-workout	25 g whey	100	18	2	2
	300 ml skimmed milk	104	10	14	1
Dinner	125 g grilled chicken breast fillet	127	30	0	1
	75 g pasta	269	10	53	1
	1 tbsp (11 g) olive oil	99	0	0	11
	100 g broccoli	40	4	2	1
	100 g carrots	42	1	8	0
	30 g pasta sauce/tomato salsa	13	0	2	0
Evening	2 slices (80 g) wholemeal toast	190	8	32	2
	20 g peanut butter	124	5	3	10
Total		**2587**	**157**	**276**	**87**

3000 KCAL MEAL PLAN

		Kcal	Protein (g)	Carbohydrate (g)	Fat (g)
Breakfast	75 g oats	320	10	52	7
	300 ml semi-skimmed milk	140	10	13	5
	100 g blueberries	68	1	15	0
	1 slice (40 g) wholegrain toast	95	4	16	1
	10 g peanut butter	62	3	1	5
Mid-morning	25 g almonds	158	6	2	14
	100 g low-fat plain Greek yoghurt	98	8	9	4
	1 banana	99	1	22	0
Lunch	200 g baked potato or sweet potato	158	4	33	0
	10 g olive oil spread	57	0	0	6
	100 g tuna in brine	99	24	0	1
	Rocket salad	16	1	2	0
	15 g oil/vinegar dressing	69	0	0	7
	2 clementines	65	1	13	0
Mid-afternoon	1 Flapjack	265	5	24	16
Workout	Water	0	0	0	0
Post-workout	25 g whey	100	18	2	2
	300 ml semi-skimmed milk	140	10	13	5
	1 banana	99	1	22	0
Dinner	125 g grilled chicken breast fillet	127	30	0	1
	75 g pasta	269	10	53	1
	1 tbsp (11 g) olive oil	99	0	0	11
	100 g broccoli	40	4	2	1
	100 g carrots	42	1	8	0
	30 g pasta sauce/tomato salsa	13	0	2	0
Evening	2 slices (80 g) wholemeal toast	190	8	32	2
	20 g peanut butter	124	5	3	10
Total		3013	165	338	102

3500 KCAL MEAL PLAN

		Kcal	Protein (g)	Carbohydrate (g)	Fat (g)
Breakfast	75 g oats	320	10	52	7
	300 ml semi-skimmed milk	140	10	13	5
	25 g raisins	70	1	17	1
	100 g blueberries	68	1	15	0
	1 slice (40 g) wholegrain toast	95	4	16	1
	10 g peanut butter	62	3	1	5
Mid-morning	50 g mixed nuts and raisins	252	8	15	17
	100 g low fat plain Greek yoghurt	98	8	9	4
	1 banana	99	1	22	0
Lunch	200 g baked potato or sweet potato	158	4	33	0
	10 g olive oil spread	57	0	0	6
	100 g tuna in brine	99	24	0	1
	150 g sweetcorn	191	4	38	2
	Rocket salad	16	1	2	0
	15 g oil/vinegar dressing	69	0	0	7
	2 clementines	65	1	13	0
Mid-afternoon	1 Flapjack	265	5	24	16
Workout	500 ml isotonic sports drink	130	0	33	0
Post-workout	25 g whey	100	18	2	2
	300 ml semi-skimmed milk	140	10	13	5
	1 banana	99	1	22	0
Dinner	125 g grilled chicken breast fillet	127	30	0	1
	75 g pasta	269	10	53	1
	1 tbsp (11 g) olive oil	99	0	0	11
	100 g broccoli	40	4	2	1
	100 g carrots	42	1	8	0
	30 g pasta sauce/tomato salsa	13	0	2	0
Evening	2 slices (80 g) wholemeal toast	190	8	32	2
	20 g peanut butter	124	5	3	10
Total		**3500**	**172**	**438**	**107**

4000 KCAL MEAL PLAN

		Kcal	Protein (g)	Carbohydrate (g)	Fat (g)
Breakfast	100 g oats	427	13	69	9
	400 ml semi-skimmed milk	187	14	18	7
	25 g raisins	70	1	17	1
	100 g blueberries	68	1	15	0
	1 slice (40 g) wholegrain toast	95	4	16	1
	2 eggs	148	12	0	11
Mid-morning	50 g mixed nuts and raisins	252	8	15	17
	100 g low fat plain Greek yoghurt	98	8	9	4
	1 banana	99	1	22	0
Lunch	300 g baked potato or sweet potato	237	6	49	1
	20 g olive oil spread	114	0	0	13
	100 g tuna in brine	99	24	0	1
	150 g sweetcorn	191	4	38	2
	Rocket salad	16	1	2	0
	15 g oil/vinegar dressing	69	0	0	7
	2 clementines	65	1	13	0
Mid-afternoon	1 Flapjack	265	5	24	16
Workout	500 ml isotonic sports drink	130	0	33	0
Post-workout	25 g whey	100	18	2	2
	300 ml semi-skimmed milk	140	10	13	5
	1 banana	99	1	22	0
Dinner	125 g grilled chicken breast fillet	127	30	0	1
	75 g pasta	269	10	53	1
	1 tbsp (11 g) olive oil	99	0	0	11
	100 g broccoli	40	4	2	1
	100 g carrots	42	1	8	0
	30 g pasta sauce/tomato salsa	13	0	2	0
	150 g mango	98	1	20	0
Evening	2 slices (80 g) wholemeal toast	190	8	32	2
	20 g peanut butter	124	5	3	10
Total		**3973**	**192**	**496**	**123**

4500 KCAL MEAL PLAN

		Kcal	Protein (g)	Carbohydrate (g)	Fat (g)
Breakfast	100 g oats	427	13	69	9
	400 ml semi-skimmed milk	187	14	18	7
	25 g raisins	70	1	17	1
	100 g blueberries	68	1	15	0
	2 slices (80 g) wholegrain toast	190	8	32	2
	2 eggs	148	12	0	11
Mid-morning	50 g mixed nuts and raisins	252	8	15	17
	100 g low fat plain Greek yoghurt	98	8	9	4
	1 banana	99	1	22	0
	1 raw energy bar	173	5	13	11
Lunch	300 g baked potato or sweet potato	237	6	49	1
	20 g olive oil spread	114	0	0	13
	200 g tuna in brine	199	47	0	1
	150 g sweetcorn	191	4	38	2
	Rocket salad	16	1	2	0
	15 g oil/vinegar dressing	69	0	0	7
	2 clementines	65	1	13	0
Mid-afternoon	1 Flapjack	265	5	24	16
	25 g mixed nuts	149	7	3	12
Workout	500 ml isotonic sports drink	130	0	33	0
Post-workout	25 g whey	100	18	2	2
	300 ml semi-skimmed milk	140	10	13	5
	1 banana	99	1	22	0
Dinner	125 g grilled chicken breast fillet	127	30	0	1
	75 g pasta	269	10	53	1
	1 tbsp (11 g) olive oil	99	0	0	11
	150 g broccoli	59	7	3	1
	150 g carrots	63	1	11	1
	30 g pasta sauce/tomato salsa	13	0	2	0
	150 g mango	98	1	20	0
Evening	2 slices (80 g) wholemeal toast	190	8	32	2
	20 g peanut butter	124	5	3	10
Total		**4529**	234	532	148

5000 KCAL MEAL PLAN

		Kcal	Protein (g)	Carbohydrate (g)	Fat (g)
Breakfast	100 g oats	427	13	69	9
	400 ml semi-skimmed milk	187	14	18	7
	25 g raisins	70	1	17	1
	100 g blueberries	68	1	15	0
	2 slices (80 g) wholegrain toast	190	8	32	2
	2 eggs	148	12	0	11
Mid-morning	50 g mixed nuts and raisins	252	8	15	17
	100 g low fat plain Greek yoghurt	98	8	9	4
	1 banana	99	1	22	0
	1 energy bar	173	5	13	11
Lunch	300 g baked potato or sweet potato	237	6	49	1
	20 g olive oil spread	114	0	0	13
	200 g tuna in brine	199	47	0	1
	150 g sweetcorn	191	4	38	2
	Rocket salad	16	1	2	0
	15 g oil/vinegar dressing	69	0	0	7
	2 clementines	65	1	13	0
Mid-afternoon	2 Flapjacks	530	10	47	32
	25 g mixed nuts	149	7	3	12
Workout	500 ml isotonic sports drink	130	0	33	0
Post-workout	25 g whey	100	18	2	2
	300 ml semi-skimmed milk	140	10	13	5
	1 banana	99	1	22	0
Dinner	125 g grilled chicken breast fillet	127	30	0	1
	100 g pasta	359	13	71	2
	1 tbsp (11 g) olive oil	99	0	0	11
	150 g broccoli	59	7	3	1
	150 g carrots	63	1	11	1
	60 g pasta sauce/tomato salsa	27	1	5	0
	150 g mango	98	1	20	0
Evening	2 slices (80 g) wholemeal toast	190	8	32	2
	20 g peanut butter	124	5	3	10
	100 g low fat plain Greek yoghurt	98	8	9	4
Total		**4995**	**250**	**584**	**169**

2000 KCAL VEGETARIAN MEAL PLAN

		Kcal	Protein (g)	Carbohydrate (g)	Fat (g)
Breakfast	2 clementines	65	1	13	0
	1 slice (40 g) wholegrain toast	95	4	16	1
	2 tsp (10 g) olive oil spread	57	0	0	6
	2 scrambled or poached eggs	148	12	0	11
Mid-morning	100 g 0% fat Greek yoghurt	57	10	4	0
	100 g strawberries	30	1	6	0
Lunch	50 g pasta	179	7	35	1
	125 g mixed beans	144	11	17	3
	100 g chopped peppers	36	1	6	0
	100 g tomatoes	20	1	2	0
	1 tbsp (11 g) oil dressing	69	0	0	7
Mid-afternoon	25 g mixed nuts	149	7	3	12
Workout	Water	0	0	0	0
Post-workout	25 g whey protein	174	18	26	0
Dinner	Tofu with Noodles (recipe p. 322)	555	21	75	19
	100 g kale	42	3	1	2
	100 g cauliflower	39	4	3	1
	150 g mango	98	1	20	0
Total		**2010**	**89**	**251**	**68**

2500 KCAL VEGETARIAN MEAL PLAN

		Kcal	Protein (g)	Carbohydrate (g)	Fat (g)
Breakfast	75 g oats	320	10	52	7
	300 ml skimmed milk	104	10	14	1
	100 g blueberries	68	1	15	0
Mid-morning	25 g almonds	158	6	2	14
	100 g low fat plain Greek yoghurt	98	8	9	4
Lunch	200 g baked potato	158	4	33	0
	100 g cottage cheese or low fat soft cheese	100	12	3	4
	Rocket salad	16	1	2	0
	15 g oil/vinegar dressing	69	0	0	7
	2 kiwi fruit	65	1	12	1
Mid-afternoon	1 Flapjack	265	5	24	16
Workout	Water	0	0	0	0
Post-workout	25 g whey	100	18	2	2
	300 ml skimmed milk	104	10	14	1
Dinner	Chickpeas with Butternut Squash and Tomatoes (recipe p. 324)	342	15	48	10
	50 g pasta	179	7	35	1
	100 g broccoli	40	4	2	1
	100 g carrots	42	1	8	0
Evening	2 slices (80 g) wholemeal toast	190	8	32	2
	20 g peanut butter	124	5	3	10
Total		**2544**	**127**	**307**	**82**

3000 KCAL VEGETARIAN MEAL PLAN

		Kcal	Protein (g)	Carbohydrate (g)	Fat (g)
Breakfast	75 g oats	320	10	52	7
	300 ml semi-skimmed milk	140	10	13	5
	100 g blueberries	68	1	15	0
	1 slice (40 g) wholegrain toast	95	4	16	1
	10 g peanut butter	62	3	1	5
Mid-morning	25 g almonds	158	6	2	14
	100 g low fat plain Greek yoghurt	98	8	9	4
	1 banana	99	1	22	0
Lunch	200 g baked potato	158	4	33	0
	100 g cottage cheese or low fat soft cheese	100	12	3	4
	Rocket salad	16	1	2	0
	15 g oil/vinegar dressing	69	0	0	7
	2 clementines	65	1	13	0
Mid-afternoon	1 Flapjack	265	5	24	16
Workout	Water	0	0	0	0
Post-workout	25 g whey	100	18	2	2
	300 ml semi-skimmed milk	140	10	13	5
	1 banana	99	1	22	0
Dinner	Chickpeas with Butternut Squash and Tomatoes (recipe p. 324)	342	15	48	10
	75 g pasta	269	10	53	1
	100 g broccoli	40	4	2	1
	100 g carrots	42	1	8	0
Evening	2 slices (80 g) wholemeal toast	190	8	32	2
	20 g peanut butter	124	5	3	10
Total		**3060**	**139**	**387**	**97**

3500 KCAL VEGETARIAN MEAL PLAN

		Kcal	Protein (g)	Carbohydrate (g)	Fat (g)
Breakfast	75 g oats	320	10	52	7
	300 ml semi-skimmed milk	140	10	13	5
	100 g blueberries	68	1	15	0
	25 g raisins	70	1	17	1
	1 slice (40 g) wholegrain toast	95	4	16	1
	10 g peanut butter	62	3	1	5
Mid-morning	50 g mixed nuts and raisins	252	8	15	17
	100 g low fat plain Greek yoghurt	98	8	9	4
	1 banana	99	1	22	0
Lunch	200 g baked potato	158	4	33	0
	100 g cottage cheese or low fat soft cheese	100	12	3	4
	150 g sweetcorn	191	4	38	2
	Rocket salad	16	1	2	0
	15 g oil/vinegar dressing	69	0	0	7
	2 clementines	65	1	13	0
Mid-afternoon	1 Flapjack	265	5	24	16
Workout	500 ml isotonic sports drink	130	0	33	0
Post-workout	25 g whey	100	18	2	2
	300 ml semi-skimmed milk	140	10	13	5
	1 banana	99	1	22	0
Dinner	Chickpeas with Butternut Squash and Tomatoes (recipe p. 324)	342	15	48	10
	75 g pasta	269	10	53	1
	100 g broccoli	40	4	2	1
	100 g carrots	42	1	8	0
Evening	2 slices (80 g) wholemeal toast	190	8	32	2
	20 g peanut butter	124	5	3	10
Total		3546	145	487	102

4000 KCAL VEGETARIAN MEAL PLAN

		Kcal	Protein (g)	Carbohydrate (g)	Fat (g)
Breakfast	100 g oats	427	13	69	9
	400 ml semi-skimmed milk	187	14	18	7
	100 g blueberries	68	1	15	0
	25 g raisins	70	1	17	1
	1 slice (40 g) wholegrain toast	95	4	16	1
	2 eggs	148	12	0	11
Mid-morning	50 g mixed nuts and raisins	252	8	15	17
	100 g low fat plain Greek yoghurt	98	8	9	4
	1 banana	99	1	22	0
Lunch	300 g baked potato or sweet potato	237	6	49	1
	20 g olive oil spread	114	0	0	13
	100 g cottage cheese or low fat soft cheese	100	12	3	4
	150 g sweetcorn	191	4	38	2
	Rocket salad	16	1	2	0
	15 g oil/vinegar dressing	69	0	0	7
	2 clementines	65	1	13	0
Mid-afternoon	1 Flapjack	265	5	24	16
Workout	500 ml isotonic sports drink	130	0	33	0
Post-workout	25 g whey	100	18	2	2
	300 ml semi-skimmed milk	140	10	13	5
	1 banana	99	1	22	0
Dinner	Chickpeas with Butternut Squash and Tomatoes (recipe p. 324)	342	15	48	10
	75 g pasta	269	10	53	1
	100 g broccoli	40	4	2	1
	100 g carrots	42	1	8	0
Evening	2 slices (80 g) wholemeal toast	190	8	32	2
	20 g peanut butter	124	5	3	10
Total		**3978**	164	524	124

4500 KCAL VEGETARIAN MEAL PLAN

		Kcal	Protein (g)	Carbohydrate (g)	Fat (g)
Breakfast	100 g oats	427	13	69	9
	400 ml semi-skimmed milk	187	14	18	7
	100 g blueberries	68	1	15	0
	25 g raisins	70	1	17	1
	2 slices (80 g) wholegrain toast	190	8	32	2
	2 eggs	148	12	0	11
Mid-morning	50 g mixed nuts and raisins	252	8	15	17
	100 g low fat plain Greek yoghurt	98	8	9	4
	1 banana	99	1	22	0
	1 energy bar	173	5	13	11
Lunch	300 g baked potato or sweet potato	237	6	49	1
	20 g olive oil spread	114	0	0	13
	100 g cottage cheese or low fat soft cheese	100	12	3	4
	150 g sweetcorn	191	4	38	2
	Rocket salad	16	1	2	0
	15 g oil/vinegar dressing	69	0	0	7
	2 clementines	65	1	13	0
Mid-afternoon	2 Flapjacks	530	10	47	32
Workout	500 ml isotonic sports drink	130	0	33	0
Post-workout	25 g whey	100	18	2	2
	300 ml semi-skimmed milk	140	10	13	5
	1 banana	99	1	22	0
Dinner	Chickpeas with Butternut Squash and Tomatoes (recipe p. 324)	342	15	48	10
	75 g pasta	269	10	53	1
	100 g broccoli	40	4	2	1
	100 g carrots	42	1	8	0
Evening	2 slices (80 g) wholemeal toast	190	8	32	2
	20 g peanut butter	124	5	3	10
Total		**4511**	**178**	**577**	**153**

5000 KCAL VEGETARIAN MEAL PLAN

		Kcal	Protein (g)	Carbohydrate (g)	Fat (g)
Breakfast	100 g oats	427	13	69	9
	400 ml semi-skimmed milk	187	14	18	7
	100 g blueberries	68	1	15	0
	25 g raisins	70	1	17	1
	2 slices (80 g) wholegrain toast	190	8	32	2
	2 eggs	148	12	0	11
Mid-morning	50 g mixed nuts and raisins	252	8	15	17
	100 g low fat plain Greek yoghurt	98	8	9	4
	1 banana	99	1	22	0
	1 energy bar	173	5	13	11
Lunch	300 g baked potato or sweet potato	237	6	49	1
	20 g olive oil spread	114	0	0	13
	200 g cottage cheese or low fat soft cheese	200	25	6	9
	150 g sweetcorn	191	4	38	2
	Rocket salad	16	1	2	0
	15 g oil/vinegar dressing	69	0	0	7
	2 clementines	65	1	13	0
Mid-afternoon	2 Flapjacks	530	10	47	32
	25 g mixed nuts	149	7	3	12
Workout	500 ml isotonic sports drink	130	0	33	0
Post-workout	25 g whey	100	18	2	2
	300 ml semi-skimmed milk	140	10	13	5
	1 banana	99	1	22	0
Dinner	Chickpeas with Butternut Squash and Tomatoes (recipe p. 324)	342	15	48	10
	25 g Cheddar cheese	103	6	0	9
	75 g pasta	269	10	53	1
	100 g broccoli	40	4	2	1
	100 g carrots	42	1	8	0
	150 g mango	98	1	20	0
Evening	2 slices (80 g) wholemeal toast	190	8	32	2
	20 g peanut butter	124	5	3	10
	100 g low-fat plain Greek yoghurt	98	8	9	4
Total		**5059**	**212**	**611**	**182**

//The recipes

17

Breakfasts

FRUIT MUESLI

Serves 4
175 g (6 oz) oats
300 ml (½ pint) milk
40 g (1½ oz) sultanas
40 g (1½ oz) toasted flaked almonds, chopped
    hazelnuts or cashews
225 g (8 oz) fresh fruit, e.g. bananas,
    blueberries, strawberries, raspberries
1 apple, peeled and grated
1 tbsp honey

- In a large bowl, mix together the oats, milk, sultanas and nuts. Cover and leave overnight in the fridge.
- Just before serving, stir in the fruit, grated apple and honey. Spoon into cereal bowls.

Nutritional information (per serving):
Calories = 329; protein = 11 g;
carbohydrate = 52 g; fat = 10 g;
fibre = 6 g

ATHLETE'S PORRIDGE

Serves 1
50 g (2 oz) porridge oats
350 ml (12 fl oz) milk
1 banana, sliced
25 g (1 oz) dried fruit e.g. raisins, dates or figs

- Mix the oats and milk in a saucepan. Bring to the boil and simmer for approx 5 minutes, stirring frequently.
- Top with the banana and dried fruit.

Nutritional information (per serving):
Calories = 476; protein = 20 g;
carbohydrate = 85 g; fat = 5 g;
fibre = 5 g

BREAKFAST MUFFINS

Makes 8 muffins
125 g (4 oz) self-raising flour
125 g (4 oz) oatmeal
25 g (1 oz) butter or margarine
40 g (1½ oz) soft brown sugar
1 egg
150 ml (5 fl oz) milk
50 g (2 oz) chopped dates or raisins

- Preheat the oven to 220°C/425°F/Gas mark 7.
- Mix the flour and oatmeal together in a bowl.
- Add the butter, sugar, egg and milk. Mix well.
- Stir in the dried fruit.
- Spoon into a non-stick muffin tray and bake for approx 15 minutes until golden brown.

YOGHURT WITH DRIED FRUIT COMPOTE

Serves 4
Zest and juice of 1 orange
2 tbsp (30 ml) acacia honey
300 ml (½ pint) water
150 ml (5 fl oz) orange juice
75 g (3 oz) ready-to-eat dried figs, halved
75 g (3 oz) ready-to-eat dried apricots
75 g (3 oz) ready-to-eat pitted prunes
450 ml (¾ pint) whole-milk or Greek-style yoghurt

- Combine the orange zest and freshly squeezed juice, honey, water and orange juice in a saucepan.
- Bring the mixture to the boil, stirring until the honey is dissolved, then add the dried fruit and simmer, covered, for about 15 minutes until the fruit becomes plump and soft. Allow to cool and keep covered in the fridge until you are ready to serve.
- Divide the yoghurt between 4 bowls. Top with the fruit compote.

Nutritional information (per serving):
Calories = 189; protein = 5 g;
carbohydrate = 33 g; fat = 5 g;
fibre = 2 g

Nutritional information (per serving):
Calories = 223; protein = 9 g;
carbohydrate = 41 g; fat = 4 g;
fibre = 4 g

GREEK YOGHURT WITH BANANA AND HONEY

Serves 2

2 bananas

300 g (11 oz) Greek-style bio-yoghurt

1–2 level tbsp honey (to taste)

2 tbsp toasted flaked almonds (or walnuts, hazelnuts or pecans)

- Slice the bananas into two bowls. Spoon half the yoghurt on top of each bowl. Drizzle with honey and scatter over the toasted nuts.

Main meals

SALMON AND VEGETABLE PASTA

Serves 2

175 g (6 oz) pasta

175 g (6 oz) salmon steak

1 red pepper, deseeded and chopped

1 courgette, sliced

1 garlic clove, crushed

75 g (3 oz) cherry tomatoes

1 tbsp olive oil

A handful of rocket

- Cook the pasta according to the pack instructions, adding the salmon to the pan 6 minutes before the end of the cooking time.
- Heat the oil in a pan, and cook the pepper, courgette and garlic for 5 minutes until they start to soften.
- When the pasta is cooked, remove the salmon, then drain the pasta. Fork the salmon into large chunks and add to the vegetables along with the pasta, olive oil and rocket. Toss together, then serve.

Nutritional information (per serving):
Calories = 368; protein = 12 g;
carbohydrate = 43 g; fat = 18 g;
fibre = 2 g

Nutritional information (per serving):
Calories = 570; protein = 31 g;
carbohydrate = 69 g; fat = 18 g;
fibre = 6 g

FISH TAGINE WITH CHICKPEAS

Serves 2

1 tbsp light-in-colour olive oil
1 onion, chopped
1 garlic clove, crushed
½ tsp each of ground cumin, coriander,
    cinnamon and turmeric
2 small potatoes, peeled and cut into quarters
300 ml (10 fl oz) fish or chicken stock
75 g (3 oz) cherry tomatoes, halved
1 tbsp ground almonds
½ tin (200 g/7 oz) chickpeas, drained
300 g (10 oz) white fish, cut into chunks
125 g (4 oz) baby spinach
25 g (1 oz) flaked almonds
Squeeze of lemon juice
A handful of fresh coriander, chopped
Greek yoghurt, to serve

- Heat the oil in a large pan. Add the onion and cook for a few minutes until soft. Add the garlic and spices and cook for a few minutes more.
- Add the potatoes, stock, tomatoes, ground almonds and chickpeas. Simmer for 10 minutes, then add the fish. Cover and simmer on a low heat for 2–3 minutes until just cooked. Stir in the spinach, allow to wilt for 1–2 minutes, then add a squeeze of lemon juice and the coriander and scatter with the flaked almonds.
- Serve with plain Greek yogurt.

Nutritional information (per serving):
Calories = 598; protein = 46 g;
carbohydrate = 49 g; fat = 21 g;
fibre = 14 g

QUINOA AND CHICKEN SALAD WITH BEETROOT YOGURT

Serves 2

125 g (4oz) quinoa
1 small cooked beetroot, finely chopped
2 tbsp plain Greek yogurt
1 garlic clove, crushed
2 skinless cooked chicken breasts, shredded
½ red onion, chopped
½ tin (200g/7oz) flageolet beans (or other
    variety of beans)
2 tomatoes, chopped
100g (3½ oz) spinach, watercress and rocket
    salad leaves
Salt and freshly ground black pepper

- Cook the quinoa according to the pack instructions. Drain.
- Meanwhile mix the beetroot, yogurt and garlic with a little salt and freshly ground black pepper in a small bowl.
- In a large bowl, mix the quinoa, chicken, vegetables and beans. Serve with the beetroot yogurt.

Nutritional information (per serving):
Calories = 496; protein = 58 g;
carbohydrate = 58 g; fat = 6 g;
fibre = 9 g

CHICKEN AND BROCCOLI PASTA

Serves 2

175 g (6 oz) wholewheat pasta
150 g (5 oz) broccoli, cut into small florets
1–2 tbsp light-in-colour olive oil
2 skinless chicken breasts, cut into bite-sized chunks
1 garlic clove, crushed
150 g (5 oz) passata
1 tbsp tomato puree
75 g (3 oz) baby spinach
25 g (1 oz) flaked almonds, toasted

- Cook the pasta according to the pack instructions. Add the broccoli 3 minutes before the end of cooking.
- Meanwhile, fry the chicken in half the olive oil for 8–10 minutes or until cooked and golden.
- Heat the remaining olive oil, add the garlic and cook for 2 minutes, then stir in the passata and tomato puree. Simmer for 5 minutes.
- Drain the pasta and broccoli. Add to the pan with the tomato sauce then add the chicken, spinach and almonds. Allow the spinach to wilt, then serve.

Nutritional information (per serving):
Calories = 618; protein = 50 g;
carbohydrate = 62 g; fat = 16 g;
fibre = 14 g

CHICKEN AND VEGETABLE STIR FRY

Serves 2

1 tbsp light-in-colour olive oil
1 small onion, chopped
1 cm (½ inch) piece of fresh ginger, finely chopped
1 garlic clove, crushed
2 chicken thigh fillets, thinly sliced
1 red pepper, deseeded and thinly sliced
75 g (3 oz) green or white cabbage, shredded
A handful of beansprouts
1 courgette, sliced
1 tbsp soy sauce
2 nests of egg noodles

- Heat the oil in a wok or frying pan and fry the onion for 2 minutes. Add the ginger, garlic and chicken and stir-fry until the chicken is browned all over. Add the vegetables to the pan and stir-fry for 2–3 minutes until starting to soften.
- Stir in the soy sauce and a little water. Continue to stir-fry over a medium–high heat for 3–4 minutes, or until the chicken is cooked through.
- Cook the noodles according to the pack instructions. Add to the chicken and vegetables and stir to combine.

Nutritional information (per serving):
Calories = 497; protein = 29 g;
carbohydrate = 47 g; fat = 20 g;
fibre = 7 g

ONE-POT TURKEY AND CHICKPEA PILAU

Serves 2

1 tbsp light-in-colour olive oil
1 onion, chopped
1 leek, sliced
1 garlic clove, crushed
150 g (5 oz) turkey breast steaks, cut into
    1 cm (½ inch) strips
½ tin (200 g/7 oz) tinned tomatoes
½ tin (200 g/7 oz) chickpeas, drained
125 g (4 oz) brown rice
250 ml (9 fl oz) chicken stock
200 g (7 oz) broccoli, broken into florets
100 g (3½ oz) frozen peas
A handful of fresh coriander, chopped
Greek yoghurt, to serve

- Heat the oil in a large frying pan or flameproof casserole, add the onion, leek and garlic and cook gently for 5 minutes, stirring occasionally.
- Add the turkey, tomatoes, chickpeas, rice and stock. Bring to the boil, cover and cook on a low heat for 20 minutes, or until the rice has absorbed all the liquid. Stir in the broccoli and peas and continue to cook for 5 minutes, adding a little more water if necessary.
- Stir in the coriander and serve with a spoonful of plain Greek yoghurt.

Nutritional information (per serving):
Calories = 606; protein = 40 g; carbohydrate = 76 g; fat = 13 g; fibre = 17 g

MOROCCAN FISH STEW

Serves 4

225 g (8 oz) basmati rice
2 tbsp light-in-colour olive oil
1 red onion, finely chopped
2 garlic cloves, crushed
1 tsp freshly grated ginger
½ tsp each ground cinnamon and cumin
1 tbsp harissa paste
1 tbsp tomato puree
500 ml (16 fl oz) fish or vegetable stock
400 g (14 oz) tin chopped tomatoes
500 g (1 lb 2 oz) white fish fillets, cut into chunks
400 g (14 oz) tin cannellini beans, rinsed and drained

- Cook the rice according to the pack instructions.
- Meanwhile, heat the oil in a pan and fry the onion until soft. Add the garlic, ginger, spices, harissa and tomato puree and cook for 1 minute. Add the stock and tomatoes and bring to the boil. Cook for 10 minutes.
- Add the fish chunks and beans to the stew and continue cooking for 5 minutes. Serve with the cooked rice.

Nutritional information (per serving):
Calories = 471; protein = 40 g; carbohydrate = 58 g; fat = 8 g; fibre = 6 g

SPICY CHICKEN WITH RICE

Serves 2
2 chicken breasts (approx. 175 g/6 oz each)
175 g (6 oz) brown rice
2 tsp (10 ml) sunflower oil
1 onion, chopped
2 garlic cloves, crushed
1–2 tsp curry powder (to taste)
1 tbsp tomato purée
1 tbsp water
Green vegetables, to serve

- Cook the chicken breasts under a hot grill for 10–15 minutes, turning a few times.
- Boil the rice for 20–25 minutes until cooked. Drain.
- Meanwhile, heat the oil in a large non-stick pan and cook the onion for 5 minutes, until golden.
- Add the garlic and curry powder and cook for a further 2 minutes.
- Cut the chicken into chunks and add to the pan with the tomato purée and water.
- Cover and cook for a further 5–10 minutes.
- Serve with rice and green vegetables.

Nutritional information (per serving):
Calories = 657; protein = 58 g;
carbohydrate = 74 g; fat = 16 g;
fibre = 2 g

CHICKEN WITH BUTTERNUT SQUASH

Serves 4
400 g (14 oz) butternut squash
1 tbsp extra virgin olive oil
2 tbsp chopped fresh thyme (or 2 tsp dried thyme)
4 chicken breasts, on the bone
A little salt and freshly ground black pepper

- Heat the oven to 200°C/400°F/gas mark 6.
- Peel the butternut squash and cut the flesh into 5 mm (¼ inch) slices. Cover the base of a baking tin with the squash slices, drizzle over a little of the oil, then scatter with the thyme and season to taste.
- Place the chicken breasts over the squash, drizzle with the remaining olive oil and turn so that they are well coated with oil.
- Cook the chicken and the squash in the oven for 20–30 minutes, depending on the size of the chicken breasts, until the chicken is golden. The squash should be soft but not mushy.

Nutritional information (per serving):
Calories = 252; protein = 40 g;
carbohydrate = 8 g; fat = 7 g;
fibre = 2 g

MOROCCAN CHICKEN WITH RICE

Serves 1

1 skinless chicken breast

1 garlic clove, crushed

½ red chilli, deseeded and chopped (use according to taste)

A pinch of paprika

A pinch of ground cumin

Juice of ½ a lemon

1 tbsp chopped fresh mint leaves

75 g (3 oz) wholegrain rice

1 tbsp toasted pumpkin seeds

- Slash the chicken breast 3 or 4 times.
- Place the garlic, chilli, paprika, cumin, the juice of half the lemon and the chopped mint in a bowl and mix well. Add the chicken and turn a few times. Leave to marinate, ideally for 30 minutes.
- Meanwhile, boil the rice according to the pack instructions, approx 25 minutes. Drain and mix with the toasted pumpkin seeds.
- Preheat the grill. Place the chicken on a baking tray and grill for 6 or 7 minutes on each side, until cooked through.
- Spoon the rice on to a plate and place the chicken on top. Serve with green vegetables.

SALMON AND BEAN SALAD

Serves 4

150 g (5 oz) salad leaves

400 g (14 oz) can mixed beans, drained and rinsed

4 tbsp French dressing

2 tbsp chopped fresh parsley

200 g (7 oz) can wild red salmon, drained

200 g (7 oz) cherry tomatoes, halved

4 spring onions, chopped

Freshly ground black pepper

- Arrange the salad leaves on 4 plates.
- Mix the beans with the vinaigrette, parsley and freshly ground black pepper to taste.
- Remove the skin and bones from the salmon and lightly flake the flesh. Mix with the tomatoes, spring onions and the bean mixture. Heap on top of the salad leaves.

Nutritional information (per serving):
Calories = 545; protein = 48 g;
carbohydrate = 63 g; fat = 13 g;
fibre = 2 g

Nutritional information (per serving):
Calories = 219; protein = 17 g;
carbohydrate = 14 g; fat = 9 g;
fibre = 7 g

SWEET AND SOUR CHICKEN WITH MANGO

Serves 4
For the sweet and sour sauce:
4 tbsp water
2 tbsp each dry sherry, sesame oil and white wine vinegar
1 tbsp light soy sauce
2 tsp honey

1 large mango peeled and cubed
2 tbsp sunflower oil
4 chicken breast fillets, cut into 1 cm (½ inch) pieces
2 onions, sliced
250 g (9 oz) broccoli, divided into small florets
1 tsp grated fresh ginger
Basmati rice, to serve

- For the sauce, combine the water, sherry, sesame oil, vinegar, soy sauce and honey.
- Heat half the sunflower oil in a wok or large frying pan, add the chicken and quickly brown on all sides for 2–3 minutes. Transfer to a warm plate.
- Heat the remaining oil, add the onions and cook for 1–2 minutes until softened. Add the broccoli and ginger followed by the sauce and the mango.
- Bring to the boil and then simmer gently for 3 minutes. Return the chicken to the wok and continue to cook for a further 2–3 minutes until thoroughly cooked. Serve with basmati rice.

Nutritional information (per serving):
Calories = 255; protein = 23 g;
carbohydrate = 9 g; fat = 14 g;
fibre = 3 g

CHICKEN AND LENTIL SALAD

Serves 4
2 tbsp olive oil
4 chicken breast fillets, sliced
1 garlic clove, crushed
1 small onion, chopped
400 g (14 oz) can lentils, drained and rinsed
3–4 tomatoes, finely chopped
2 tbsp lemon juice
1 tbsp clear honey
2 tbsp roughly chopped fresh flat-leaf parsley

- Heat 1 tablespoon of the olive oil in a large frying pan over a high heat and sauté the chicken for 5–6 minutes or until cooked and there is no pink meat.
- Add the garlic, onion, lentils and tomatoes and cook, stirring, for about 2 minutes until heated.
- For the dressing, shake together the remaining olive oil with the lemon juice and honey in a bottle or screw-top jar.
- Stir the dressing and half the parsley into the lentils in the pan. Transfer to a serving dish, scatter over the remaining parsley and serve warm.

Nutritional information (per serving):
Calories = 347; protein = 45 g;
carbohydrate = 20 g; fat = 10 g;
fibre = 2 g

PILAFF WITH PLAICE

Serves 2
175 g (6 oz) brown rice
600 ml (1 pint) water
1 small onion, chopped
Pinch of turmeric (or mild curry powder)
1 courgette, sliced
1 small red pepper, deseeded and chopped
350 g (12 oz) plaice fillets, cut into strips
Salt and freshly ground black pepper
1 tbsp sunflower seeds (optional)

- Place the rice, water, onion and turmeric in a large saucepan.
- Bring to the boil, cover and simmer for 20 minutes.
- Add the courgette, red pepper and plaice and season to taste.
- Cook for a further 5 minutes or until the fish is cooked and the water absorbed.
- Scatter the sunflower seeds over before serving.

Nutritional information (per serving):
Calories = 530; protein = 40 g;
carbohydrate = 76 g; fat = 10 g;
fibre = 3 g

NOODLES WITH PRAWNS AND GREEN BEANS

Serves 2
225 g (8 oz) frozen or fresh whole green beans
175 g (6 oz) egg noodles
1 tsp sunflower oil
175 g (6 oz) peeled prawns
1 tbsp soy sauce

- Cook the green beans in a little boiling water for 5 minutes, then drain.
- Cook the noodles in a large pan for 10 minutes.
- Meanwhile, heat the oil in a wok or frying pan and stir-fry the prawns for 2 minutes.
- Add the beans, noodles and soy sauce, and heat through.

Nutritional information (per serving):
Calories = 483; protein = 32 g;
carbohydrate = 66 g; fat = 12 g;
fibre = 5 g

POTATO AND FISH PIE

Serves 2
450 g (1 lb) potatoes
200 g (7 oz) white fish fillets (e.g. cod or plaice)
3 tbsp skimmed milk
2 eggs
1 tbsp parsley
1 tbsp lemon juice
Green vegetables, to serve

- Cut the potatoes into chunks and boil until tender.
- Drain, then mash with the flaked fish, milk, eggs, parsley and lemon juice.
- Place in a dish, then cook either in microwave at full power for 5 minutes, or in oven at 200°C/400°F/gas mark 6 for 20 minutes.
- Serve with green vegetables.

Nutritional information (per serving):
Calories = 352; protein = 33 g;
carbohydrate = 39 g; fat = 8 g;
fibre = 3 g

Vegetarian main meals

BAKED EGGS WITH ROASTED MEDITERRANEAN VEGETABLES

Serves 2
½ aubergine, sliced
1 courgette, sliced
½ yellow pepper, sliced
½ red pepper, sliced
½ bulb of fennel, cut into wedges
1 small onion, sliced
1 tbsp olive oil
1 garlic clove, crushed
A few sprigs of rosemary
A handful of black olives
2 large eggs
Crusty bread, to serve

- Preheat the oven to 200°C/400°F/gas mark 6.
- Place all the vegetables in an ovenproof dish.
- Drizzle over the olive oil, add the garlic and rosemary, then toss lightly so that the vegetables are well coated in the oil. Roast in the oven for about 20 minutes, until the vegetables are just tender.
- Mix in the black olives. Make two wells in the middle of the vegetables. Crack an egg into each indentation. Bake for a further 8–10 minutes or until the eggs are set.
- Serve with crusty bread.

Nutritional information (per serving):
Calories = 201; protein = 10 g;
carbohydrate = 9 g; fat = 14 g;
fibre = 4 g

SWEET POTATO AND LENTIL CURRY

Serves 2
1 tbsp light-in-colour olive oil or rapeseed oil
1 small onion, chopped
1 garlic clove, crushed
½ tsp ground cumin
1 tsp ground coriander
½ tsp turmeric
100 g (3½ oz) red lentils
1 medium sweet potato, peeled and cut into chunks
250 ml (9 fl oz) vegetable stock
½ tin (200 g/7 oz) chopped tomatoes
50 g (2 oz) baby spinach
25 g (1 oz) cashew nuts, toasted
Juice of ½ lemon
Salt
Small handful of fresh coriander, finely chopped
Brown rice, to serve

- Heat the oil in a large pan, add the onion and cook for a few minutes until softened. Add the garlic and spices and cook for 1 minute more.
- Add the lentils, sweet potato, stock and chopped tomatoes. Bring to the boil, cover and simmer for 20 minutes until the lentils and sweet potatoes are tender. Then turn off the heat and stir in the spinach.
- Stir in the cashew nuts, lemon juice, salt to taste and coriander. Serve with cooked brown rice.

Nutritional information (per serving):
Calories = 414; protein = 18 g;
carbohydrate = 52 g; fat = 13 g fat;
fibre = 9 g

VEGETABLE TAGINE WITH CHICKPEAS

Serves 2
1 tbsp light-in-colour olive oil or rapeseed oil
1 small onion, thinly sliced
2 garlic cloves, thinly sliced
½ tsp each of ground coriander and cumin
1 sweet potato, peeled and cut into chunks
½ aubergine, cut into chunks
1 courgette, sliced
½ red pepper, seeds removed and chopped
½ tin (200 g/7 oz) tomatoes
1 tsp harissa paste
½ tin (200 g/7 oz) chickpeas, drained and rinsed
150 ml (5 fl oz) vegetable stock
50 g/2 oz ready-to-eat dried apricots, halved
A handful of fresh coriander, chopped
Couscous, to serve

- Heat the oil in a large non-stick pan. Add the onion and cook gently for 4–5 minutes, stirring occasionally, until softened. Add the garlic and spices and stir for a few moments. Add the vegetables and continue cooking for a few minutes, then add the tinned tomatoes, harissa paste, chickpeas, vegetable stock and apricots.
- Stir and bring to the boil. Cover then simmer for 15 minutes or until the vegetables are tender. Stir in the chopped coriander and serve with couscous.

Nutritional information (per serving):
Calories = 346; protein = 11 g;
carbohydrate = 49 g; fat = 9 g fat;
fibre = 15 g

VEGETARIAN SHEPHERD'S PIE WITH SWEET POTATO MASH

Serves 4

1 tbsp light-in-colour olive oil
1 onion, chopped
2 garlic cloves, crushed
4 carrots, chopped
1 red pepper, chopped
125 g (4 oz) mushrooms, sliced
2 tbsp chopped fresh thyme (or 2 tsp dried)
400 g (14 oz) tin green or brown lentils
400 g (14 oz) tin chopped tomatoes
1 tsp vegetable bouillon
2 tbsp tomato puree
1 kg (2.2 lb) sweet potatoes, peeled and cut into chunks
2 tbsp olive oil
Salt and freshly ground black pepper
Beoccoli and green beans, to serve

- Preheat the oven to 190 C/170 C fan/gas 5.
- Heat the olive oil in a large pan and fry the onion and garlic for 3–4 minutes until softened. Add the vegetables and thyme and cook for 10 minutes. Add the lentils, tomatoes, vegetable bouillon and tomato puree, cover and simmer for 10 minutes.
- Meanwhile, boil the sweet potatoes for 15–20 minutes until tender, drain, then mash with the olive oil and salt and pepper to taste.
- Spoon the lentil mixture into an ovenproof dish, top with the mash, then bake for 20 minutes.

Nutritional information (per serving):
Calories = 490; protein = 13 g;
carbohydrate = 78 g; fat = 10 g fat;
fibre = 18 g

SWEET POTATO SPANISH TORTILLA

Serves 1

1 small sweet potato (175 g/6 oz), peeled and thickly sliced
1 tbsp olive oil
1 small onion, chopped
2 large eggs, beaten
1 tbsp chopped fresh parsley
Salt and freshly ground black pepper
Salad, to serve

- Cook the sweet potato in a small pan of boiling water for 5–6 minutes, until just tender. Drain and set aside.
- Preheat the grill to medium.
- Heat the oil in an ovenproof frying pan and fry the onion over a medium heat for 3–4 minutes, or until softened. Add the sweet potato and season to taste with salt and pepper.
- Pour in the eggs and cook for 1–2 minutes, until the egg starts to set. Transfer to the grill and cook for 3–4 minutes or until the top is golden and the tortilla is cooked through.
- Slide the tortilla onto a plate, scatter over the parsley and cut into wedges. Serve with a simple salad.

Nutritional information (per serving):
Calories = 447; protein = 18 g;
carbohydrate = 42 g; fat = 25 g fat;
fibre = 5 g

STIR-FRIED VEGETABLE OMELETTE

Serves 1
2 tsp vegetable oil
1 small onion, sliced
1 garlic clove, crushed
1 tsp chopped fresh root ginger
Vegetables, e.g. carrot, cut into strips; red
    pepper, deseeded and sliced; mangetout,
    trimmed and halved; button mushrooms,
    sliced
1 tbsp soy sauce
Juice of ½ lime
2 large eggs
2 tsp vegetable oil
Salt and freshly ground black pepper
Noodles or rice, to serve

- For the stir-fried vegetables, heat the oil in a wok or heavy-based pan, and then add the onion, garlic and ginger. Cook for 2 minutes and add the vegetables. Stir-fry for 3–4 minutes, until softened. Stir in the soy sauce and lime juice and set aside.
- For the omelette, beat the eggs in a small bowl and season to taste with salt and pepper. Heat the oil in a medium non-stick frying pan, add the eggs and cook for 2–3 minutes over a medium heat until the egg is almost set.
- Pile the stir-fried vegetables on one half of the omelette and fold the other half over the top. Slide on to a plate and serve with boiled noodles or rice.

> **Nutritional information (per serving):**
> Calories = 372; protein = 20 g;
> carbohydrate = 16 g; fat = 26 g;
> fibre = 4 g

TOFU WITH NOODLES

Serves 2
For the marinade:
2 tbsp soy sauce
2 tbsp dry sherry
1 tbsp wine vinegar
For the dish:
225 g (8 oz) tofu (bean curd), cubed
1 tbsp olive oil
1 garlic clove, crushed
1 piece fresh root ginger, chopped
1 red pepper, sliced
100 g (3½ oz) mangetout
1 tsp cornflour
175 g (6 oz) noodles, cooked in water

- Mix the ingredients for the marinade together. Add the tofu and leave for at least 30 minutes in the fridge (or overnight).
- Heat the oil in a wok and stir-fry the garlic, ginger and vegetables for 4 minutes.
- Remove the tofu from the marinade.
- Blend the marinade with the cornflour and pour over the vegetables. Stir until the sauce has thickened. Place the vegetables and sauce in a serving dish.
- Stir-fry the tofu for 2 minutes and add to the vegetables. Serve with noodles.

> **Nutritional information (per serving):**
> Calories = 533; protein = 21 g;
> carbohydrate = 75 g; fat = 19 g;
> fibre = 4 g

POTATO, PEA AND SPINACH FRITTATA

Serves 2

1 potato (175 g/6 oz), peeled and sliced
75 g (3 oz) frozen peas
2 tsp olive oil
1 onion, finely sliced
1 garlic clove, crushed
4 large eggs
200 g (7 oz) fresh baby leaf spinach
Salt and freshly ground black pepper
Salad, to serve

- Cook the potato in a small pan of boiling water for 5–6 minutes, or until just tender. Add the peas during the last 3 minutes. Drain.
- Heat the olive oil in a frying pan, add the onion and garlic and sauté for 4–5 minutes or until they are softened.
- Beat the eggs in a large bowl and season to taste with salt and freshly ground pepper. Add to the pan, stir in the potatoes, peas and spinach and cook over a medium heat for a few minutes until the eggs are almost set. Place the pan underneath a hot grill to finish cooking. The frittata should be set and golden on top.
- Slide a knife around the edge and slide the frittata on to a large plate. Serve in wedges with a simple salad.

HUMMUS WITH PINE NUTS

Serves 4

400 g (14 oz) tinned chickpeas or 125 g (4 oz) dried chickpeas, soaked overnight and then boiled for 45 minutes
1–2 garlic cloves, crushed
2 tbsp extra virgin olive oil
1 tbsp tahini (sesame seed paste)
Juice of ½ lemon
2–4 tbsp water
1–2 tbsp pine nuts
Salt and freshly ground black pepper

- Drain and rinse the chickpeas. Reserve 1–2 tablespoons and put the remainder in a food processor or blender with the garlic, olive oil, tahini, lemon juice and 2 tablespoons of water. Whizz until smooth, add a little salt and freshly ground black pepper and process again. Taste to check the seasoning. Add extra water if necessary to give the desired consistency.
- Meanwhile, lightly toast the pine nuts under a hot grill for 3–4 minutes until they are lightly coloured but not brown (watch carefully because they colour quickly).
- Stir in the reserved whole chickpeas. Spoon into a shallow dish. Scatter over the pine nuts and drizzle over a few drops of olive oil. Chill in the fridge for at least 2 hours before serving.

Nutritional information (per serving):
Calories = 347; protein = 23 g;
carbohydrate = 27 g; fat = 18 g;
fibre = 6 g

Nutritional information (per serving):
Calories = 193; protein = 7 g;
carbohydrate = 12 g; fat = 13 g;
fibre = 4 g

CHICKPEAS WITH BUTTERNUT SQUASH AND TOMATOES

Serves 4

2 tbsp extra virgin olive oil
2 onions, chopped
1 red pepper, deseeded and chopped
225 g (8 oz) butternut squash, peeled and chopped
400 g (14 oz) tinned chopped tomatoes
250 ml (8 fl oz) vegetable stock
2 × 400 g (14 oz) tins chickpeas, drained and rinsed
225 g (8 oz) potatoes, peeled and chopped
Grated cheese, to serve

- Heat the oil in a heavy-based pan, add the onion and pepper and cook over a moderate heat for 5 minutes.
- Add the squash, tomatoes, vegetable stock, chickpeas and potatoes, stir and then bring to the boil. Lower the heat and simmer for 20 minutes, stirring occasionally.
- Serve sprinkled with a little grated cheese.

Nutritional information (per serving):
Calories = 331; protein = 15 g;
carbohydrate = 48 g; fat = 10 g;
fibre = 10 g

SPICY COUSCOUS

Serves 4

250 g (9 oz) couscous
400 ml (14 fl oz) hot vegetable stock or water
½ red pepper, deseeded
½ yellow pepper, deseeded
1 red onion, sliced
10–12 cherry tomatoes, halved
2 tbsp extra virgin olive oil
½ tsp cumin seeds
A small handful of fresh coriander, chopped
1 tbsp lemon juice
Salt and freshly ground black pepper

- Preheat the oven to 200°C/400°F/gas mark 6
- Put the couscous in a large bowl and cover with the hot stock or water. Stir briefly, cover and allow to stand for 5 minutes until the stock has been absorbed. Fluff up with a fork.
- Cut the pepper into wide strips. Place in a large roasting tin with the onion slices and cherry tomatoes, drizzle over the olive oil, scatter over the cumin seeds and toss lightly so that the vegetables are well coated in the oil.
- Roast in the oven for about 15 minutes until the peppers are slightly charred on the outside and tender in the middle. Allow to cool, then roughly chop the peppers.
- Add the roasted vegetables (with the cumin seeds), coriander and lemon juice to the couscous. Season to taste. Stir well to combine and serve.

Nutritional information (per serving):
Calories = 224; protein = 5 g;
carbohydrate = 39 g; fat = 7 g;
fibre = 2 g

VEGETABLE RISOTTO WITH CASHEW NUTS

Serves 2

2 tbsp olive oil
1 onion, chopped
1 red pepper, chopped
1 garlic clove, crushed
1 bay leaf
150 g (5 oz) wholegrain rice
500 ml (18 fl oz) hot vegetable stock
75 g (3 oz) green beans, cut into 2 cm (¾ inch) lengths
125 g (4 oz) sugar snap peas
2 tomatoes, deseeded and chopped
50 g (2 oz) baby spinach leaves
50 g (2 oz) cashew nuts, lightly toasted
Freshly ground black pepper

- Heat the olive oil in a large heavy-based pan and cook the onion with the red pepper, garlic and bay leaf over a moderate heat, stirring frequently.
- Stir in the rice and cook for 1–2 minutes, stirring constantly until the grains are coated with oil and translucent.
- Add half the hot vegetable stock and bring to the boil. Reduce the heat and simmer gently until the liquid is absorbed. Stir in the remaining stock, a ladleful at a time, and continue to simmer until the rice is almost tender (about 25–30 minutes). Add the green beans, peas and tomatoes and continue cooking for a further 5 minutes. As a guide, the total cooking time should be around 35 minutes.
- Add the spinach leaves to the hot risotto. Stir until the leaves have wilted. Remove the pan from the heat.
- Season to taste with freshly ground black pepper, then scatter over the cashew nuts.

Nutritional information (per serving):
Calories = 652; protein = 16 g;
carbohydrate = 84 g; fat = 29 g;
fibre = 9 g

ROASTED VEGETABLES WITH MARINATED TOFU

Serves 2
1 small red onion, roughly sliced
½ red pepper, cut into strips
½ yellow pepper, cut into strips
½ orange pepper, cut into strips
1 small courgette, trimmed and thickly sliced
¼ aubergine, cut into 2 cm (¾ inch) cubes
2 garlic cloves, crushed
2 tbsp extra virgin olive oil
200 g (7 oz) marinated tofu pieces
A small handful of fresh basil, roughly torn
Freshly ground black pepper

- Preheat the oven to 200°C/400°F/gas mark 6.
- Place the prepared vegetables in a large roasting tin and scatter over the crushed garlic. Pour over the olive oil and toss lightly, thoroughly coating the vegetables.
- Roast in the oven for 25 minutes, turning them occasionally. Scatter the tofu pieces over and continue roasting for 5 minutes until the vegetables are slightly charred on the outside and tender in the middle.
- Remove from the oven and spoon on to a serving dish. Grind over black pepper to taste and sprinkle with the torn basil.

Nutritional information (per serving):
Calories = 245; protein = 11 g;
carbohydrate = 14 g; fat = 16 g;
fibre = 4 g

PASTA WITH CHICKPEAS AND SPINACH

Serves 4
400 g (14 oz) can chickpeas, drained and rinsed
350 g (12 oz) tub fresh tomato pasta sauce
400 g (14 oz) fresh penne pasta
200 g (7 oz) bag fresh spinach
25 g (1 oz) parmesan shavings
Olive oil, to drizzle
Freshly ground black pepper

- Place the chickpeas in a medium pan with the tomato sauce and 100 ml (3½ fl oz) cold water. Bring to the boil over a low heat. Turn off the heat and cover.
- Meanwhile, bring a large pan of water to the boil. Add the pasta and return to the boil for 5 minutes or until the pasta is just tender. Drain thoroughly. Stir in the spinach and allow to wilt.
- Place the pasta in a serving dish and pour the hot pasta sauce and chickpea mixture over the top, then toss together and season to taste with black pepper. Top each serving with Parmesan shavings and a drizzle of olive oil.

Nutritional information (per serving):
Calories = 434; protein = 20 g;
carbohydrate = 76 g; fat = 8 g;
fibre = 7 g

VEGETABLE STIR-FRY WITH SESAME NOODLES

Serves 4

1 tsp clear honey
Juice of 1 large orange
3 tbsp soy sauce
2 tbsp oil
1 onion, sliced
1 large carrot, peeled and cut into thin strips
225 g (8 oz) pak choi or spring cabbage, shredded
2.5 cm (1 inch) piece root ginger, peeled and grated
1 garlic clove, crushed
225 g (8 oz) ready-cooked egg noodles
3 tbsp sesame seeds, toasted

• In a small bowl, mix together the honey, orange juice and soy sauce and set aside.
• Heat the oil in a wok or large frying pan.
• Add the onion and carrot and stir-fry for 2–3 minutes. Add the pak choi or cabbage, ginger and garlic and stir-fry for a further 2–3 minutes.
• Add the ready-cooked egg noodles to the wok and pour in the sauce mix. Toss everything together and cook for a further 2–3 minutes, or until piping hot. Scatter with the toasted sesame seeds and serve at once.

RICE, BEAN AND VEGETABLE STIR FRY

Serves 2

175 g (6 oz) brown rice
1 tbsp olive oil
1 onion, chopped
2 garlic cloves, crushed
1 piece fresh root ginger, chopped
125 g (4 oz) large mushrooms, sliced
2 stalks celery, chopped
125 g (4 oz) peas
½ can (200 g/ 7 oz) can red kidney beans, rinsed and drained

• Cover the rice with plenty of boiling water. Bring to the boil and simmer for 25–30 minutes.
• Meanwhile, heat the oil in a wok over a high heat.
• Add the onion, and stir-fry for 1 minute.
• Add the garlic, ginger, mushrooms, celery and peas and stir-fry for 3 minutes.
• Tip in the red kidney beans and cooked rice.
• Cook for a further 2 minutes, until all the ingredients are thoroughly heated through.

Nutritional information (per serving):
Calories = 330; protein = 9 g;
carbohydrate = 44 g; fat = 14 g;
fibre = 4 g

Nutritional information (per serving):
Calories = 526; protein = 18 g;
carbohydrate = 94 g; fat = 11 g;
fibre = 11 g

VEGETARIAN CHILLI

Serves 2

1 garlic clove, crushed
1 onion, chopped
1 green or red pepper, deseeded and chopped
½ tsp chilli powder (or to taste)
225 g (8 oz) can tomatoes
50 g (2 oz) red lentils
175 g (6 oz) rice
300 ml (½ pint) water
½ can (200 g/ 7 oz) can red kidney beans, rinsed and drained
Salt and freshly ground black pepper
Broccoli or green salad, to serve

- Place the garlic, onion, pepper, chilli, tomatoes, lentils, rice and water in a large pan.
- Bring to the boil and simmer for 20 minutes.
- Add the kidney beans and cook for a further 5 minutes.
- Season to taste.
- Serve with broccoli or green salad.

MIXED BEAN HOTPOT

Serves 2

400 g (14 oz) can of beans (e.g. red kidney beans, chickpeas or haricot beans), rinsed and drained
125 g (4 oz) green beans
225 g (8 oz) can tomatoes
1 tbsp tomato purée
1 tsp mixed herbs
450 g (1 lb) potatoes, boiled and cooled
Green vegetables or salad, to serve

- Place the beans in a large casserole dish and mix in the green beans, tomatoes, purée and herbs.
- Thinly slice the potatoes and arrange on top.
- Bake at 170°C/325°F/gas mark 3 for 30 minutes until the potatoes are cooked, or microwave on full for 8 minutes.
- Serve with green vegetables or salad.

Nutritional information (per serving):
Calories = 550; protein = 21 g;
carbohydrate = 119 g; fat = 2 g;
fibre = 10 g

Nutritional information (per serving):
Calories = 346; protein = 17 g;
carbohydrate = 71 g; fat = 2 g;
fibre = 14 g

LENTIL AND VEGETABLE LASAGNE

Serves 2
6 sheets ready-cooked lasagne
For the lentil and vegetable sauce:
100 g (4 oz) red lentils
1 onion, chopped
400 g (14 oz) tin of tomatoes
2 carrots, chopped
1 tsp oregano
150 ml (¼ pint) water
For the topping:
125 g (4 oz) fromage frais
2 eggs
1 tbsp freshly grated parmesan cheese
Mixed salad, to serve

- Place all the ingredients for the lentil and vegetable sauce in a saucepan and bring to the boil.
- Simmer for 20 minutes or cook in a pressure cooker for 3 minutes (release the steam slowly).
- Place half of the sauce in a dish, with 3 lasagne sheets on top. Then add the rest of the sauce, followed by the remaining lasagne sheets. For the topping, beat the eggs with the fromage frais, then spoon the mixture on top of the lasagne. Sprinkle with the parmesan cheese. Bake at 200°C/400°F/gas mark 6 for 40 minutes, until the topping is golden. Serve with a large mixed salad.

BEAN BURGERS

Serves 2
1 small onion, finely chopped
1 garlic clove, crushed
2 tsp oil
400 g (14 oz) tin red kidney beans, rinsed and drained
1 tbsp parsley
1 tbsp lemon juice
Flour (optional)
Oats, for coating
Wholemeal bap or pitta and salad, to serve

- Cook the onion and garlic in the oil for 5 minutes.
- Mash with a fork or blend in a food processor with the other ingredients, except the oats, until a coarse purée is formed.
- Add a little flour if necessary for a firmer texture.
- Place the oats in a dish.
- Using your hands, form the mixture into 4 large burgers, coating them with oats.
- Grill for about 2 minutes on each side, fry in a small amount of hot oil, or barbecue.
- Serve in a wholemeal bap or pitta bread with lots of salad.

Nutritional information (per serving):
Calories = 513; protein = 33 g;
carbohydrate = 75 g; fat = 11 g;
fibre = 6 g

Nutritional information (per serving):
Calories = 234; protein = 12 g;
carbohydrate = 34 g; fat = 7 g;
fibre = 10 g

Desserts

BANANA PANCAKES

Makes 8 pancakes
100 g (3½ oz) wholemeal flour, or fine
   oatmeal
300 ml (½ pint) milk
2 eggs
1 tsp oil
3 ripe bananas
Low fat yoghurt, to serve

- Blend all the ingredients, except the bananas, in a liquidiser for 30 seconds.
- Heat a non-stick frying pan and add the oil.
- Pour in 1 tablespoon of the batter, tilting the pan to coat it evenly.
- Cook until the underside of the pancake is brown.
- Turn, and cook for a further 10 seconds until the other side is brown.
- Repeat until the batter is used up.
- Stack the pancakes on an ovenproof plate and keep them warm in the oven on a very low heat.
- Mix one mashed banana with two sliced bananas.
- Place a spoonful on each pancake and fold into quarters.
- Serve with low fat yoghurt.

BAKED APPLES

Serves 1
1 large cooking apple
1 tbsp raisins or sultanas
1 tsp honey
1 tsp toasted, chopped hazelnuts (optional)
Yoghurt, low fat custard or fromage frais, to
   serve

- Remove the core from the apple.
- Score the skin lightly around the middle. Place the apple in a small dish.
- Mix together the raisins or sultanas, honey and nuts and fill the centre of the apple.
- Cover loosely with foil and bake at 180°C/ 350°F/gas mark 4 for 45–60 minutes or cover with another dish and microwave on medium power for 5–7 minutes (depending on the size of the apple), until tender.
- Serve with yoghurt, low fat custard or fromage frais.

Nutritional information (per serving):
Calories = 103; protein = 5 g;
carbohydrate = 17 g; fat = 2 g;
fibre = 2 g

Nutritional information (per serving):
Calories = 144; protein = 1 g;
carbohydrate = 33 g; fat = 2 g;
fibre = 1 g

WHOLEMEAL BREAD AND BUTTER PUDDING

Serves 4
8 slices wholemeal bread
40 g (1½ oz) low fat spread
75 g (3 oz) sultanas
1 tbsp brown sugar
3 eggs
600 ml (1 pint) milk
Freshly ground nutmeg

• Spread the bread with the low fat spread.
• Cut each slice into 4 squares and layer in a 1 litre (2 pint) dish, scattering sultanas between each layer.
• Beat together the sugar, eggs and milk and pour over the bread.
• Sprinkle with a little grated nutmeg.
• Leave to soak for 30 minutes, if time allows.
• Bake at 350°F/180°C/gas mark 4 for 1 hour, until the top is golden.

OAT APPLE CRUMBLE

Serves 6
700 g (1½ lb) cooking apples, peeled and sliced
75 g (3 oz) clear honey
½ tsp cinnamon
4 tbsp water
Topping
125 g (4 oz) plain flour
75 g (3 oz) olive oil margarine
50 g (2 oz) oats
50 g (2 oz) brown sugar

• Preheat the oven to 190°C/375°C/gas mark 5.
• Place the apples, honey and cinnamon in a deep baking dish. Combine well and pour the water over.
• For the crumble topping, put the flour in a bowl and rub in the margarine until the mixture resembles coarse breadcrumbs. Mix in the oats and sugar. Alternatively, mix in a food mixer or processor.
• Sprinkle the crumble mixture over the fruit.
• Bake for 20–25 minutes, until the topping is golden and the fruit is tender.

Nutritional information (per serving):
Calories = 345; protein = 17 g; carbohydrate = 49 g; fat = 11g; fibre = 4 g

Nutritional information (per serving):
Calories = 311; protein = 3 g; carbohydrate = 52 g; fat = 11 g; fibre = 3 g

SPICED FRUIT SKEWERS

Serves 4
50 g (2 oz) clear honey
1 tbsp lemon juice
Juice of 1 orange
8 cardamom pods, lightly crushed
1 cinnamon stick, halved
8 Medjool dates, pitted
8 apricots, halved and stoned
4 plums, halved and stoned

- Place the honey, lemon juice, orange juice, cardamom pods and cinnamon stick in a shallow dish. Add the dates, apricots and plums. Marinate for at least 30 minutes.
- Drain the fruits, reserving the honey syrup, and thread on to 4 long wooden skewers. Cook under a preheated grill (or over a prepared barbecue) for 10–15 minutes, or until beginning to colour.
- Remove the cardamom pods and cinnamon sticks from the honey syrup. Serve the fruit skewers drizzled with the syrup.

EXOTIC FRUIT WITH LIME

Serves 4
2 tbsp clear honey
100 ml (3½ fl oz) hot water
Zest of 1 lime
20 g (⅔ oz) pack fresh mint leaves
1 pineapple, skin removed, quartered and cored
3 kiwi fruit, peeled and cut into chunks
1 mango, peeled and sliced
Yoghurt, to serve

- Place the honey, water, lime zest and half the mint in a jug. Allow to infuse for 1 hour, then strain.
- Cut the pineapple into small wedges and toss gently in a large bowl with the kiwi fruit and mango pieces. Pour the cooled syrup over and combine well.
- Divide the fruit between 4 bowls, decorate with the remaining mint and serve with natural yoghurt.

Nutritional information (per serving):
Calories = 147; protein = 2 g;
carbohydrate = 37 g; fat = 1 g;
fibre = 3 g

Nutritional information (per serving):
Calories = 124; protein = 1 g;
carbohydrate = 30 g; fat = 1 g;
fibre = 4 g

ROASTED PEACHES AND PLUMS WITH YOGHURT

Serves 4
4 ripe peaches
4 ripe plums
1 cinnamon stick, broken in half
Zest and juice of 2 oranges
2 tbsp clear honey
400 g (14 oz) Greek-style yoghurt

- Preheat the oven to 200°C/400°F/gas mark 6.
- Halve and stone the peaches and plums and arrange, cut sides up, in a shallow dish large enough to hold them all in one layer.
- Put the cinnamon stick, orange zest and juice and honey in a small pan. Heat gently until the honey has melted. Pour evenly over the fruit. Roast in the oven for 25–30 minutes, basting halfway through the cooking time, until the fruit is tender.
- Cool for 10 minutes, then divide between serving plates. Place a dessertspoonful of yoghurt into the cavity of each fruit and drizzle some of the honey syrup over. Serve the rest of the yoghurt separately.

Nutritional information (per serving):
Calories = 179; protein = 6 g;
carbohydrate = 26 g; fat = 6 g;
fibre = 3 g

Snacks

FRUIT SCOTCH PANCAKES

Serves 2–4
100 g (3½ oz) plain flour
1 tbsp sugar
1 tsp baking powder
2 medium eggs
150 ml (5 fl oz) semi-skimmed milk
50 g (2 oz) raisins
50 g (2 oz) ready-to-eat dried apricots, chopped
Oil, for brushing
Fresh fruit and honey, to serve

- Mix together the dry ingredients in a bowl.
- Add the eggs and a splash of milk and whisk until smooth. Stir in the raisins and apricots.
- Heat a large griddle or heavy-based non-stick frying pan and brush it lightly with oil. Drop small spoonfuls of the batter on to the griddle to make 8–10 cm (3–4 inch) rounds and cook for about 2 minutes or until air bubbles start to form on the surface. Turn and cook the other side for 1–2 minutes or until golden. You may need to cook in 2 batches.
- Serve with fresh fruit and honey.

Nutritional information (per serving):
For 2 servings: Calories = 423;
protein = 25 g; carbohydrate = 76 g;
fat = 9 g; fibre = 4 g

For 4 servings: Calories = 212;
protein = 8 g; carbohydrate = 38 g;
fat = 5 g; fibre = 2 g

BANANA MUFFINS

Makes 10 muffins
50 g (2 oz) butter
75 g (3 oz) brown sugar
1 egg
225 g (8 oz) flour (wholemeal or half
  wholemeal, half white)
2 mashed bananas
Pinch of salt
1 tsp baking powder
1 tsp vanilla essence
5 tbsp milk

- Combine all the ingredients in a large bowl until just mixed.
- Spoon into 10 non-stick bun tins (or paper cases).
- Bake at 190°C/375°F/gas mark 5 for approx. 20 minutes, until well risen and golden.

Variations:
- Add 50 g (2 oz) chocolate chips to the mixture (recommended!).
- Substitute 225 g (8 oz) fresh blueberries or 75 g (3 oz) dried blueberries for the bananas.
- Substitute 225 g (8 oz) fresh cranberries or 75 g (3 oz) dried cranberries for the bananas.
- Substitute 100 g (3½ oz) chopped dried apricots for the bananas. Add the grated rind of 1 lemon instead of the vanilla essence.
- Add 50 g (2 oz) chopped walnuts.

Nutritional information (per serving):
Calories = 164; protein = 4 g;
carbohydrate = 27 g; fat = 5 g;
fibre = 2 g

RAISIN BREAD

Makes 1 loaf (10 slices)
225 g (8 oz) strong flour (half wholemeal,
  half white)
½ tsp salt
1½ tbsp sugar
1 sachet easy-blend yeast
1 tbsp melted butter
180 ml (6 fl oz) warm water
100 g (3½ oz) raisins

- Mix together the flour, salt, sugar, yeast and butter.
- Add the warm water to form a dough.
- Turn out on to a floured surface and knead for 5–10 minutes until smooth and silky.
- Knead in the raisins.
- Place in a bowl, cover and leave in a warm place or at room temperature to rise until doubled in size (approximately 1 hour).
- Knead for a few minutes then shape into a round loaf.
- Place on an oiled baking tray and bake at 220°C/ 425°F/gas mark 7 for 20 minutes or until the bread sounds hollow when tapped underneath.

Variations:
- Add 2 tsp cinnamon to the flour mixture.
- Substitute 100 g (3½ oz) chopped dried apricots for the raisins.
- Substitute 100 g (3½ oz) sultanas for the raisins.
- Add 1 tsp grated orange rind.
- Add 50 g (2 oz) toasted chopped hazelnuts with the raisins.

Nutritional information (per serving):
Calories = 120; protein = 3 g;
carbohydrate = 25 g; fat = 2 g;
fibre = 2 g

APPLE AND CINNAMON OAT BARS

Makes 12 bars

2 apples, sliced and cooked, or 175 g (6 oz)
   apple purée
175 g (6 oz) oats
2 tsp cinnamon
4 egg whites
1 tbsp honey
50 g (2 oz) raisins
6 tbsp skimmed milk

- Mix all the ingredients together in a bowl.
- Transfer to a non-stick baking tin 23 cm × 15
  cm (approx. 9" × 6").
- Bake at 200°C/400°F/gas mark 6 for 15
  minutes.
- When cool, cut into squares.

SULTANA FLAPJACKS

Makes 12 slices

200 g (7 oz) butter or margarine
200 g (7 oz) sugar
200 g (7 oz) honey or golden syrup
400 g (14 oz) porridge oats
75 g (3 oz) sultanas

- Preheat the oven to 180°C/350°F/gas mark 4.
- Butter a 20 cm × 30 cm cake tin.
- Put the butter, sugar and honey in a saucepan
  and heat, stirring occasionally, until the butter
  has melted and the sugar has dissolved. Add
  the oats and sultanas and mix well.
- Transfer the oat mixture to the prepared cake
  tin and spread to about 2 cm (¾ inch) thick.
  Smooth the surface with the back of a spoon.
- Bake in the oven for 15–20 minutes, until
  lightly golden around the edges, but still
  slightly soft in the middle. Let cool in the tin,
  then turn out and cut into squares.

Nutritional information (per serving):
Calories = 87; protein = 3 g;
carbohydrate = 17 g; fat = 1 g;
fibre = 1 g

Nutritional information (per serving):
Calories = 389; protein = 5 g;
carbohydrate = 59 g; fat = 17 g;
fibre = 2 g

BANANA AND WALNUT LOAF

Makes 10 slices or 12 muffins
2 medium bananas
125 g (4 oz) butter
125 g (4 oz) dark brown sugar
2 eggs
1 tsp vanilla essence
1 tsp ground cinnamon
250 g (9 oz) plain flour
1 tsp baking powder
3 tbsp milk
125 g (4 oz) walnuts

- Preheat the oven to 180°C/350°F/gas mark 4.
- Butter a 1 (2 lb) kg loaf tin or use 12 large muffin cases.
- Mash the bananas. Cream the butter and sugar until smooth and then beat in the mashed bananas. Add the eggs, vanilla and cinnamon and mix well.
- Add the flour, baking powder and milk, and mix until smooth. Fold in the walnuts.
- Spoon the mixture into the tin and bake for about 50 minutes, until the loaf is crusty on the top and a skewer inserted into the middle comes out clean. Cool in the tin, and then turn out on to a cooling rack. For muffins, cook for 20–25 minutes.

Nutritional information (per serving):
Calories = 348; protein = 6 g;
carbohydrate = 37 g; fat = 217 g;
fibre = 1 g

BLUEBERRY MUFFINS

Makes 18
250 g (9 oz) flour
1 tsp baking powder
100 g (3½ oz) caster sugar
2 eggs
50 g (2 oz) melted butter
200 ml (7 fl oz) buttermilk or yoghurt
125 g (4 oz) blueberries

- Preheat the oven to 200°C/400°F/gas mark 6. Line 2 × 12-hole muffin trays with paper cases.
- Sift the flour and baking powder into a large bowl and stir in the sugar.
- In another bowl, whisk together the eggs, melted butter and buttermilk or yoghurt. Fold this mixture into the flour and stir the blueberries through. Spoon into paper cases and bake for 20–25 minutes until cooked and golden.

Nutritional information (per serving):
Calories = 164; protein = 4 g;
carbohydrate = 26 g; fat = 6 g;
fibre = 1 g

RASPBERRY MUFFINS

Makes 10

4 tbsp sunflower oil
5 tbsp milk
1 large egg
150 g (5 oz) self-raising flour
100 g (4 oz) caster sugar
175 g (6 oz) fresh or thawed frozen
    raspberries
4 tbsp icing sugar, sifted
2 tsp lemon juice

- Preheat the oven to 200°C/400°F/gas mark 6.
- Line a 12-hole deep muffin tray with paper cases.
- Mix the oil, milk and egg together. Sift the flour and sugar into a bowl. Add the liquid and half the raspberries to the flour and briefly mix until just coming together. Spoon into the muffin cases and scatter over the remaining raspberries. Bake for 25–30 minutes.
- Cool the muffins on a wire rack.
- Sift the icing sugar into a bowl and stir in the lemon juice to make a runny icing. Drizzle the icing over the muffins and leave to set.

CHERRY, ALMOND AND OAT COOKIES

Makes 15

125 g (4 oz) butter or margarine
125 g (4 oz) granulated or caster sugar
1 tbsp golden syrup
½ tsp vanilla essence
150 g (5 oz) plain white flour
100 g (3½ oz) rolled oats
100 g (3½ oz) ground almonds
100 g (3½ oz) glacé cherries, chopped
Oil, for greasing

- Preheat the oven to 170°C/350°F/gas mark 3 and oil two baking sheets (or use baking parchment).
- Cream together the butter or margarine and the sugar until light and smooth.
- Beat in the golden syrup and vanilla.
- Add the flour, oats and almonds to the mixture, mixing well. Stir in the cherries.
- Place spoonfuls on to the baking sheets, about 2.5 cm (1 inch) apart, then flatten with your hand. Bake for 10–12 minutes or until light golden.

Nutritional information (per serving):
Calories = 131; protein = 3 g;
carbohydrate = 19 g; fat = 5 g;
fibre = 1 g

Nutritional information (per serving):
Calories = 216; protein = 3 g;
carbohydrate = 27 g; fat = 11 g;
fibre = 1 g

APPENDIX ONE
THE GLYCAEMIC INDEX AND GLYCAEMIC LOAD

Food	Portion size	GI	Carbohydrate (g) per portion	GL per portion
High GI (> 70)				
Dates	6 (60 g)	103	40	42
Glucose	2 tsp (10 g)	99	10	10
French baguette	5 cm slice (30 g)	95	15	15
Lucozade	250 ml bottle	95	42	40
Baked potato	1 average (150 g)	85	30	26
Rice krispies	Small bowl (30 g)	82	26	22
Cornflakes	Small bowl (30 g)	81	26	21
Gatorade	250 ml bottle	78	15	12
Rice cakes	3 (25 g)	78	21	17
Chips	Average portion (150 g)	75	29	22
Shredded wheat	2 (45 g)	75	20	15
Bran flakes	Small bowl (30 g)	74	18	13
Cheerios	Small bowl (30 g)	74	20	15
Mashed potato	4 tbsp (150 g)	74	20	15
Weetabix	2 (40 g)	74	22	16
Bagel	1 (70 g)	72	35	25
Breakfast cereal bar (crunchy nut cornflakes)	1 bar (30 g)	72	26	19
Watermelon	1 slice (120 g)	72	6	4
Golden Grahams	Small bowl (30 g)	71	25	18
Millet	5 tbsp (150 g)	71	36	25
Water biscuit	3 (25 g)	71	18	13
Wholemeal bread	1 slice (30 g)	71	13	9
Isostar	250 ml can	70	18	13

Food	Portion size	GI	Carbohydrate (g) per portion	GL per portion
White bread	1 slice (30 g)	70	14	10
Moderate GI (56–69)				
Fanta	262 ml	68	34	23
Sucrose	2 tsp (10 g)	68	10	7
Croissant	1 (57 g)	67	26	17
Instant porridge	250 g bowl	66	26	17
Cantaloupe melon	1 slice (120 g)	65	6	4
Couscous	5 tbsp (150 g)	65	35	23
Mars bar	1 bar (60 g)	65	40	26
Raisins	3 tbsp (60 g)	64	44	28
Rye crispbread	2 (25 g)	64	16	11
Shortbread	2 (25 g)	64	16	10
White rice	5 tbsp (150 g)	64	36	23
Tortillas/corn chips	1 bag (50 g)	63	26	17
Ice cream	1 scoop (50 g)	61	13	8
Muesli bar	1 bar (30 g)	61	21	13
Sweet potato	1 medium (150 g)	61	28	17
Just Right cereal	1 small bowl (30 g)	60	22	13
Pizza	1 slice (100 g)	60	35	21
Digestive biscuit	2 (25 g)	59	16	10
Pineapple	2 slices (120 g)	59	13	7
Basmati rice	5 tbsp (150 g)	58	38	22
Porridge	250 g bowl	58	22	13
Squash (diluted)	250 ml glass	58	29	17
Apricots	3 (120 g)	57	9	5
Pitta bread	1 small (30 g)	57	17	10
Power Bar	1 bar (65 g)	56	42	24
Sultanas	3 tbsp (60 g)	56	45	25

Food	Portion size	GI	Carbohydrate (g) per portion	GL per portion
Rich tea biscuit	2 (25 g)	55	19	10
Potato – boiled, old	2 medium (150 g)	54	27	15
Low GI (< 55)				
Brown rice	5 tbsp (150 g)	55	33	18
Honey	1 tsbp (25 g)	55	18	10
Muesli (Alpen)	1 small bowl (30 g)	55	19	10
Buckwheat	5 tbsp (150 g)	54	30	16
Crisps	1 large packet (50 g)	54	21	11
Sweetcorn	4 tbsp (150 g)	54	17	9
Kiwi fruit	3 (120 g)	53	12	6
Banana	1 (120 g)	52	24	12
Orange juice	1 large glass (250 ml)	52	23	12
Mango	½ (120 g)	51	17	8
Strawberry jam	1 tbsp (30 g)	51	20	10
Rye bread	1 slice (30 g)	50	12	6
Muesli	1 small bowl (30 g)	49	20	10
Baked beans	1 small tin (150 g)	48	15	7
Bulgar wheat	5 tbsp (150 g)	48	26	12
Peas	2 tbsp (80 g)	48	7	3
Carrots	2 tbsp (80 g)	47	6	3
Macaroni	5 tbsp (180 g)	47	48	23
Grapes	Small bunch (120 g)	46	18	8
Pineapple juice	1 large glass (250 ml)	46	34	15
Sponge cake	1 slice (63 g)	46	36	17
Muffin, apple	1 (60 g)	44	29	13
Milk chocolate	1 bar (50 g)	43	28	12
All Bran	1 small bowl (30 g)	42	23	9
Orange	1 (120 g)	42	11	5

Food	Portion size	GI	Carbohydrate (g) per portion	GL per portion
Peach	1 (120 g)	42	11	5
Apple juice	1 large glass (250 ml)	40	28	11
Strawberries	21 (120 g)	40	3	1
Spaghetti	5 tbsp (180 g)	38	48	18
Plum	3 (120 g)	39	12	5
Apples	1 (120 g)	38	15	6
Pear	1 (120 g)	38	11	4
Protein bar	1 bar (80 g)	38	13	5
Tinned peaches – tinned in fruit juice	½ tin (120 g)	38	11	4
Yoghurt drink	1 glass (200 ml)	38	29	11
Plain yoghurt, low fat	1 large carton (200 g)	36	9	3
Custard	2 tbsp (100 g)	35	17	6
Chocolate milk	1 large glass (250 ml)	34	26	9
Fruit yoghurt, low fat	1 large carton (200 g)	33	31	10
Protein shake	1 carton (250 ml)	32	3	1
Skimmed milk	1 large glass (250 ml)	32	13	4
Apricot (dried)	5 (60 g)	31	28	9
Butter beans	4 tbsp (150 g)	31	20	6
Meal replacement bar	1 bar (40 g)	31	19	6
Lentils (green/ brown)	4 tbsp (150 g)	30	17	5
Chickpeas	4 tbsp (150 g)	28	30	8
Red kidney beans	4 tbsp (150 g)	28	25	7
Whole milk	1 large glass (250 ml)	27	12	3
Lentils (red)	4 tbsp (150 g)	26	18	5
Grapefruit	½ (120 g)	25	11	3
Cherries	Small handful (120 g)	22	12	3
Fructose	2 tsp (10 g)	19	10	2
Peanuts	Small handful (50 g)	14	6	1

Vitamin	Function(s)	Sources	RNI and SUL*	
A	Essential for normal colour vision and for the cells in the eye that enable us to see in dim light; promotes healthy skin and mucous membranes lining the mouth, nose, digestive system, etc.	Liver, meat, eggs, whole milk, cheese, oily fish, butter, margarine	Men: 700 µg/day Women: 600 mcg/day SUL: 1500 µg/day (800 mcg for pregnant women)	
Beta-carotene	Converted into vitamin A (6 µg produces 1 µg vitamin A): a powerful antioxidant and free radical scavenger	Brightly coloured fruit and vegetables (e.g. carrots, spinach, apricots, tomatoes)	No official carotene RNI. 15 mg is suggested intake SUL: 7 mg	
B (Thiamin)	Forms a co-enzyme essential for the conversion of carbohydrates into energy; used for the normal functioning of nerves, brain and muscles	Wholemeal bread and cereals, liver, kidneys, red meat, pulses (beans, lentils, peas)	Men: 0.4 mg/1000 calories Women: 0.4 mg/1000 calories No SUL. FSA recommends 100 mg	
B_2 (Riboflavin)	Required for the conversion of carbohydrates to energy; promotes healthy skin and eyes and normal nerve functions	Liver, kidneys, red meat, chicken, milk, yoghurt, cheese, eggs	Men: 1.3 mg/day Women: 1.1 mg/day No SUL. FSA recommends 40 mg	

*RNI = Reference nutrient intake (Department of Health, 1991)

**NV = no value published.

SUL = Safe Upper Limit recommended by the Expert Group on Vitamins and Minerals, an independent advisory committee to the Food Standards Agency (Food Standards Agency, 2003)

Claim(s) of supplements	The evidence	Possible dangers of high doses
Maintains normal vision, healthy skin, hair and mucous membranes; may help to treat skin problems such as acne and boils; may affect protein manufacture	Not involved in energy production; little evidence to suggest it can improve sporting performance	Liver toxicity from taking supplements: symptoms include liver and bone damage; abdominal pain; dry skin; double vision; vomiting; hair loss; headaches. May also cause birth defects. Pregnant women should avoid liver. Never exceed 9000 µg/day (men), 7500 µg/day (women)
Reduces risk of heart disease, cancer and muscle soreness	As an antioxidant, may help prevent certain cancers. Other carotenoids in food may also be important	Orange tinge to the skin – probably harmless and reversible
May optimise energy production and performance; is usually present within a B-complex or multivitamin	Involved in energy (ATP) production, so the higher the energy expenditure, the higher the thiamin requirement; increased needs can normally be met in the diet; there is no evidence to suggest that high intakes enhance performance; supplements are probably unnecessary	Cannot be stored – excess is excreted, therefore unlikely to be toxic; toxic symptoms (rare) may include insomnia, rapid pulse, weakness and headaches. Avoid taking more than 3 g/day
Sportspeople may need more B_2 because they have higher energy needs – supplements may optimise energy production; usually present within a B-complex or multivitamin	Forms part of the enzymes involved in energy production, so exercise may increase the body's requirements; however, these can usually be met by a balanced diet; there is no evidence that supplements improve performance; if you take the contraceptive pill you may need extra B_2	Rarely toxic as it cannot be stored; any excess is excreted in the urine (a bright yellow colour)

Vitamin	Function(s)	Sources	RNI and SUL*
Niacin	Helps to convert carbohydrates into energy; promotes healthy skin, normal nerve functions and digestion	Liver, kidneys, red meat, chicken, turkey, nuts, milk, yoghurt and cheese, eggs, bread, cereals	Men: 6.6 mg/1000 calories Women: 6.6 mg/1000 calories SUL: 17 mg
B_6 (Pyridoxine)	Involved in the metabolism of fats, proteins and carbohydrates; promotes healthy skin, hair and normal red blood cell formation; is actively used in many chemical reactions of amino acids and proteins	Liver, nuts, pulses, eggs, bread, cereals, fish, bananas	Men: 1.4 mg/day Women: 1.2 mg/day SUL: 80 mg
Pantothenic acid (B vitamin)	Involved in the metabolism of fats, proteins and carbohydrates; promotes healthy skin, hair and normal growth; helps in the manufacture of hormones and antibodies, which fight infection; helps energy release from food	Liver, wholemeal bread, brown rice, nuts, pulses, eggs, vegetables	No RNI in the UK No SUL
Folic acid (B vitamin)	Essential in the formation of DNA; necessary for red blood cell manufacture	Liver and offal, green vegetables, yeast extract, wheatgerm, pulses	Men: 200 µg/day Women: 200 µg/day SUL: 1000 µg (1 mg)
B_{12}	Needed for red blood cell manufacture and to prevent some forms of anaemia; used in fat, protein and carbohydrate metabolism; promotes cell growth and development; needed for normal nerve functions	Meat, fish, offal, milk, cheese, yoghurt; vegan sources (fortified foods) are soya protein and milk, yeast extract, breakfast cereals	Men: 1.5 µg/day Women: 1.5 µg/day SUL: 2 mg

Claim(s) of supplements	The evidence	Possible dangers of high doses
Sportspeople need more niacin since it is involved in metabolism; higher doses may help to reduce blood cholesterol levels	Not enough evidence to prove that high doses can help to improve performance; requirements can be met by a balanced diet	Excess is excreted in the urine; doses of more than 200 mg of niacin may cause dilation of the blood vessels near the skin's surface (hot flushes)
Sportspeople may need higher doses to meet their increased energy requirements	Requirements are related to protein intake, so sportspeople on high protein diets may need extra B_6; endurance work may cause greater than normal losses; there is no evidence to suggest that high doses improve performance; extra doses may help to alleviate PMS (premenstrual syndrome)	Excess is excreted in the urine; very high doses (over 2 g/day) over months or years may cause numbness and unsteadiness
Since it is involved in protein, fat and carbohydrate metabolism, sportspeople may need higher doses; usually present within a B-complex or multivitamin – for overall well-being	No evidence to suggest that high doses improve performance	Excess is excreted in the urine
Supplements help overall well-being, and also prevent folic acid deficiency and anaemia; these would, in theory, hinder aerobic performance	No studies have been carried out on athletic performance and folic acid	Dangers of toxicity are very small, though high doses may reduce zinc absorption and disguise a deficiency of vitamin B_{12}
Since it is involved in the development of red blood cells, the implication is that B_{12} can improve the body's oxygen carrying capacity (and therefore its aerobic performance); athletes have been known to use injections of vitamin B_{12} before competition in the hope that it will improve their endurance; usually present within a B-complex or multivitamin	Extra vitamin B_{12} has no effect on endurance or strength; there is no benefit to be gained from taking supplements (deficiencies are very rare)	Excess is excreted in the urine

Vitamin	Function(s)	Sources	RNI and SUL*
Biotin	Involved in the manufacture of fatty acids and glycogen, and in protein metabolism; needed for normal growth and development	Egg yolk, liver and offal, nuts, whole grains (whole grains), oats	No RNI in the UK; 10–200 µg/day is thought to be a safe and adequate range SUL: 900 µg
C	Growth and repair of body cells; collagen formation (in connective tissue) and tissue repair; promotes healthy blood vessels, gums and teeth; haemoglobin and red blood cell production; manufacture of adrenalin; powerful antioxidant	Fresh fruit (especially citrus), berries and currants, vegetables (especially dark green, leafy vegetables, tomatoes, peppers)	Men: 40 mg/day Women: 40 mg/day SUL: 1000 mg
D	Controls absorption of calcium from the intestine and helps to regulate calcium metabolism; prevents rickets in children and osteomalacia in adults; helps to regulate bone formation	Sunlight (UV light striking the skin), fresh oils, oily fish, eggs, vitamin-D-fortified cereals, margarines and some yoghurts	10 mcg SUL: 25 mcg
E	As an antioxidant, it protects tissues against free radical damage; promotes normal growth and development; helps in normal red blood cell formation	Pure vegetable oils, wheatgerm, wholemeal bread and cereals, egg yolk, nuts, sunflower seeds, avocado	No RNI in the UK; FSA suggests 4 mg (men) 3 mg (women) (10 mg in EU) SUL: 540 mg

Mineral	Function(s)	Sources	RNI and SUL*
Calcium	Important for bone and teeth structure; helps with blood clotting; acts to transmit nerve impulses; helps with muscle contraction	Milk, cheese, yoghurt, soft bones of small fish, seafood, green leafy vegetables, fortified white flour and bread, pulses	700 mg SUL: 1500 mg

Claim(s) of supplements	The evidence	Possible dangers of high doses
Although biotin was once known among bodybuilders as the 'dynamite vitamin', no specific role for this vitamin in sporting performance has been claimed; it is usually present within a B-complex or multivitamin	The body can make its own biotin, so supplements are unnecessary	There are no known cases of biotin toxicity
Vitamin C may help to increase oxygen uptake and aerobic energy production; exercise causes an increased loss so extra may be needed; intense exercise tends to cause greater free radical damage, so sportspeople need higher doses	A deficiency reduces physical performance; exercise may increase requirements to approximately 80 mg/day – these can be met by including 5 portions of fresh fruit and vegetables in the diet each day; intakes of 100–150 mg may help prevent heart disease and cancer	Excess is excreted, so toxic symptoms are unlikely; high doses may lead to diarrhoea and increase the risk of kidney stones in people who are prone to them
No specific claims for athletic performance	So far not shown to be beneficial to performance	Fat-soluble and can be stored in the body; toxicity is rare but symptoms may include high blood pressure, nausea, and irregular heart beat and thirst
Since it is an antioxidant, it may improve oxygen utilisation in the muscle cells; it may also help to protect the cells from the damaging effects of intense exercise; may help to protect against heart disease and cancer	Supplements may have a beneficial effect on performance at high altitudes, and may help reduce heart disease, cancer risk, and post-exercise muscle soreness; requirements are related to intake of polyunsaturated fatty acids	Although it cannot be excreted, toxicity is extremely rare
Claim(s) of supplements	The evidence	Possible dangers of high doses
May help to prevent calcium deficiency and, in some cases, osteoporosis (brittle bone disease)	There is no evidence that extra calcium prevents osteoporosis; exercise (with adequate calcium intake) prevents bone loss, so supplements would seem to be unnecessary; sportspeople who eat few or no dairy products may find calcium supplements useful for meeting basic dietary requirements; extra calcium may help to reduce the risk of stress fractures in sportswomen with menstrual irregularities	The balance of calcium in the bones and blood is finely controlled by hormones – calcium toxicity is thus virtually unknown. Very high intakes may interfere with the absorption of iron and with kidney function

Mineral	Function(s)	Sources	RNI and SUL*
Sodium	Helps to control body fluid balance; involved in muscle and nerve functions	Table salt, tinned vegetables, fish, meat, ready-made sauces and condiments, processed meats, bread, cheese	Men: 1.6 g/day (= 4 g salt) Women: 1.6 g/day (= 4 g salt) FSA recommends a maximum daily intake of 2.5 g (= 6 g salt)
Potassium	Works with sodium to control fluid balance and muscle and nerve functions	Vegetables, fruit and fruit juices, unprocessed cereals	Men: 3.5 g/day Women: 3.5 g/day SUL: 3.7 g
Iron	Involved in red blood cell formation and oxygen transport and utilisation	Red meat, liver, offal, fortified breakfast cereals, shellfish, wholegrain bread, pasta and cereals, pulses, green leafy vegetables	Men: 6.7 mg/day Women: 16.4 mg/day SUL: 17 mg
Zinc	A component of many enzymes involved in the metabolism of proteins, carbohydrates and fats; helps to heal wounds; assists the immune system; needed for building cells	Meat, eggs, wholegrain cereals, milk and dairy products	Men: 9.5 mg/day Women: 7 mg/day SUL: 25 mg
Magnesium	Involved in the formation of new cells, in muscle contraction and nerve functions; assists with energy production; helps to regulate calcium metabolism; forms part of the mineral structure of bones	Cereals, vegetables, fruit, potatoes, milk	Men: 300 mg/day Women: 270 mg/day SUL: 400 mg
Phosphorus	Assists in bone and teeth formation; involved in energy metabolism as a component of ATP	Cereals, meat, fish, milk and dairy products, green vegetables	550 mg/day SUL: 250 mg from supplements

Claim(s) of supplements	The evidence	Possible dangers of high doses
It has been claimed that extra salt is needed if you sweat a lot or exercise in hot, humid conditions; advocated for treating cramp	Excessive sweating during exercise may cause a marked loss of sodium, but as salt is present in most foods, supplements are usually unnecessary; extra salt is more likely to cause, rather than prevent, cramp – dehydration is normally the cause of cramp (together possibly with a shortage of potassium)	High salt intakes may increase blood pressure, risk of stroke, fluid retention and upset the electrolyte balance of the body
May help to reduce blood pressure and encourage sodium excretion	Extra potassium is not known to enhance performance; may help to prevent cramp	Excess is excreted, therefore toxicity is very rare
Extra iron can improve the oxygen-carrying capacity of red blood cells, and therefore improve aerobic performance; can prevent or treat anaemia	Iron-deficiency anaemia can impair performance, especially in aerobic activity; exercise destroys red blood cells and haemoglobin and increases loss of iron, therefore iron requirements of sportspeople may be slightly higher than those of sedentary people; iron is lost through menstruation, so supplements may be sensible for sportswomen	High doses may cause constipation and stomach discomfort; they may also interact with zinc, reducing its absorption
Suggest a possible role in high intensity and strength exercises; may help to boost the immune system	Studies have failed to show that extra zinc is of any benefit to performance; sportspeople with a zinc deficiency may have an impaired immune system, so an adequate intake is important	High doses may cause nausea and vomiting; daily doses of more than 50 mg also interfere with the absorption of iron and other minerals, leading to iron-deficiency anaemia
Magnesium status may be related to aerobic capacity	Studies have failed to show that magnesium supplements are beneficial to performance	May cause diarrhoea
It has been claimed that phosphate loading enhances aerobic performance and delays fatigue	The consensus is that phosphate loading is of little benefit to performance	High intakes over a long period of time may lower blood calcium levels

LIST OF ABBREVIATIONS

ACSM	American College of Sports Medicine
ADP	adenosine diphosphate
ALA	alpha-linolenic acid
ATP	adenosine triphosphate
BCAA	branched-chain amino acids
BMI	Body Mass Index
BMR	basal metabolic rate
BV	Biological Value
EAA	essential amino acid
DHA	docosahexanoic acid
DHEA	dehydroepiandrosterone
DoH	Department of Health
DRV	Dietary Reference Value
EFA	essential fatty acid
EPA	eicosapentanoic acid
FT	fast-twitch (type II) muscle fibres
GI	glycaemic index
GL	glycaemic load
HDL	high density lipoprotein
HMB	beta-hydroxy beta-methylbutyrate
IGF-I	insulin-like growth factor-I
IOC	International Olympic Committee
LDL	low density lipoprotein
MRP	Meal Replacement Product
NEAA	non-essential amino acid
PC	phosphocreatine
NRV	Nutrient Reference Value (on supplement labels)
RMR	resting metabolic rate
RNI	Reference Nutrient Intake
ST	slow-twitch (type I) muscle fibres
SUL	safe upper limit
VO_2max	maximal aerobic capacity

SYMBOLS USED AND CONVERSIONS

FURTHER READING

SYMBOLS USED

g	gram
h	hour
kcal	kilocalorie
kJ	kilojoule
m	metre
min	minute
mcg	microgram
mg	milligram (1000 g = 1 g)
ml	millilitre
mmol	millimole
mph	miles per hour
sec	seconds
tbsp	tablespoon
tsp	teaspoon
dl	decilitre (10 dl = 1 l)
μg	microgram (1000 μg = 1 mg)
<	less than
>	greater than
°C	degree Celsius

CONVERSIONS

1 kcal	=	4.2 kJ
25 g	=	1 oz
450 g	=	1 lb
1 kg	=	2.2 lb
5 ml	=	1 tsp
15 ml	=	1 tbsp
25 ml	=	1 fl oz
600 ml	=	1 pint

Antonio J., Kalman, D. *et al.* (eds) (2008), *Essentials of Sports Nutrition and Supplements*, Humana Press.

Benardot, D. (2012), *Advanced Sports Nutrition*, 2nd edn, Human Kinetics.

Burke, L. (2007), *Practical Sports Nutrition*, Human Kinetics.

Burke, L. and Deakin, V. (2015), *Clinical Sports Nutrition*, McGraw-Hill Medical.

Dunford, M. (2010), *Fundamentals of Sport and Exercise Nutrition*, Human Kinetics.

Food Standards Agency (2002), *McCance and Widdowson's The Composition of Foods*, 6th summary ed., Royal Society of Chemistry.

Jeukendrup, A. and Glesson, M. (2010), *Sport Nutrition*, 2nd ed., Human Kinetics.

Lanham-New, S. *et al.* (eds) (2011), *Sport and Exercise Nutrition*, Wiley-Blackwell.

McArdle, W. *et al.* (2006), *Exercise Physiology: Energy, Nutrition, and Human Performance*, 6th ed., Lippincott, Williams and Wilkins.

Wilmore, J. and Costill, D. (2005), *Physiology of Sport and Exercise*, 3rd ed., Human Kinetics.

REFERENCES

Aceto, C. (1997), *Everything You Need to Know about Fat Loss* (Adamsville TN: Fundco).

Achten J. *et al.* (2004), 'Higher dietary carbohydrate content during intensified running training results in better maintenance of performance and mood state'. *J. Appl. Physiol.*, vol. 96(4), pp. 1331–40.

Ackland T. *et al.* (2012), 'Current Assessment of Body Composition in Sport'. *Sports Med.*, vol. 42(3): 227–49.

ACSM (1996), 'Position stand on exercise and fluid replacement'. *Med. Sci. Sports and Ex.*, vol. 28, pp. i–vii.

ACSM (2007), Armstrong, L.E., Casa, D.J. *et al.* 'American College of Sports Medicine position stand. Exertional heat illness during training and competition'. *Med. Sci. Sports and Ex.*, vol. 39(3): 556–72.

ACSM/AND/DC (2016), 'Nutrition and Athletic Performance'. Med Sci in Sports and Ex, vol. 48 (3) pp. 543–568.

Adams, R. B., Egbo, K. N., & Demmig-Adams, B. (2014) 'High-dose vitamin C supplements diminish the benefits of exercise in athletic training and disease prevention', *Nutrition & Food Science*, vol. 44(2), pp. 95–101

Ahlborg, B. *et al.* (1967), 'Human muscle glycogen content and capacity for prolonged exercise after different diets'. *Forsvarsmedicin*, vol. 3, pp. 85–99.

Ainsworth, B. E. *et al.* (2011) 'Compendium of physical activities: A second update of codes and MET values'. *Med. Sci. Sports and Ex.*, vol. 43. p. 1575. Accessed from http://www.shapesense.com/fitness-exercise/calculators/activity-based-calorie-burn-calculator.aspx#change-activity-category, March 2016.

Alexander, D., Ball, M. J. and Mann, J. (1994), 'Nutrient intake and hematological status of vegetarians and age-sex matched omnivores'. *Eur. J. Clin. Nutr.*, vol. 48, pp. 538–46.

Alghannam, A. F. *et al.* (2016), 'Impact of muscle glycogen availability on the capacity for repeated exercise in man'. *Med. Sci. Sports and Ex.*, vol. 48(1), pp. 123–31.

American Dietetic Association (1997), 'Vegetarian diets – ADA position'. *J. Am. Diet. Assoc.*, vol. 97, pp. 1317–21.

Anderson, M. *et al.* (2000), 'Improved 2000m rowing performance in competitive oarswomen after caffeine ingestion'. *Int. J. Sport Nutr.*, vol. 10, pp. 464–75.

Anthony, J. C. *et al.* (2001) 'Signaling pathways involved in translational control of protein synthesis in skeletal muscle by leucine'. *J. Nutr.*, vol. 131(3), pp. 856S–860S.

Antonio, J. and Street, C. (1999), 'Glutamine: a potentially useful supplement for athletes'. *Can.*

J. Appl. Physiol., vol. 24(1): S69–77.

Appleby, P. N. *et al.* (1999), 'The Oxford Vegetarian Study: an overview'. *Am. J. Clin. Nutr.*, vol. 70 (3 Suppl), pp. 525S–31S.

Areta J. L. *et al.* (2013), 'Timing and distribution of protein ingestion during prolonged recovery from resistance exercise alters myofibrillar protein synthesis'. *J. Physiol.*, vol. 591(9), pp. 2319–31.

Armstrong, L. E. (2002), 'Caffeine, body fluid-electrolyte balance and exercise performance'. *Int. J. Sport Nutr.*, vol. 12, pp. 189–206.

Armstrong, L. E. *et al.* (1985), 'Influence of diuretic induced dehydration on competitive running performance'. *Med. Sci. Sports Ex.*, vol. 17, pp. 456–61.

Armstrong, L. E. *et al.* (1998), 'Urinary indices during dehydration, exercise and rehydration'. *Int. J. Sport Nutr.*, vol. 8, pp. 345–55.

Armstrong, L. E. *et al.* (2005), 'Fluid, electrolyte and renal indices of hydration during 11 days of controlled caffeine consumption'. *Int. J. Sport Nutr. Exerc. Metab.*, vol. 15, pp. 252–65.

Ashwell, M. *et al.* (2011), 'Waist-to-height ratio is a better screening tool than waist circumference and BMI for adult cardiometabolic risk factors: systematic review and meta-analysis'. *Obes. Rev.* vol 13(3), pp. 275–86.

Astrand, P. O. (1952), *Experimental studies of physical working capacity in relation to sex and age* (Copenhagen, Munksgaard).

Astrup, A., *et al.* (2010), 'The role of reducing intakes of saturated fat in the prevention of cardiovascular disease: where does the evidence stand in 2010?' *Am. J. Clin. Nutr.*, vol. 93, pp. 684–8.

Atallah, R. *et al.* (2014), 'Long-term effects of 4 popular diets on weight loss and cardiovascular risk factors: a systematic review of randomized controlled trials'. *Circ. Cardiovasc. Qual. Outcomes*, vol. 7(6), pp. 815–27.

Bacon, L. *et al.* (2005), 'Size acceptance and intuitive eating improve health for obese, female chronic dieters'. *J. Am. Diet. Assoc.*, vol. 105 (6), pp. 929–36.

Barr, S. I. and Costill, D. L. (1989), 'Water. Can the endurance athlete get too much of a good thing?' *J. Am. Diet. Assoc.*, vol. 89, pp. 1629–32.

Barr, S. I. and Rideout, C. A. (2004), 'Nutritional considerations for vegetarian athletes'. *Nutrition*, vol. 20 (7–8), pp. 696–703.

Bartlett, J. D. *et al.* (2015), 'Carbohydrate availability and exercise training adaptation: too much of a good thing?' *Eur. J. Sport Sci.*, vol. 15(1), pp. 3–12.

Bates *et al.* (2014), National Diet and Nutrition Survey. Headline results from years 1, 2, 3, 4 of the Rolling Programme (2208/9–2011/12) (Public Health England, London).

Bauer, J. *et al.* (2013), 'Evidence-based recommendations for optimal dietary protein intake in older people: a position paper from the PROT-AGE Study Group'. *J. Am. Med. Dir. Assoc.*, vol. 14, pp. 542–59.

Bazzare, T. L. *et al.* (1986), 'Incidence of poor nutritional status among triathletes, endurance athletes and controls'. *Med. Sci. Sports Ex.*, vol. 18, p. 590.

BDA (British Dietetic Association) (2014) https://www.bda.uk.com/foodfacts/vegetarian foodfacts.pdf, accessed March 2016.

Beals, K. A. and Hill, A. K. (2006), 'The prevalence of disordered eating, menstrual dysfunction and low bone mineral density among US collegiate athletes'. *Int. J. Sports Nutr. Exerc. Metab.*, vol. 16, pp. 1–23.

Beals, K. A. and Manore, M. M. (1994), 'The prevalence and consequences of subclinical eating disorders in female athletes'. *Int. J. Sport Nutr.*, vol. 4, pp. 157–95.

Beals, K. A. and Manore M. M. (2002), 'Disorders of the female athlete triad among collegiate athletes'. *Int. J. Sport Nutr. Exerc. Metab.*, vol. 12, pp. 281–93.

Beelen, M. *et al.* (2008), Protein coingestion stimulates muscle protein synthesis during resistance type exercise'. *Am. J. Physiol. Endocrinol Metab.*, vol. 295, pp. E70–7.

Beelen, M. *et al.* (2010), 'Nutritional strategies to promote postexercise recovery'. *Int. J. Sport Nutr. Exerc. Metab.*, vol. 20, pp. S15–32.

Beis, L. Y. *et al.* (2011), 'Food and macronutrient intake of elite Ethiopian distance runners'. *J. Int. Soc. Sports Nutr.*, vol. 8 pp. 7–11.

Bell, D. G. *et al.* (2001), 'Effect of caffeine and ephedrine ingestion on anaerobic exercise performance'. *Med. Sci. Sport Exerc.*, vol. 33 (8), pp. 1399–1403.

Bell, P. G. *et al.* (2015), 'Recovery facilitation with Montmorency cherries following high-intensity, metabolically challenging exercise'. *Appl. Physiol. Nutr. Metab.*, vol. 40, pp. 414–23.

Below, P. R. *et al.* (1995), 'Fluid and carbohydrate ingestion independently improve performance during one hour of intense exercise'. *Med. Sci. Sports Exerc.*, vol. 27, pp. 200–10.

Belza, A., Ritz, C., Sørensen, M. Q. *et al.* (2013), 'Contribution of gastroenteropancreatic appetite hormones to protein-induced satiety'. *Am. J. Clin. Nutr.*, vol. 97(5), pp. 980–9.

Bennell K. L. *et al.* (1995), 'Risk factors for stress fractures in female track and field athletes: a retrospective anaysis'. *Clin. J. Sports Med.*, vol. 5, pp. 229–35.

Beradi, J. M. *et al.* (2008), 'Recovery from a cycling time trial is enhanced with carbohydrate-protein supplementation vs. isoenergetic carbohydrate supplementation'. *J. Int. Soc. Sports Nutr.* 2008, vol. 5, p. 24.

Berg, A. and Keul, J. (1988), 'Biomechanical changes during exercise in children'. *Young athletes: Biological, psychological and educational perspectives*, ed. R. M. Malina (Champaign, IL, Human Kinetics) pp. 61–77.

Bergstrom, J. *et al.* (1967), 'Diet, muscle glycogen and physical performance'. *Acta. Physiol. Scand.*, vol. 71, pp. 140–50.

Bescos, R. *et al.* (2012), 'The effect of nitric oxide related supplements on human performance'. *Sports Med.*, vol. 42(2), pp. 99–117.

Betts, J. *et al.* (2007), 'The influence of carbohydrate and protein ingestion during recovery from prolonged exercise on subsequent endurance performance'. *J. Sports Sci.*, vol. 25(13), pp. 1449–60.

Betts, J. *et al.* (2014), 'The causal role of breakfast in energy balance and health: a randomized controlled trial in lean adults'. *Am. J. Clin. Nutr.*, vol. 100(2), pp. 539–47.

Bishop, N. C. *et al.* (2002), 'Influence of carbohydrate supplementation on plasma cytokine and neutrophil degranulation responses to high intensity intermittent exercise'. *Int. J. Sport Nutr.*, vol. 12, pp. 145–56.

Bloomer, R. J. *et al.* (2000), 'Effects of meal form and composition on plasma testosterone, cortisol and insulin following resistance exercise'. *Int. J. Sport Nutr.*, vol. 10, pp. 415–24.

Boirie, Y. *et al.* (1997), 'Slow and fast dietary proteins differently modulate postprandial protein accretion'. *Proc. Nat. Acad. Sci. USA.*, vol. 94(26), pp. 14930–5.

Bompa, T. O. and Cornacchia, L. J. (2013), *Serious Strength Training* (Champaign, IL, Human Kinetics).

Booth, F. and Zwetsloot, K. (2010), 'Basic concepts about genes, inactivity and aging'. *Scand. J. Med. Sci. Sports*, vol. 20, pp. 1–4.

Borsheim E *et al.* (2004), 'Effect of an amino acid, protein, and carbohydrate mixture on net muscle protein balance after resistance training'. *Int. J. Sport. Nutr. Exerc. Metab.*, vol. 14, pp. 255–71.

Bosch, A. N. *et al.* (1994), 'Influence of carbohydrate ingestion on fuel substrate turnover and oxidation during prolonged exercise'. *J. Appl. Physiol.*, vol. 76, pp. 2364–72.

Bounous, G. and Gold, P. (1991), 'The biological activity of un-denatured whey proteins: role of glutathione'. *Clin. Invest. Med.*, vol. 4, pp. 296–309.

Bouvard, V. *et al.* (2015), 'Carcinogenicity of consumption of red and processed meat', *The Lancet Oncology*, Oct. 26.

Bowtell, J. L., Sumners, D. P., Dyer, A. *et al.* (2011), 'Montmorency cherry juice reduces muscle damage caused by intensive strength exercise', *Medicine and Science in Sports Exercise*, vol. 43(8), pp. 1544–51.

Brand-Miller, J., Foster-Powell, K. and McMillan Price J. (2005), *The Low GI Diet.* (Hodder Mobius).

Brand-Miller, J. *et al.* (2003), 'Low GI diet in the management of diabetes'. *Diabetes Care,* vol. 26, pp. 2261–7.

Brilla, L. R. and Conte, V. (2000), 'Effects of a novel zinc-magnesium formulation on hormones and strength'. *J. Exerc. Physiol. Online*, vol. 3(4), pp. 1–15.

Brinkworth, G. D. and Buckley, J. D. (2003), 'Concentrated bovine colostrum protein supplementation reduces the incidence of self-reported symptoms of upper respiratory tract infection in adult males'. *Eur. J. Nutr.*, vol. 42, pp. 228–32.

Brinkworth, G. D. *et al.* (2004), 'Effect of bovine colostrum supplementation on the composition of resistance trained and untrained limbs in healthy young men'. *Eur. J. Appl. Physiol.*, vol. 91, pp. 53–60.

British Nutrition Foundation (1999), Briefing paper: *n-3 Fatty acids and health.*

Broeder, C. E. *et al.* (2000), 'The Andro Project'. *Arch. Intern. Med.*, vol. 160(20), pp. 3093–104.

Brouns, F. *et al.* (1998), 'The effect of different rehydration drinks on post-exercise electrolyte excretion in trained athletes'. *Int. J. Sports Med.*, vol. 19, pp. 56–60.

Brown, E. C. *et al.* (2004), 'Soy versus whey protein bars: Effects of exercise training impact on lean body mass and antioxidant status'. *J. Nutr.*, vol. 3, pp. 22–7.

Brown, G. A. *et al.* (2000), 'Effects of anabolic precursors on serum testosterone concentrations and adaptations to resistance training in young men'. *Int. J. Sport Nutr.*, vol. 10, pp. 340–59.

Brownlie, T., *et al.* (2004) 'Tissue iron deficiency without anemia impairs adaptation in endurance capacity after aerobic training in previously untrained women'. *Am. J. Clin. Nutr.*, vol. 79(3), pp. 437–43.

Bryce-Smith, D. and Simpson, R. (1984), 'Anorexia, depression and zinc deficiency'. *Lancet*, vol. 2, p. 1162.

Bryer S. C. and Goldfarb, A. H. (2006), 'Effect of high dose vitamin C supplementation on muscle soreness, damage, function and oxidative stress to eccentric exercise'. *Int. J. Sport Nutr. Exerc. Metab.*, vol. 16, pp. 270–80.

Buckley, J. D. *et al.* (2003), 'Effect of bovine colostrum on anaerobic exercise performance and plasma insulin-like growth factor'. *J. Sports Sci.,* vol. 21, pp. 577–88.

Buford, T. W., *et al.* (2007). 'International Society of Sports Nutrition position stand: creatine supplementation and exercise'. *J. Int. Soc. Sports Nutr.*, vol. 4, p. 6.

Burd, N. A. *et al.* (2009), 'Exercise training and protein metabolism: influences of contraction, protein intake, and sex-based differences'. *J. Appl. Physiol.*, vol. 106(5), pp. 1692–701.

Burd, N. A. *et al.* (2011), 'Enhanced amino acid sensitivity of myofibrillar protein synthesis persists for up to 24 h after resistance exercise in young men'. *J. Nutr.*, vol. 141(4), pp. 568–73.

Burd, N. A. *et al.* (2013), 'Anabolic resistance of muscle protein synthesis with aging'. *Exerc. Sport Sci. Rev.*, vol. 41, pp. 169–73.

Burke, D. G. *et al.* (1993), 'Muscle glycogen storage after prolonged exercise: effect of glycaemic index of carbohydrate feedings'. *J. Appl. Physiol.*, vol. 75, pp. 1019–23.

Burke, D. G. *et al.* (1998), 'Glycaemic index – a new tool in sports nutrition'. *Int. J. Sport Nutr.*, vol. 8, pp. 401–15.

Burke, D. G. *et al.* (2000), 'The effect of continuous low dose creatine supplementation on force, power and total work'. *Int. J. Sport Nutr.*, vol. 10, pp. 235–44.

Burke, D. G. *et al.* (2001a), 'The effect of alpha lipoic supplementation on resting creatine during acute creatine loading' (conference abstract). *FASEB Journal*, vol. 15(5), p. A814.

Burke, D. G. *et al.* (2001b), 'The effect of whey protein supplementation with and without creatine monohydrate combined with resistance training on lean tissue mass and muscle strength'. *Int. J. Sport Nutr.*, vol. 11, pp. 349–64.

Burke, L. M. (2001) 'Nutritional practices of male and female endurance cyclists'. *Sports Med.*, vol. 31(7), pp. 521–32.

Burke, L. M. (2007), *Practical Sports Nutrition* (Champaign, IL, Human Kinetics).

Burke, L. M. (2010) 'Fueling strategies to optimize performance: training high or training low?' *Scand. J. Med. Sci. Sports*, vol. 20, Suppl. 2, pp. 48–58.

Burke, L. M. *et al.* (2004), 'Carbohydrates and fat for training and recovery'. *J. Sports Sci.*, vol. 22(1), pp. 15–30.

Burke L. M. *et al.* (2011), 'Carbohydrates for training and competition'. *J. Sports Sci.*, vol. 29, Suppl. 1, pp. S17–27.

Burke, L. M. *et al.* (2012), 'Effect of intake of different dietary protein sources on plasma amino acid profiles at rest and after exercise'. *Int. J. Sport Nutr. and Exerc. Metab.*, vol. 22, pp. 452–62.

Burke, L. M. *et al* (2017), 'Low carbohydrate, high fat diet impairs exercise economy and negates the performance benefit from intensified training in elite race walkers'. *J. Physiol.*, doi:10.1113/JP273230

Bussau, V. A. *et al.*, (2002), 'Carbohydrate loading in human muscle: an improved 1-day protocol'. *Eur. J. Appl. Physiol.*, vol. 87, pp. 290–5.

Butterfield G. E. (1996), 'Ergogenic Aids: Evaluating sport nutrition products'. *Int. Sport Nutr.*, vol. 6, pp. 191–7.

Cahill, C. F. (1976), 'Starvation in Man'. *J. Clin. Endocrinol. Metab.*, vol. 5, pp. 397–415.

Cameron S. L. *et al.* (2010), 'Increased blood pH but not performance with sodium bicarbonate supplementation in elite rugby union players'. *Int. J. Sport Nutr. Exerc. Metab.*, vol. 20(4), pp. 307–21.

Campbell, W. W. *et al.* (1995), 'Effects of resistance training and dietary protein intake in protein metabolism in older adults'. *Am. J. Physiol.*, Vol 268, pp. 1143–53.

Candow, D. G. *et al.* (2001), 'Effect of glutamine supplementation combined with resistance training in young adults'. *Eur. J. Appl. Physiol.*, vol. 86(2), pp. 142–9.

Candow, D. G. *et al.* (2006), 'Effect of whey and soy protein supplementation combined with resistance training in young adults'. *Int. J. Sports Nutr. Exerc. Metab.*, vol. 16, pp. 233–44.

Cann, C. E. *et al.* (1984), 'Decreased spinal mineral content in amenhorreic women'. *JAMA*, vol. 251, pp. 626–9.

Cannell, J. *et al.* (2009), 'Athletic performance and vitamin D'. *Med. Sci. Sports Exerc.*, vol. 41, pp. 1102–10.

Carbon, R. (2002), 'The female athlete triad does not exist'. *Sports Care News*, 26, pp. 3–5.

Carr, A. J. (2011), 'Effects of acute alkalosis and acidosis on performance: a meta-analysis'. *Sports Med.*, vol. 41(10), pp. 801–14.

Carter, J. M. *et al.* (2004), 'The effect of carbohydrate mouth rinse on 1-h cycle time-trial performance'. *Med. Sci. Sports Exerc.*, vol. 36, pp. 2107–11.

Castell, L. M. and Newsholme, E. A. (1997), 'The effects of oral glutamine supplementation on athletes after prolonged exhaustive exercise'. *Nutrition*, vol. 13, pp. 738–42.

Cermak N. M. *et al.* (2012), 'Nitrate supplementation's improvement of 10 km time trial performance in trained cyclists'. *Int. J. Sport Nutr. Exerc. Metab.*, vol. 1, pp. 64–71.

Cheung, S. S. *et al.* (2015), 'Separate and combined effects of dehydration and thirst sensation on exercise performance in the heat'. *Scand. J. Med. Sci. Sports*, vol. 25, Suppl. 1, pp. 104–11.

Cheuvront, S. N., Carter, R., and Sawka, M. N. (2003), 'Fluid balance and endurance exercise performance', *Current Sports Medicine Reports*, vol. 2 pp. 202–8.

Chowdhury, E. A. *et al.* (2015), 'Carbohydrate-rich breakfast attenuates glycaemic, insulinaemic and ghrelin response to *ad libitum* lunch relative to morning fasting in lean adults'. *Br. J. Nutr.*, vol. 114(1), pp. 98–107.

Chowdhury R. *et al.* (2014), 'Association of dietary, circulating, and supplement fatty acids with coronary risk: A systematic review and meta-analysis'. *Ann. Intern. Med.*, vol. 160(6), pp. 398–406.

Christensen, E. H. and Hansen, O. (1939), 'Arbeitsfähigheit und Ernährung'. *Skand. Arch. Physiol.*, vol. 81, pp. 160–71.

Chryssanthopoulos, C. *et al.* (2002), 'The effect of a high carbohydrate meal on endurance running capacity'. *Int. J. Sport Nutr.*, vol. 12, pp. 157–71.

Clark, J. F. (1997), 'Creatine and phosphocreatine: a review'. *J. Athletic Training*, vol. 32(1), pp. 45–50.

Clark, N. (1995), 'Nutrition quackery: when claims are too good to be true'. *Phys. Sports Med.*, vol. 23, pp. 7–8.

Clayton, D. J. and James, L. (2015), 'The effect of breakfast on appetite regulation, energy balance and exercise performance'. *Proc. Nutr. Soc.*, vol. 14, pp. 1–9 (Epub ahead of print).

Clayton D. J. *et al.* (2015), 'Effect of breakfast omission on energy intake and evening exercise performance'. *Med. Sci. Sports Exerc.*, vol. 47(12), pp. 2645–52.

Close, G. L., Cobley, R. J., Owens, D. J. *et al.* (2013a), 'Assessment of vitamin D concentration in non-supplemented professional athletes and healthy adults during the winter months in the UK: implications for skeletal muscle function'. *J. Sports Sci.*, vol. 31(4), pp. 344–53.

Close, G. L., *et al.* (2013b), 'The effects of vitamin D3 supplementation on serum total 25(OH) D concentration and physical performance: a randomised dose-response study'. *Br. J. Sports Med.*, vol. 47, pp. 692–6.

Cobb, K. L. *et al.* (2003), 'Disordered eating, menstrual irregularity and bone mineral density in female runners'. *Med. Sci. Sports Exerc.*, vol. 35, pp. 711–19.

Cockburn, E., Robson-Ansley, P., Hayes, P. R., Stevenson, E. (2012), 'Effect of volume of milk consumed on the attenuation of exercise-induced muscle damage'. *Eur. J. Appl. Physiol.*, Jan 7. (Epub ahead of print.)

Cockburn, E. *et al.* (2008), 'Acute milk-based protein-CHO supplementation attenuates exercise-induced muscle damage'. *Appl. Physiol. Nutr. Metab.*, Aug; 33(4): 775–83.

Coggan, A. R. and Coyle, E. F. (1987), 'Reversal of fatigue during prolonged exercise by carbohydrate infusion or ingestion'. *J. Appl. Physiol.*, vol. 63, pp. 2388–95.

Coggan, A. R. and Coyle, E. F. (1991), 'Carbohydrate ingestion during prolonged exercise: effects on metabolism and performance'. In J. Holloszy (ed.), *Exercise and Sports Science Reviews*, vol. 19 (Williams and Wilkins), pp. 1–40.

Cole, T. J., Bellizzi, M., Flegal, K. and Dietz, W. H. (2000), 'Establishing a standard definition for child overweight and obesity worldwide: international survey'. *British Medical Journal*, vol. 320, pp. 1240–3.

Cook, M. D. *et al.* (2015), 'New Zealand blackcurrant extract improves cycling performance and fat oxidation in cyclists'. *Eur. J. Appl. Physiol.*, vol. 115(11), pp. 2357–65.

Cooper, R. *et al.* (2012), 'Creatine supplementation with specific view to exercise/sports performance: an update'. *J. Int. Soc. Sports Nutr.*, vol. 9, p. 33.

Corder, K. E. *et al.* (2016), 'Effects of short-term docosahexaenoic acid supplementation on markers of inflammation after eccentric strength exercise in women'. *J. Sports Sci. Med.*, vol 15, pp. 176–83.

Costill, D. L. (1985), 'Carbohydrate nutrition before, during and after exercise'. *Fed. Proc.*, vol. 44, pp. 364–368.

Costill, D. L. (1986), *Inside Running: Basics of Sports Physiology* (Benchmark Press), p. 189.

Costill, D. L. (1988), 'Carbohydrates for exercise: dietary demands for optimal performance'. *Int. J. Sports Med.*, vol. 9, pp. 1–18.

Costill, D. L. and Hargreaves, M. (1992), 'Carbohydrate nutrition and fatigue'. *Sports Med.*, vol. 13, pp. 86–92.

Costill, D. L. *et al.* (1971), 'Muscle glycogen utilisation during prolonged exercise on successive days'. *J. Appl. Physiol.*, vol. 31, pp. 834–8.

Cox, A. J., Pyne, D. B., Saunders, P. U., and Fricker, P. A. (2008), 'Oral administration of the probiotic Lactobacillus fermentum VRI-003 and mucosal immunity in endurance athletes'. Br. *J. Sports Med.* (Epub Feb. 13).

Cox, G. *et al.* (2002), 'Acute creatine supplementation and performance during a field test simulating match play in elite female soccer players'. *Int. J. Sport Nutr.*, vol. 12, pp. 33–46.

Coyle, E. F. (1988), 'Carbohydrates and athletic performance'. *Sports Sci. Exch. Sports Nutr.*, Gatorade Sports Science Institute, vol. 1.

Coyle, E. F. (1991), 'Timing and method of increased carbohydrate intake to cope with heavy training, competition and recovery'. *J. Sports Sci.*, vol. 9 (suppl.), pp. 29–52.

Coyle, E. F. (1995), 'Substrate utilization during exercise in active people'. *Am. J. Clin. Nutr.*, vol. 61 (suppl), pp. 968–79.

Coyle, E. (2004), 'Fluid and fuel intake during exercise'. *J. Sports Sci.*, vol. 22, pp. 39–55.

Craddock, J. *et al.* (2015), 'Vegetarian and omnivorous nutrition – comparing physical performance'. *Int. J. Sport Nutr. Exerc. Metab.*, Nov 16 (Epub ahead of print).

Craig, W. J., Mangels, A. R.; American Dietetic Association (2009), Position of the American Dietetic Association: vegetarian diets'. *J. Am. Diet. Assoc.*, vol. 109(7), pp. 1266–82.

Cribb P. J. *et al.* (2006), 'The effect of whey isolate and resistance training on strength, body composition and plasma glutamine'. *Int. J. Sports Nutr. Exerc. Metab.*, vol. 16, pp. 494–509.

Crooks, C. V. *et al.* (2006), 'The effect of bovine colostrum supplementation on salivary IgA in distance runners'. *Int. J. Sport Nutr. Exerc. Metab.*, vol. 16, pp. 47–64.

Crowe, M. J., Weatherson, J. N., Bowden, B. F. (2006), 'Effects of dietary leucine supplementation on exercise performance'. *Eur. J. Appl. Physiol.*, vol. 97(6), p. 664.

Cupisti, A. *et al.* (2002), 'Nutrition knowledge and dietary composition in Italian female athletes and non-athletes'. *Int. J. Sport Nutr.*, vol. 12, pp. 207–19.

Currell, K. and Jeukendrup, A. E. (2008), 'Superior endurance performance with ingestion of multiple transportable carbohydrates'. *Med. Sci. Sports Exerc.*, vol. 40(2), pp. 275–81.

Dangin, M. *et al.* (2001), 'The digestion rate of protein is an independent regulating factor of postprandial protein retention'. *Am. Physiol. Soc. Abstracts,* vol. 7: 022E.

Dansinger, M. *et al.* (2005), 'Comparison of the Atkins, Ornish, Weight Watchers, and Zone diets for weight loss and heart disease risk reduction: a randomized trial'. *JAMA*, vol. 293(1), pp. 43–53.

Danz, M. *et al.* (2016), 'Hyponatremia among triathletes in the Ironman European Championship'. *N. Engl. J. Med.*, vol. 374, pp. 997–9.

Davey, G. K. *et al.* (2003), 'EPIC-Oxford: Lifestyle characteristics and nutrient intakes in a cohort of 33,883 meat-eaters and 31,546 non meat-eaters in the UK'. *Public Health Nutrition*, vol. 6(3), pp. 259–68.

Davis, C. (1993), 'Body image, dieting behaviours and personality factors: a study of high-performance female athletes'. *Int. J. Sport Psych.*, vol. 23, pp. 179–92.

Davis, J. M. *et al.* (1988), 'Carbohydrate-electrolyte drinks: effects on endurance cycling in the heat'. *Am. J. Clin. Nutr.*, vol. 48, pp. 1023–30.

Davison, G. (2012), 'Bovine colostrum and immune function after exercise'. *Med. Sport Sci.* vol. 59, pp. 62–9.

de Ataide e Silva, T. *et al.* (2013), 'Can carbohydrate mouth rinse improve performance during exercise? A systematic review'. *Nutrients.* Dec 19, 6(1), pp. 1–10. doi: 10.3390/nu6010001.

DeMarco, H. M. *et al.* (1999), *Med. Sci. Sports Ex.*, vol. 31(1), pp. 164–70.

de Oliveira, E. P., Burini, R. C., Jeukendrup, A. (2014), 'Gastrointestinal complaints during exercise: prevalence, etiology, and nutritional recommendations'. *Sports Med.* vol. 44 Suppl 1, pp. S79–85.

de Oliveira Otto, M. C., Mozaffarian, D., Kromhout, D. *et al.* (2012), 'Dietary intake of saturated fat by food source and incident cardio vascular disease: the multi-ethnic study of atherosclerosis'. *Am. J. of Clin. Nutr.*, vol. 96(2), pp. 397–404.

De Souza, R. J. *et al.* (2015), 'Intake of saturated and trans unsaturated fatty acids and risk of all cause mortality, cardiovascular disease, and type 2 diabetes:

systematic review and meta-analysis of observational studies'. *BMJ*, vol. 351, h3978.

Department of Health (1991), 'Dietary Reference Values for Food Energy and Nutrients for the United Kingdom'. London: HMSO.

Department of Health (1994), *Nutritional Food Guide* (HMSO).

Department of Health (2004), *At least five a week: Evidence on the impact of physical activity and its relationship to health. A report from the Chief Medical Officer.*

Derave, W. *et al.* (2007), 'Beta-alanine supplementation augments muscle carnosine content and attenuates fatigue during repeated isokinetic contraction bouts in trained sprinters'. *J. Appl. Physiol.*, vol. 103, pp. 1736–43.

Desbrow, B. *et al.* (2004), 'Carbohydrate-electrolyte feedings and 1 h time trial cycling performance'. *Int. J. Sport Nutr. Exerc. Metab.*, vol. 14, pp. 541–9.

Desbrow, B. *et al.* (2014), 'Comparing the rehydration potential of different milk-based drinks to a carbohydrate-electrolyte beverage'. *Appl. Physiol. Nutr. Metab.*, vol. 39(12), pp. 1366–72.

Deutz, N. E. P. *et al.* (2014), 'Protein intake and exercise for optimal muscle function with aging: Recommendations from the ESPEN Expert Group'. *Clin. Nutr.*, vol. 33(6), pp. 929–36.

Dodd, H. *et al.* (2011), 'Calculating meal glycaemic index by using measured and published food values compared with directly measured meal glycaemic index'. *Am. J. Clin. Nutr.*, vol. 95, pp. 992–6.

Dodd, S. L. *et al.* (1993), 'Caffeine and exercise performance'. *Sports Med.*, vol. 15, pp. 14–23.

Doherty, M. and Smith, P. M. (2004), 'Effects of caffeine ingestion on exercise testing: a meta-analysis'. *Int. J. Sport Nutr. Exerc. Metab.*, vol. 14, pp. 626–46.

Donnelly, J. E. *et al.* (2009), 'American College of Sports Medicine Position Stand. Appropriate physical activity intervention strategies for weight loss and prevention of weight regain for adults'. *Med. Sci. Sports Exerc.*, pp. 459–71.

Downes, J. W. (2002), 'The master's athlete: Defying aging'. *Topics in Clinical Chiropractic*, vol. 9(2), pp. 53–9.

Drinkwater, B. L. (1986), 'Bone mineral content after resumption of menses in amenorrheic athletes'. *JAMA*, vol. 256, pp. 380–2.

Drinkwater, B. L. *et al.* (1984), 'Bone mineral content of amenorrheic and eumenorrheic athletes'. *New England. J. Med.*, vol. 311, pp. 277–81.

Drummond, M. J. and Rasmussen, B. B. (2008), 'Leucine-enriched nutrients and the regulation of mammalian target of rapamycin signalling and human skeletal muscle protein synthesis. *Curr. Opin. Clin. Nutr. Metab. Care*, vol. 11, pp. 222–6

Ducker, K. J., Dawson, B., Wallman, K. E. (2013), 'Effect of beta-alanine supplementation on 800-m running performance'. *Int. J. Sport Nutr. Exerc. Metab.*, vol. 23(6), pp. 554–61.

Dueck, C. A. *et al.* (1996), 'Role of energy balance in athletic menstrual dysfunction'. *Int. J. Sport Nutr.*, vol. 6, pp. 165–90.

Dulloo, A. G. *et al.* (1999), 'Efficacy of a green tea extract rich in catechin polyphenols and caffeine in increasing 24 hour energy expenditure and fat oxidation in humans'. *Am. J. Clin. Nutr.*, vol. 70, pp. 1040–5.

Durnin, J. V. G. A. and Womersley, J. (1974), 'Body fat assessed from total body density and its estimation from skinfold thickness: measurements on 481 men and women ages from 16 to 72 Years'. *Brit. J. Nutr.*, vol. 32, p. 77.

Easton, C. *et al.* (2007), 'Creatine and glycerol hyperhydration in trained subjects before exercise in the heat'. *Int. J. Sports Nutr. Exerc. Metab.*, vol. 17, pp. 70–91.

Eckerson, J. M., Bull, A. J., Baechle, T. R., Fischer, C. A., O'Brien, D. C., Moore, G. A., Yee, J. C., Pulverenti, T. S. (2013), 'Acute ingestion of sugar-free Red Bull energy drink has no effect on upper body strength and muscular endurance in resistance trained men'. *J. Strength Cond. Res.*, vol. 27(8), pp. 2248–54.

Edwards, J. R. *et al.* (1993), 'Energy balance in highly trained female endurance runners'. *Med. Sci. Sports Ex.*, vol. 25(12), pp. 1398–404.

EFSA Panel on Dietetic Products, Nutrition, and Allergies (2010), 'Scientific opinion on Dietary Reference Values for water'. *EFSA Journal*, vol. 8(3), p. 1459.

EFSA (2015), 'Scientific and technical assistance on food intended for sportspeople'. http://www.efsa.europa.eu/sites/default/files/scientific_output/files/main_documents/871e.pdf accessed March 2016.

Egli, L. *et al.* (2013), 'Exercise prevents fructose-induced hypertriglyceridemia in healthy young subjects'. *Diabetes*, vol. 62(7), pp. 2259–65.

Eisinger, M. (1994), 'Nutrient intake of endurance runners with lacto-ovo vegetarian diet and regular Western diet'. *Z. Ernährungswiss*, vol. 33, pp. 217–29.

Elliot, T. A. *et al.* (2006), 'Milk ingestion stimulates net muscle protein synthesis following resistance exercise,' *Med. Sci. Sports Exer.*, vol. 38(4) pp. 667–74.

Erlenbusch, M. *et al.* (2005), 'Effect of high fat or high carbohydrate diets on endurance exercise: a meta-analysis'. *Int. J. Sport Nutr. Exerc. Metab.*, vol. 14, pp. 1–14.

Estruch, R. *et al.* (2013), 'Primary prevention of cardiovascular disease with a Mediterranean diet'. *N. Engl. J. Med.*, vol. 368, pp. 1279–90.

Fairchild, T. J. *et al.* (2002), 'Rapid carbohydrate loading after a short bout of near maximal-intensity exercise'. *Med. Sci. Sports Exer.*, pp. 980–6.

Farajian, P. *et al.* (2004), 'Dietary intake and nutritional practices of elite Greek aquatic athletes'. *Int. J. Sport Nutr. Exerc. Metab.*, vol 14, pp. 574–85.

Febbraio, M. A. and Stewart, K. L. (1996), 'CHO feeding before prolonged exercise: effect of glycaemic index on muscle glycogenolysis and exercise performance'. *J. Appl. Phsyiol.*, vol. 81, pp. 1115–20.

Febbraio, M. A. *et al.* (2000), 'Effects of carbohydrate ingestion before and during exercise on glucose kinetics and performance'. *J. Appl. Physiol.*, vol. 89, pp. 2220–6.

Ferguson-Stegall, L. *et al.* (2011), 'Aerobic exercise training adaptations are increased by post-exercise carbohydrate-protein supplementation'. *J. Nutr. Metab.*, Epub Jun 9.

Fiala, K. A. *et al.* (2004), 'Rehydration with a caffeinated beverage during the non-exercise periods of 3 consecutive days of 2-a-day practices'. *Int. J. Sport Nutr. Exerc. Metab.*, vol 14. pp. 419–29.

Fleck, S. J. and Reimers, K. J. (1994), 'The practice of making weight: does it affect performance?' *Strength and Cond.*, vol. 1, pp. 66–7.

Fogelholm, M. (1994), 'Effects of bodyweight reduction on sports performance'. *Sports Med.*, vol. 18(14), pp. 249–67.

Fogelholm, M. (1995), 'Indicators of vitamin and mineral status in athletes' blood: a review'. *Int. J. Sports Nutr.*, vol. 5, pp. 267–84.

Food Standards Agency (2003), *Safe upper levels for vitamins and minerals* (HMSO).

Food Standards Agency and Department of Health (2004). *National diet and nutrition survey of adults aged 19–64*, vol. 5 (HMSO).

Forbes, S. C., Candow, D. G., Little, J. P., *et al.* (2007), 'Effect of Red Bull energy drink on repeated Wingate cycle performance and bench-press muscle endurance'. *Int. J. Sport Nutr. Exerc. Metab.*, vol. 17(5), pp. 433–44.

Foster-Powell, K. and Brand-Miller, J. C. (1995), 'International tables of glycaemic index'. *Am. J. Clin. Nutr.*, vol. 62 (suppl), pp. 871S–90S.

Foster-Powell, K., Holt, S. and Brand-Miller, J. C. (2002), 'International table of glycaemic index and glycaemic load values: 2002'. *Am. J. Clin. Nutr.*, vol. 76, pp. 5–56.

Frankenfield D. C. *et al.* (2005), 'Comparison of predictive equations for Resting Metabolic Rate in healthy nonobese and obese adults: a systematic review'. *J. Am. Diet. Assoc.*, vol. 105, pp. 775–89.

Frentsos, J. A. and Baer, J. T. (1997), 'Increased energy and nutrient intake during training and competition improves elite triathletes' endurance performance'. *Int. J. Sport Nutr.*, vol. 7, pp. 61–71.

Gaeini, A. A., Rahnama, N., Hamedinia, M. R. (2006), 'Effects of vitamin E supplementation on oxidative stress at rest and after exercise to exhaustion in athletic students'. *J. Sports Med. Phys. Fitness*, vol. 46(3), pp. 458–61.

Galloway, S. D. R. and Maughan, R. (2000), 'The effects of substrate and fluid provision on thermoregulatory and metabolic responses to prolonged exercise in a hot environment'. *J. Sports Sci.*, vol. 18(5), pp. 339–51.

Gant, N., Ali, A. and Foskett, A. (2010), 'The influence of caffeine and carbohydrate coingestion on simulated soccer performance'. *Int. J. Sport Nutr. Exerc. Metab.*, vol. 20, pp. 191–7.

Gardner, C. D. *et al.* (2007), 'Comparison of the Atkins, Zone, Ornish, and LEARN Diets for change in weight and related risk factors among overweight premenopausal women: the A to Z weight loss study: a randomized trial'. *JAMA*, vol. 297(9), pp. 969–77.

Garfinkel, P. E. and Garner, D. M. (1982), *Anorexia nervosa: a multidimensional perspective*. (Brunner/ Mazel).

GSSI (1995), 'Roundtable on methods of weight gain in athletes'. *Sports Science Exchange*, vol. 6(3), pp. 1–4.

German, J. B. *et al.* (2009), 'A reappraisal of the impact of dairy foods and milk fat on cardiovascular disease risk'. *European Journal of Nutrition*, vol. 48(4), pp. 191–203.

Geyer, H., Parr. M. K., Mareck, U., *et al.*, (2004), 'Analysis of non-hormonal nutritional supplements for anabolic-androgenic steroids – results of an international study'. *Int. J. Sports Med.*, vol. 25(2), pp. 124–9.

Gibala, M. J. (2000), 'Nutritional supplementation and resistance exercise: what is the evidence for enhanced skeletal muscle hypertrophy?' *Can. J. Appl. Physiol.*, vol. 25(6), pp. 524–35.

Gilchrist, M., Winyard, P. G., and Benjamin, N. (2010), 'Dietary nitrate – good or bad?' *Nitric Oxide*, vol. 22, pp. 104–9.

Gilson, S. F. *et al.* (2009), 'Effects of chocolate milk consumption on markers of muscle recovery during intensified soccer training'. *Medicine and Science in Sports and Exercise*, vol. 41, p. S577.

Gisolphi, C. V. *et al.* (1992), 'Intestinal water absorption from select carbohydrate solutions in humans'. *J. Appl. Physiol.*, vol. 73, pp. 2142–50.

Gisolphi, C. V. *et al.* (1995), 'Effect of sodium concentration in a carbohydrate-electrolyte solution on intestinal absorption'. *Med. Sci. Sports Ex.*, vol. 27(10), pp. 1414–20.

Gleeson, M. (2011), 'Nutrition and immunity'. In *Diet, Immunity and Inflammation*, Calder, P. C. and Yaqoob, P (eds) (Woodhead Publishing).

Gleeson, M. *et al.* (2008), 'Exercise and immune function: is there any evidence for probiotic benefit for sportspeople?' *Complete Nutrition*, vol. 8, pp. 35–7.

Goldstone, A. P. *et al.* (2009), 'Fasting biases brain reward systems towards high-calorie foods'. *Eur. J. Neurosci.*, vol 30(8), pp. 1625–35.

Gomez-Cabrera *et al.* (2008), 'Oral administration of vitamin C decreases muscle mitochondrial biogenesis and hampers training-induced adaptations in endurance performance'. *Am. J. Clin. Nutr.* 87(1), pp. 142–9.

Gontzea, I. *et al.* (1975), 'The influence of adaptation to physical effort on nitrogen balance in man'. *Nutr. Rep. Int.*, vol. 22, pp. 213–16.

Gonzalez-Alonzo, J. *et al.* (1992), 'Rehydration after exercise with common beverages and water'. *Int. J. Sports Med.*, vol. 13, pp. 399–406.

Goulet, E. D. B. (2011), 'Effects of exercise-induced dehydration on time trial exercise performance: a meta-analysis'. *Brit. J. Sports Med.*, vol. 45, pp. 1149–56.

Goulet, E. D. B. (2013), 'Effect of exercise-induced dehydration on endurance performance: evaluating the impact of exercise protocols on outcomes using a meta-analytic procedure'. *Br. J. Sports Med.*, vol. 47(11), pp. 679–86.

Graham, T. E. and Spriet, L. L. (1991), 'Performance and metabolic responses to a high caffeine dose during prolonged exercise'. *J. Appl. Physiol.*, vol. 71(6), pp. 2292–8.

Graham, T. E. and Spriet, L. L. (1995), 'Metabolic, catecholamine and exercise performance responses to various doses of caffeine'. *J. Appl. Physiol.*, vol. 78: pp. 867–74.

Grandjean, A. (2000), 'The effect of caffeinated, non-caffeinated, caloric and non-caloric beverages on hydration'. *J. Am. Coll. Nutr.*, vol. 19, pp. 591–600.

Gray-Donald, K. *et al.* (2014), 'Protein intake protects against weight loss in healthy community-dwelling older adults'. *J. Nutr.* vol. 144, pp. 321–6.

Green, A. L. *et al.* (1996), 'Carbohydrate augments creatine accumulation during creatine supplementation in humans'. *Am. J. Physiol.*, vol. 271, E821–6.

Greenhaff, P. L. (1997), 'Creatine supplementation and implications for exercise performance and guidelines for creatine supplementation'. In A. Jeukendrup *et al.* (eds), *Advances in Training and Nutrition for Endurance Sports* (Maastricht: Novertis Nutrition Research Unit), pp. 8–11.

Greenwood, M., *et al.* (2003), 'Creatine cramps. Not'. *J. Athletic Training*, vol. 38(3), pp. 216–19.

Greer B. K. *et al.* (2007), 'Branched chain amino acid supplementation and indicators of muscle damage after endurance exercise'. *Int. J. Sports Nutr. Exerc. Metab.*, vol. 17, pp. 595–607.

Gregory, J. *et al.* (2000), *The National Diet and Nutrition Survey: young people aged 4–18 years*, vol. 1, (HMSO).

Groen, B. *et al.* (2012), 'Intragastric protein administration stimulates overnight muscle protein synthesis in elderly men'. *Am. J. Physiol. Endocrinol. Metab.*, vol. 302, pp. 52–60.

Gualano, B., *et al.* (2012), 'In sickness and in health: The widespread application of creatine supplementation'. *Amino Acids*, vol. 43, pp. 519–29.

Guest, N. S. and Barr, S. (2005), 'Cognitive dietary restraint is associated with stress fractures in women runners'. *Int. J. Sports Nutr. Exerc. Metab.*, vol. 15, pp. 147–59.

Hall, Kevin D. *et al.* (2015), 'Calorie for calorie, dietary fat restriction results in more body fat loss than carbohydrate restriction in people with obesity'. *Cell Metabolism*, vol. 22(3), pp. 427–36.

Halliday, T. *et al.* (2011), 'Vitamin D status relative to diet, lifestyle, injury and illness in college athletes'. *Med. Sci. Sports Exerc.*, vol. 43, pp. 335–43.

Halliwell, B. and Gutteridge, J. M. C. (1985), *Free Radicals in Biology and Medicine* (Clarendon Press), pp. 162–4.

Hamilton, B. (2011), 'Vitamin D and athletic performance: the potential role of muscle'. *Asian J. Sports Med.*, vol. 2(4), pp. 211–19.

Hanne, N., Dlin, R. and Rotstein, A. (1986), 'Physical fitness, anthropometric and metabolic parameters in vegetarian athletes'. *J. Sports Med. Phys. Fitness.*, vol. 26, pp. 180–5.

Hansen, A. K. *et al.* (2005), 'Skeletal muscle adaptation: training twice every second day vs. training once daily'. *J. Appl. Physiol.*, vol 98(1), pp. 93–9.

Hao, Q. *et al.* (2011), 'Probiotics for preventing acute upper respiratory tract infections'. *Cochrane Database Syst. Rev.*, 7(9).

Hargreaves, M. and Snow, R. (2001), 'Amino acids and endurance exercise'. *Int. J. Sport Nutr.*, vol. 11, pp. 133–145.

Hargreaves, M. *et al.* (2004), 'Pre-exercise carbohydrate and fat ingestion: effects on metabolism and performance'. *J. Sports Sci.*, vol. 22(1), pp. 31–38.

Harris, R. C. (1998), 'Ergogenics 1'. *Peak Performance*, vol. 112, pp. 2–6.

Harris, R. C. *et al.* (2006), 'The absorption of orally supplied beta-alanine and its effect on muscle carnosine synthesis in human vastus lateralis'. *Amino Acids*, vol. 30(3), pp. 279–89.

Hartman, J. W. *et al.* (2007), 'Consumption of fat-free fluid milk after resistance exercise promotes greater lean mass accretion than does consumption of soy or carbohydrate in young, novice, male weightlifters'. *Am. J. Clin. Nutr.*, vol. 86(2), pp. 373–81.

Haub, M. D. (1998), 'Acute l-glutamine ingestion does not improve maximal effort exercise'. *J. Sport Med. Phys. Fitness*, vol. 38, pp. 240–4.

Haub, M. D. *et al.* (2002), 'Effect of protein source on resistive-training-induced changes in body composition and muscle size in older men'. *Am. J. Clin. Nutr.*, vol. 76, pp. 511–17.

Haussinger, D. *et al.* (1996), 'The role of cellular hydration in the regulation of cell functioning'. *Biochem. J.*, vol. 31, pp. 697–710.

Havemann, L. *et al.* (2006), 'Fat adaptation followed by carbohydrate loading compromises high-intensity sprint performance'. *J. Appl. Physiol.*, vol. 100(1), pp. 194–202.

Hawley, J. A. and Burke, L. M. (2010), 'Carbohydrate availability and training adaptation: effects on cell metabolism'. *Exerc. Sports Sci. Rev.*, vol. 38, pp. 152–160.

Hawley, J. A. and Leckey, J. (2015), 'Carbohydrate dependence during prolonged, intense endurance exercise'. *Sports Med.*, vol 45 (Suppl 1), pp. S5–S12.

Hawley, J. A. and Lessard, S. J. (2008), 'Exercise training-induced improvements in insulin action'. *Acta Physiol* (Oxf), vol 192(1), pp. 127–35.

Hawley, J. *et al.* (1997), 'Carbohydrate loading and exercise performance'. *Sports Med.*, vol. 24(1), pp. 1–10.

Hawley, J. *et al.* (2011) 'Nutritional modulation of training-induced skeletal muscle adaptations'. *J. Appl. Physiol.*, vol. 100, pp. 834–45.

Heaney, R. P. (2011), 'Assessing vitamin D status'. *Curr. Opin. Clin. Nutr. Metab. Care*, vol. 14, pp. 440–4.

Heaney, R. P. (2013), 'Health is better at serum 25(OH)D above 30ng/mL'. *J. Steroid Biochem. Mol. Biol.*, vol. 136, pp. 224–8.

Helge, J. W. *et al.* (2001), 'Fat utilisation during exercise: adaptation to a fat rich diet increases utilisation of plasma fatty acids and very low density lipoprotein-triacylglycerol in humans'. *J. Physiol.*, vol. 537; 3, pp. 1009–20.

Helms, E. R. *et al.* (2014), 'A systematic review of dietary protein during caloric restriction in resistance trained lean athletes: a case for higher intakes'. *Int. J. Sport Nutr. Exerc. Metab.*, vol. 24(2), pp. 127–38.

Hemilä, H. (2011). Zinc lozenges may shorten the duration of colds: a systematic review. The open respiratory medicine journal, 5(1).

Herman, P. and Polivy, J. (1991), 'Fat is a psychological issue'. *New Scientist*, 16 Nov., pp. 41–5.

Hickey, H. S. *et al.* (1994), 'Drinking behaviour and exercise-thermal stress: role of drink carbonation'. *Int. J. Sport Nutr.*, vol. 4, pp. 8–12.

Higgins, S. *et al.* (2015), 'The effects of pre-exercise caffeinated-coffee ingestion on endurance performance: an evidence-based review'. *Int. J. Sport Nutr. Exerc. Metab.*, Nov 16 (Epub ahead of print).

Hill, A. M. *et al.* (2007), 'Combining fish-oil supplements with regular aerobic exercise improves body composition and cardiovascular disease risk factors'. *Am. J. Clin. Nutr.*, vol. 85(5), pp. 1267–74.

Hitchins, S. *et al.* (1999), 'Glycerol hyperhydration improves cycle time trial performance in hot humid conditions'. *Eur. J. Appl. Physiol. Occup. Physiol.*, vol. 80(5), pp. 494–501.

Hobson, R. M. *et al.* (2012), 'Effects of -alanine supplementation on exercise performance: a meta-analysis'. *Amino Acids*, vol. 43(1), pp. 25–37.

Hoffman, J. R. *et al.* (2008), 'Short-duration beta-alanine supplementation increases training volume and reduces subjective feelings of fatigue in college football players'. *Nutr. Res.*, vol. 28, pp. 31–5.

Holt, S. J. (1992), 'Relationship of satiety to postprandial glycaemic, insulin and cholecystokinin responses'. *Appetite*, vol. 18, pp. 129–41.

Hoon, MW1, Johnson NA, Chapman PG, Burke LM (2013) The effect of nitrte supplementation on exercise performance in healthy individuals: a systematic review and meta-analysis. Int J Sport Nutr Exerc Metab. 2013 Oct; 23(5):522-32. Epub 2013 Apr 9.

Hoon, M. W. *et al.* (2014), 'Nitrate supplementation and high-intensity performance in competitive cyclists'. *Applied Physiology, Nutrition, and Metabolism*, 0, 0, 10.1139/apnm-2013-0574.

Hooper, L. *et al.* (2012), 'Reduced or modified dietary fat for preventing cardiovascular disease'. *Cochrane Database Syst. Rev.*, May 16;5.

Hooper, L. *et al.* (2015), 'Reduction in saturated fat intake for cardiovascular disease'. *Cochrane Database Syst. Rev.*, Jun 10;6.

Hord N. G., Tang, Y. and Bryan, N. S. (2009), 'Food sources of nitrates and nitrites: the physiologic context for potential health benefits'. *Am. J. Clin. Nutr.*, vol. 90(1), pp. 1–10.

Houtkooper, L. B. (2000), 'Body composition', in Manore, M. M. and Thompson, J. L., *Sport Nutrition for Health and Performance*, Human Kinetics, pp. 199–219.

Howarth, K. R. *et al.* (2009), 'Coingestion of protein with carbohydrate during recovery from endurance exercise stimulates skeletal muscle protein synthesis in humans'. *J. Appl. Physiol.*, vol. 106, pp. 1394–1402.

Howatson, G., McHugh, M. P., Hill, J. A., *et al.* (2010), 'Influence of tart cherry juice on indices of recovery following marathon running'. *Scand. J. Med. Sci. Sports*, vol. 20(6), pp. 843–52.

Howe, S. T. *et al.* (2013), 'The effect of beta-alanine supplementation on isokinetic force and cycling performance in highly trained cyclists'. *Int. J. Sport Nutr. Exerc. Metab.* Dec, vol. 23(6), pp. 562–70 (Epub 2013 Apr 18).

Hu, T. *et al.* (2012), 'Effects of low-carbohydrate diets versus low-fat diets on metabolic risk factors: a meta-analysis of randomized controlled clinical trials'. Am. J. Epidemiol., vol 176 Suppl 7, pp. S44–54.

Hulston CJ *et al.* (2010), 'Training with low muscle glycogen enhances fat metabolism in well-trained cyclists'. *Med. Sci. Sports Exerc.*, vol. 42, pp. 2046–55.

Hultman, E. *et al.* (1996), 'Muscle creatine loading in man'. *J. Appl. Physiol.*, vol. 81, pp. 232–9.

Hunter, A. M. *et al.* (2002), 'Caffeine ingestion does not alter performance during a 100-km cycling time trial performance'. *Int. J. Sport Nutr.*, vol. 12, pp. 438–52.

Hytten, F. E. and Leitch, I. (1971), *The Physiology of Human Pregnancy*, 2nd ed. (Blackwell Scientific Publications).

IMMDA (2006), 'International Marathon Medical Director's Association's revised fluid recommendations for runners & walkers'. http://www.aims-association.org/guidelines_fluid_replacement.htm, accessed March 2016.

International Association of Athletic Federations (IAAF) (2007), Nutrition for athletics: The 2007 IAAF Consensus Statement.

International Olympic Committee (IOC) (2005) 'IOC Position Stand on the female athlete triad' http://www.olympic.org/assets/importednews/documents/en_report_917.pdf (Accessed March 2016).

International Olympic Committee (IOC) (2011), Consensus Statement on Sports Nutrition 2010, Sports Sci 4,29 Suppl 1: S3-4. http://

www.olympic. org/Documents/Reports/EN/CONSENSUSFINAL-v8-en.pdf.

Ivy, J. L. *et al.* (1988), 'Muscle glycogen synthesis after exercise: effect of time of carbohydrate ingestion'. *J. Appl. Physiol.*, vol. 64, pp. 1480–5.

Ivy, J. L. *et al.* (2002), 'Early post-exercise muscle glycogen recovery is enhanced with carbohydrate-protein supplement'. *J. Appl. Physiol.*, vol. 93, pp. 1337–44.

Ivy, J. L. *et al.* (2003), 'Effect of a carbohydrate-protein supplement on endurance performance during exercise of varying intensity'. *Int. J. Sport Nutr. Exerc. Metab.*, vol. 13, pp. 388–401.

Ivy, J. L. *et al.* (2009), 'Improved cycling time-trial performance after ingestion of a caffeine energy drink'. *Int. J. Sport Nutr. Exerc. Metab.*, vol. 19(1), pp. 61–78.

Jacobs, K. A. and Sherman, W. M. (1999), 'The efficacy of carbohydrate supplementation and chronic high-carbohydrate diets for improving endurance performance'. *Int. J. Sport Nutr.*, vol. 9, pp. 92–115.

Jäger, R. *et al.*, (2011), 'Analysis of the efficacy, safety, and regulatory status of novel forms of creatine'. *Amino Acids*, vol. 40(5), pp. 1369–83.

Jakobsen, M. U. *et al.* (2009), 'Major types of dietary fat and risk of coronary heart disease: a pooled analysis of 11 cohort studies'. *Am. J. Clin. Nutr.*, vol. 89, pp. 1425–32.

Jamurtas, A. Z. *et al.* (2011), 'The effects of low and high glycemic index foods on exercise performance and beta-endorphin responses'. *J. Int. Soc. Sports Nutr.*, vol. 8, p. 15.

Janelle, K. C. and Barr, S. I. (1995), 'Nutrient intakes and eating behavior scores of vegetarian and non-vegetarian women'. *J. Am. Diet. Assoc.*, vol. 95, pp. 180–6, 189.

Janssen, I. *et al.* (2000), 'Skeletal muscle mass and distribution in 468 men and women aged 18–88 yr'. *J. Appl. Physiol.*, vol. 89(1), pp. 81–8.

Jebb, S. *et al.* (2004), 'New body fat reference curves for children'. *Obesity Reviews* (NAASO Suppl), A146.

Jenkins, D. J. *et al.* (1987), 'Metabolic effects of a low GI diet'. *Am. J. Clin. Nutr.*, vol. 46, pp. 968–75.

Jeukendrup, A. (2004), 'Carbohydrate intake during exercise and performance'. *Nutrition*, vol. 20, pp. 669–77.

Jeukendrup, A. (2008), 'Carbohydrate feeding during exercise'. *Eur. J. Sports Sci.*, vol. 8(2), pp. 77–86.

Jeukendrup, A. (2010), 'Carbohydrate and exercise performance: the role of multiple transportable carbohydrates'. *Curr. Opin. Clin. Nutr. Metab. Care*, vol. 13(4), pp. 452–57.

Jeukendrup, A. (2014), 'A step towards personalized sports nutrition: carbohydrate intake during exercise'. *Sports Med.*, vol. 44 (Suppl 1), pp. 25–33.

Jeukendrup, A. *et al.* (1997), 'Carbohydrate-electrolyte feedings improve 1-hour time trial cycling performance'. *Int. J. Sports Med.*, vol. 18, pp. 125–9.

Jeukendrup, A., *et al.* (2000), 'Relationship between gastro-intestinal complaints and endotoxaemia, cytokine release and the acute-phase reaction during and after a long-distance triathlon in highly trained men'. *Clin. Sci.* (Lond.), vol. 98(1), pp. 47–55.

Johnston, C. S. *et al.* (2006), 'Ketogenic low-carbohydrate diets have no metabolic advantage over nonketogenic low-carbohydrate diets'. *Am. J. Clin. Nutr.*, vol 83(5), pp. 1055–61.

Jonnalagadda, S. S. *et al.* (2004), 'Food preferences, dieting behaviours, and body image perceptions of elite figure skaters'. *Int. J. Sports Nutr. Exerc. Metab.*, vol. 14, pp. 594–606.

Josse A. R. *et al.* (2010), 'Body composition and strength changes in women with milk and resistance exercise'. *Med. Sci. Sports Exerc.*, vol. 42(6), pp. 1122–30.

Jouris K. *et al.* (2011), 'The effect of omega-3 fatty acid supplementation on the inflammatory response to eccentric strength exercise'. *J. Sports Sci. Med.*, vol. 10, pp. 432–38.

Jowko, E. *et al.*, (2001) 'Creatine and HMB additively increase lean body mass and muscle strength during a weight training programme'. *Nutrition*, vol. 17(7), pp. 558–66.

Joyce, S., *et al.*, (2012), 'Acute and chronic loading of sodium bicarbonate in highly trained swimmers'. *Eur. J. Appl. Physiol.*, vol. 112(2), pp. 461–9.

Judkins, C. (2008), 'Investigation into supplementation contamination levels in the UK market'. *HFL Sport Science*. www.informed-sport.com

Kamber, M. *et al.* (2001), 'Nutritional supplements as a source for positive doping cases?' *Int. J. Sports Nutr.*, vol. 11, pp. 258–63.

Kammer L. *et al.* (2009), 'Cereal and non-fat milk support muscle recovery following exercise'. *J. Int. Soc. Sports Nutr.*, vol. 6, p. 11.

Karlsson, J. and Saltin, B. (1971), 'Diet, muscle glycogen and endurance performance'. *J. Appl. Physiol.*, vol. 31, pp. 201–6.

Karp, J. R. *et al.* (2006), 'Chocolate milk as a post-exercise recovery aid'. *Int. J. Sport Nutr. Exerc. Metab.*, vol. 16, pp. 78–91.

Karsch–Völk, M., Barrett, B., Kiefer, D., Bauer, R., Ardjomand–Woelkart, K., & Linde, K. (2014). Echinacea for preventing and treating the common cold. The Cochrane Library.

Kasper, A. M. *et al.* (2015), 'Carbohydrate mouth rinse and caffeine improves high-intensity interval running capacity when carbohydrate restricted'. *Eur. J. Sport Sci.*, vol. 2, pp. 1–9 (Epub ahead of print).

Katsanos, C. S. *et al.* (2006), 'A high proportion of leucine is required for optimal stimulation of the rate of muscle protein synthesis by essential amino acids in the elderly'. *Am. J. Physiol. Endocrinol. Metab.*, vol. 291, pp. E381–E387.

Keizer, H. A. *et al.* (1986), 'Influence of liquid or solid meals on muscle glycogen resynthesis, plasma fuel hormone response and maximal physical working capacity'. *Int. J. Sports Med.*, vol. 8, pp. 99–104.

Kennerly, K. *et al.* (2011), Influence of banana versus sports beverage ingestion on 75 km cycling performance and exercise-induced inflammation'. *Med. Sci. Sports Exerc.*, vol. 43(5), pp. 340–341.

Kenney, W. L. and Chiu, P. (2001), 'Influence of age on thirst and fluid intake'. *Med. Sci. Sports Exerc.*, vol. 33(9), pp. 1524–32.

Key, T. J. A. *et al.* (1996), 'Dietary habits and mortality in a cohort of 11,000 vegetarians and health conscious people: results of a 17-year follow-up'. *Br. Med. J.*, vol. 313, pp. 775–9.

Keys, A.B. (1980), Seven Countries: A Multivariate Analysis of Death and Coronary Heart Desease (Harvard University Press, 1980).

Kiens, B. *et al.* (1990), 'Benefit of simple carbohydrates on the early post-exercise muscle glycogen repletion in male athletes'. *Med. Sci. Sports Ex.* (suppl.), S88.

Killer, S.C. *et al* (2014), 'No Evidence of Dehydration with Moderate Daily Coffee Intake: A Counterbalanced Cross-Over Study in a Free-Living Population'. *PLoS ONE*, vol. 9 (1): e84154.

King, D. S. *et al.* (1999), 'Effects of oral androstenedione on serum testosterone and adaptations to resistance training in young men'. *J. Am. Med. Assoc.*, vol. 281 (21), pp. 2020–8.

Knez, W. L. and Peake, J. M. (2010), 'The prevalence of vitamin supplementation in ultra-endurance triathletes'. *Int. J. Sport Nutr. Exerc. Metab.*, vol. 20(6), pp. 507–14.

Koopman, R. (2011), 'Dietary protein and exercise training in ageing'. *Proc. Nutr. Soc.*, vol. 70, pp. 104–13.

Koopman, R. *et al.* (2005), 'Combined ingestion of protein and free leucine with carbohydrate increases post-exercise muscle protein synthesis in vivo in male subjects'. *Am. J. Physiol. Endocrinol. Metab.*, vol. 288(4), pp. E645–653.

Kreider, R. (2003) 'Effects of whey protein supplementation with casein or BCAA and glutamine on training adaptations: body composition'. *Med. Sci. Sport Exerc.*, vol. 35(5), suppl. 1, p. S395.

Kreider, R. B. (2003), 'Effects of creatine supplementation on performance and training adaptations'. *Mol. Cell Biochem.*, vol. 244(1–2), pp. 89–94.

Kreider, R. B. *et al.* (1996), 'Effects of ingesting supplements designed to promote lean tissue accretion on body composition during resistance training'. *Int. J. Sport Nutr.*, vol. 63, pp. 234–46.

Kreider, R. B. *et al.* (2000), 'Effects of calcium-HMB supplementation during training on markers of catabolism, body composition, strength and sprint. performance'. *J. Exerc. Physiol.*, vol. 3 (4), pp. 48–59.

Kreider, R. B. *et al.* (2002), 'Effects of conjugated linoleic acid supplementation during resistance training on body composition, bone density, strength, and selected hematological markers'. *J. Strength Cond. Res.*, vol. 16(3), pp. 325–34.

Kristiansen, M. *et al.* (2005), 'Dietary supplement use by varsity athletes at a Canadian University'. *Int. J. Sport Nutr. Exerc. Metab.*, vol. 15, pp. 195–210.

Lambert, E. V. *et al.* (1994), 'Enhanced endurance in trained cyclists during moderate intensity exercise following 2 weeks adaptation to a high fat diet'. *Eur. J. Appl. Physiol*, vol. 69, pp. 287–293.

Lane, S. C. *et al.* (2013), 'Caffeine ingestion and cycling power output in a low or normal muscle glycogen state'. *Med. Sci. Sports Exerc.*, Aug. 45(8), pp. 1577–84.

Lane, S. C. *et al.* (2013), 'Single and combined effects of beetroot juice and caffeine supplementation on cycling time trial performance'. *Appl. Physiol. Nutr. Metab.*, 10.1139/apnm-2013-0336

Lane, S. C. *et al.* (2015), 'Effects of sleeping with reduced carbohydrate availability on acute training responses'. *J. Appl. Physiol.*, vol. 119(6), pp. 643–55.

Lansley, K. I. *et al.* (2011), 'Dietary nitrate supplementation reduces the O2 cost of walking and running: a placebo-controlled study'. *J. Appl. Physiol.*, vol. 110, pp. 591–600.

Lansley, K. I., *et al.* (2011), 'Acute dietary nitrate supplementation improves cycling time trial performance'. *Med. Sci. Sports Exerc.*, vol. 43, pp. 1125–31.

Lanza, I. R. *et al.* (2008), 'Endurance exercise as a countermeasure for aging'. *Diabetes*, vol. 57(11), pp. 2933–42.

Larson-Meyer, D. E. and Willis, K. S. (2010), 'Vitamin D and athletes'. *Curr. Sports Med. Rep.*, vol. 9(4), pp. 220–6.

Laursen, P. B. *et al.* (2006), 'Core temperature and hydration status during an Ironman triathlon'. *Br. J. Sports Med.* 2006 Apr; 40(4), pp. 320–5; discussion 325.

Layman, D. K. *et al.* (2005), 'Dietary protein and exercise have additive effects on body composition during weight loss in adult women'. *J. Nutr.* vol. 35(8), pp. 1903–10.

Lean, M. E. J. *et al.* (1995), 'Waist circumference as a measure for indicating need for weight management'. *BMJ*, vol. 311, pp. 158–61.

Leckey, J. J. *et al.* (2016), 'Altering fatty acid availability does not impair prolonged, continuous running to fatigue: Evidence for carbohydrate dependence'. *J. Appl. Physiol.*, vol. 120(2), pp. 107–13.

Leeds, A., Brand Miller, J., Foster-Powell, K. and Colagiuri, S. (2000), *The Glucose Revolution* (London: Hodder and Stoughton), p. 29.

Leenders, M. *et al.* (2013), 'Elderly men and women benefit equally from prolonged resistance-type exercise training'. *J. Gerontol. A. Biol. Sci. Med. Sci.*, vol. 68(7), pp. 769–79.

Lehnen, T. E. *et al.* (2015), 'A review on effects of conjugated linoleic fatty acid (CLA) upon body composition and energetic metabolism'. *J. Int. Soc. Sports Nutr.*, vol. 12, p. 36.

Lemon, P. W. R. (1992), 'Protein requirements and muscle mass/strength changes during intensive training in novice bodybuilders, *J. Appl. Physiol.*, vol. 73, pp. 767–75.

Lemon, P. W. R. (1995), 'Do athletes need more dietary protein and amino acids?'. *Int. J. Sport Nutr.*, vol. 5 pp. s39–61.

Lemon, P. W. R. (1998), 'Effects of exercise on dietary protein requirements'. *Int. J. Sport Nutr.*, vol. 8, pp. 426–47.

Lenn, J. *et al.* (2002), 'The effects of fish oil and isoflavones on delayed onset muscle soreness'. *Med. Sci. Sports Exerc.*, vol. 34(10), pp. 1605–13.

Levitsky, D. A. and Pacanowski, C. R. (2013), 'Effect of skipping breakfast on subsequent energy intake'. *Physiol Behav.* vol. 119, pp. 9–16.

LGC (2015), Clean Sport http://www.informed-sport.com/sites/default/files/LGC_Clean_Sport_trifold_0315_EN_4336_digital2_0.pdf. Accessed March 2016.

Li, Y., Hruby, A., Bernstein, A. M., *et al.* (2015), 'Saturated fats compared with unsaturated fats and sources of carbohydrates in relation to risk of coronary heart disease: a prospective cohort study'. *J. Am. Coll. Cardiol.*, vol. 66(14), pp. 1538–48.

Lloyd, T. *et al.* (1986), 'Women athletes with menstrual irregularity have increased musculoskeletal injuries'. *Med. Sci. Sports Ex.*, vol. 18, pp. 3427–9.

Lohman, T. G. (1992), 'Basic concepts in body composition assessment'. In *Advances in Body Composition Assessment*, Human Kinetics, pp. 109–118.

Longland, T. M. *et al.* (2016), 'Higher compared with lower dietary protein during an energy deficit combined with intense exercise promotes greater lean mass gain and fat mass loss: a randomized trial'. *Am. J. Clin. Nutr.* Jan 27 (Epub ahead of print).

Loucks, A. B. *et al.* (1989), 'Alterations in the hypothalamic-pituitary-ovarian and the hypothalamic-pituitary axes in athletic women'. *J. Clinical Endocrinol. Metab.*, vol. 68, pp. 402–22.

Loucks, A. B. (2003), 'Energy availability, not body fatness, regulates reproductive function in women'. *Exerc. Sport Sci. Rev.*, vol. 31, pp. 144–148.

Lovell, G. (2008), 'Vitamin D status of females in an elite gymnastic programme'. *Clin. J. Sports Med.*, vol. 18, pp. 159–61.

Luden, N. D. *et al.* (2007), 'Post-exercise carbohydrate-protein-antioxidant ingestion increase CK and muscle soreness in cross-country runners'. *Int. J. Sports Exerc. Metab.*, vol. 17, pp. 109–122.

Lukaski, H.C. (2004), 'Vitamin and mineral status: effects on physical performance'. *Nutrition*, vol. 20, 632–44.

Lun, V. *et al.* (2012), 'Dietary supplementation practices in Canadian high-performance athletes'. *Int. J. Sport Nutr. Exerc. Metab.*, vol. 22(1), pp. 31–7.

Lyall, K. A. *et al.* (2009), 'Short-term blackcurrant extract consumption modulates exercise-induced oxidative stress and lipopolysaccharide-stimulated inflammatory responses'. Am. J. Physiol. Regul. Integr. Comp. Physiol., vol, 297(1), pp. R70–81.

Macintosh, B. R. *et al.* (1995), 'Caffeine ingestion and performance of a 1500-metre swim'. *Can. J. Appl. Physiol.*, vol. 20 (2): pp. 168–77.

Macnaughton, L. S. *et al* (2016), 'The response of muscle protein synthesis following whole-body resistance exercise is greater following 40 g than 20 g of ingested whey protein'. *Physiol. Rep.* vol. 4 (15). pii: e12893.

Madsen, K. *et al.* (1996), 'Effects of glucose and glucose plus branched chain amino acids or placebo on bike performance over 100 km'. *J. Appl. Physiol.*, vol. 81, pp. 2644–50.

MAFF/RSC (1991), McCance and Widdowson's *The Composition of Foods*, 5th ed. (Cambridge: MAFF/RSC).

Maffucci, D. M. and McMurray, R. G. (2000), 'Towards optimising the timing of the pre-exercise meal'. *Int. J. Sport Nutr.*, vol. 10, pp. 103–13.

Mamerow, M. M. *et al.* (2014), 'Dietary Protein Distribution Positively Influences 24-h Muscle Protein Synthesis in Healthy Adults'. *J. Nutrition*, vol. 144, pp. 876–80.

Marquet, L. A. *et al.* (2016), 'Enhanced endurance performance by periodization of cho intake: 'sleep low' strategy'. Med. Sci. Sports Exerc., vol. 48(4), pp. 663–72.

Marquet, L. A. *et al* (2016), 'Periodization of Carbohydrate Intake: Short-Term Effect on Performance'. *Nutrients*, vol. 8 (12), e 755.

Martinez, L. R. and Haymes, E. M. (1992), 'Substrate utilisation during treadmill running in prepubescent girls and women'. *Med. Sci. Sports Exerc.*, vol. 24, pp. 975–83.

Mason, W. L. *et al.* (1993), 'Carbohydrate ingestion during exercise: liquid vs solid feedings'. *Med. Sci. Sports Ex.*, vol. 25, pp. 966–9.

Maughan, R. J. (1995), 'Creatine supplementation and exercise performance'. *Int. J. Sport Nutr.*, vol. 5, pp. 94–101.

Maughan, R. J. *et al.* (1996), 'Rehydration and recovery after exercise'. *Sports Sci. Ex.*, vol. 9(62), pp. 1–5.

Maughan, R. J. and Shireffs, S. M. (2012) 'Nutrition for sports performance: issues and opportunities'. *Proc. Nutr. Soc.*; vol. 71 (1), pp. 112–19.

Maughan, R. J. *et al* (2016), 'A randomized trial to assess the potential of different beverages to affect hydration status: development of a beverage hydration index'. *Am J. Clin. Nutr.*, vol. 103, pp. 717–23.

Mayhew, D. L. *et al.* (2002), 'Effects of long term creatine supplementation on liver and kidney function in American Football players'. *Int. J. Sport Nutr.*, vol. 12, pp. 453–60.

McConnell, G. K. *et al.* (1997), 'Influence of ingested fluid volume on physiological responses during prolonged exercise'. *Acta. Phys. Scand.*, vol. 160, pp. 149–56.

McGlory, Chris *et al.* (2016), 'Fish oil supplementation suppresses resistance exercise and feeding-induced increases in anabolic signaling without affecting myofibrillar protein synthesis in young men'. *Physiological Reports*, March 2016, vol, 4 no. e12715.

MacLean, D. A. *et al.* (1994), 'Branch-chain amino acids augment ammonia metabolism while attenuating protein breakdown during exercise'. *Am. J. Physiol.*, vol. 267, E1010–22.

Meier, C. *et al.* (2004), 'Supplementation with oral vitamin D and calcium during winter prevents seasonal bone loss: a randomnised controlled openlabel prospective trial'. *J. Bone Mineral Res.*, vol. 19, pp. 1221–30.

Melby, C. *et al.* (1993), 'Effect of acute resistance exercise on resting metabolic rate'. *J. Appl. Physiol.*, vol. 75, pp. 1847–53.

Mensink, R.P et al. (2003), 'Effects of dietary fatty acids and carbohydrate on the ratio of serum total to HDL cholesterol and on serum lipids and apolipo proteins: a meta-analysis of 60 controlled trials', American Journal of Clinical Nutrition, 77 (5), pp. 1146–1155.

MHRA (2012) http://webarchive.nationalarchives.gov.uk/20141205150130/http://www.mhra.gov.uk/home/groups/comms-po/documents/news/con174847.pdf

Miescher, E. and Fortney, S. M. (1989), 'Responses to dehydration and rehydration during heat exposure in young and older men'. *Am. J. Physiol.*, vol. 257, pp. R1050–R1056.

Mifflin, M. D. *et al.* (1990), 'A new predictive equation for resting energy expenditure in healthy individuals'. *J. Am. Diet. Assoc.*, vol. 51, pp. 241–7.

Mihic, S. *et al.* (2000), 'Acute creatine loading increases fat free mass but does not affect blood pressure, plasma creatinine or CK activity in men and women'. *Med. Sci. Sport. Exerc.*, vol. 32, pp. 291–6.

Millard-Stafford, M. L. *et al.* (2005), 'Should carbohydrate concentration of a sports drink be less than 8% during exercise in the heat?'. *Int. J. Sport Nutr. Exerc. Metab.*, vol. 15, pp. 117–130.

Miller, S. L. *et al.* (2002), 'Metabolic responses to provision of mixed protein-carbohydrate supplementation during endurance exercise attenuate the increases in cortisol'. *Int. J. Sport Nutr.*, vol. 12, pp. 384–97.

Minehan, M. R. *et al.* (2002), 'Effect of flavour and awareness of kilojoule content of drinks on preference and fluid balance in teAm. sports'. *Int. J. Sport Nutr.*, vol. 12, pp. 81–92.

Mitchell, W. K. *et al.* (2012), 'Sarcopenia, dynapenia, and the impact of advancing age on human skeletal muscle size and strength; a quantitative review'. *Front Physiol.* vol. 3, p. 260.

Montain, S. J. and Coyle, E. F. (1992), 'The influence of graded dehydration on hyperthermia and cardiovascular drift during exercise'. *J. Appl. Physiol.*, vol. 73, pp. 1340–50.

Moore, D. R. *et al.* (2009), 'Ingested protein dose response of muscle and albumin protein synthesis after esistence exercise in young men'. *Am. J. Clin. Nutr.*, vol. 89, pp. 161–8.

Moore, D. R. *et al.* (2014), 'Beyond muscle hypertrophy: why dietary protein is important for endurance athletes'. *Appl. Physiol. Nutr. Metab.*, vol 39(9), pp. 987–97

Moore, D. R. *et al.* (2015), 'Protein ingestion to stimulate myofibrillar protein synthesis requires greater relative protein intakes in healthy older versus younger men'. *J. Gerontol. A. Biol. Sci. Med. Sci.* vol. 70(1), pp. 57–62.

Morrison, L. J. *et al.* (2004), 'Prevalent use of dietary supplements among people who exercise at a commercial gym'. *Int. J. Sport Nutr. Exerc. Metab.*, vol. 14, pp. 481–92.

Morton, J. P. *et al.* (2009), 'Reduced carbohydrate availability does not modulate training–induced heat shock protein adaptations but does upregulate oxidative enzyme activity in human skeletal muscle'. *J. Appl. Physiol.*, vol. 106 (5), pp. 1513–21 (Epub 2009 Mar 5).

Mozaffarian, D. *et al.* (2006), 'Trans fatty acids and cardiovascular disease'. *New Eng. J. Med.*, vol. 354, pp. 1601–13.

Mozaffarian, D. *et al.* (2011), 'Components of a cardio-protective diet: new insights'. *Circulation*, vol. 123, pp. 2870–91.

Mullins, V. A. *et al.* (2001), 'Nutritional status of US elite female heptathletes during training'. *Int. J. Sport Nutr.*, vol. 11, pp. 299–314.

Muoio, D. M. *et al.* (1994), 'Effect of dietary fat on metabolic adjustments to maximal VO_2 and endurance in runners'. *Med. Sci. Sports Exerc.*, vol. 26(1), pp. 81–8.

Murphy, C.H. *et al.* 2015) 'Considerations for protein intake in managing weight loss in athletes'. *Eur. J. Sport Sci.*, vol 15(1), pp. 21–8.

Murphy, M. *et al.* (2012), 'Whole beetroot consumption acutely improves running performance'. *J. Acad. Nutr. Diet.*, vol. 112, pp. 548–52.

Murray, R. *et al.* (1999), 'A comparison of the gastric emptying characteristics of selected sports drinks'. *Int. J. Sports Nutr.*, vol. 9, pp. 263–74.

Needleman I *et al* (2014) 'Oral health and impact on performance of athletes participating in the London 2012 Olympic Games: a cross-sectional study'. *Br J Sports Med.*, vol. 47(16), pp. 1054-8.

Needleman, I. *et al.* (2015), 'Oral health and elite sport performance'. *Br. J. Sports Med.*, vol. 49, pp. 3–6.

Nattiv, A. *et al.* (2007), 'American College of Sports Medicine position stand. The female athlete triad'. *Med. Sci. Sports Exerc.*, vol. 39, pp. 1867–82.

Nelson, A. *et al.* (1997), 'Creatine supplementation raises anaerobic threshold'. FASEB J., vol. 11, A586 (abstract).

Nelson, M. E. *et al.* (1986), 'Diet and bone status in amenorrheic runners'. *Am. J. Clin. Nutr.*, vol. 43, pp. 910–16.

Neufer, P. D. *et al.* (1987), 'Improvements in exercise performance: effects of carbohydrate feedings and diet'. *J. Appl. Physiol.*, vol. 62, pp. 983–8.

Neychev, V. K. and Mitev VI. (2005), 'The aphrodisiac herb *Tribulus terrestris* does not influence the androgen production in young men'. *J. Ethnopharmacol.*, vol. 101(1–3), pp. 319–20.

Nichols, J. F. *et al.* (2007), 'Disordered eating and menstrual irregularity in high school athletes in lean-build and non lean-build sports'. *Int. J. Sport Nutr. Exerc. Metab.*, vol. 17, pp. 364–77.

Nieman, D. C. (1999), 'Physical fitness and vegetarian diets: is there a relation?' *Am. J. Clin. Nutr.*, (Sep) vol. 70 (3 suppl), pp. 570S–5S.

Nieman, D. C. *et al.* (1989), 'Hematological, anthropometric, and metabolic comparisons between vegetarian and nonvegetarian elderly women'. *Int. J. Sports Med.*, vol. 10, pp. 243–50.

Nieman, D. C., Henson, D. A., McAnulty, S. R., *et al.* (2004), 'Vitamin E and immunity after the Kona Triathlon World Championship'. *Med. Sci. Sports Exerc.*, Aug 36(8), pp. 1328–35.

Nieman, D. C. *et al.* (2007), 'Quercetin reduces illness but not immune perturbations after intense exercise'. *Med. Sci. Sports Exerc.*, vol. 39, pp. 1561–69.

Nissen, S. *et al.* (1996), 'Effect of leucine metabolite HMB on muscle metabolism during resistance exercise training'. *J. Appl. Physiol.*, vol. 81, pp. 2095–104.

Nissen, S. *et al.* (1997), 'Effect of feeding HMB on body composition and strength in women'. FASEB J., vol. 11, A150 (abstract).

Noakes, T. D. (1993), 'Fluid replacement during exercise'. *Exerc. Sport Sci. Rev.*, vol. 21, pp. 297–330.

Noakes, T. D. (2000), 'Hyponatremia in distance athletes: pulling the IV on the dehydration myth'. *Phys. Sportsmed.*, vol. 26 (Sept), pp. 71–6.

Noakes, T. D. (2007), 'Drinking guidelines for exercise: what evidence is there that athletes should drink as much as possible to replace the weight lost during exercise or ad libitum?'. *J. Sports Sci.*, vol. 25 (7), pp. 781–96.

Noakes, T. D. (2010), 'Is drinking to thirst optimum?' *Ann. Nutr. Metab.*, vol, 57, Suppl 2, pp. S9–17.

Noakes, T. D. (2012), *Waterlogged: The Serious Problem of Overhydration in Endurance Sports*, (Champaign, IL:/Human Kinetics).

Noreen, E. E. *et al.* (2010), 'Effects of supplemental fish oil on resting metabolic rate, body composition, and salivary cortisol in healthy adults'. *J. Int. Soc. Sports Nutr.*, vol. 7, p. 31.

Nosaka, K. *et al.* (2006), 'Effects of amino acid supplementation on muscle soreness and damage'. *Int. J. Sports Nutr. Exerc. Metab.*, vol. 16, pp. 620–35.

Onywera, V. O. *et al.* (2004). 'Food and macronutrient intake of elite kenyan distance runners'. *Int. J. Sport Nutr. Exerc. Metab.*, vol. 14(6), pp. 709–19.

Ostojic, S. (2004), 'Creatine supplementation in young soccer players'. *Int. J. Sport Nutr. Exerc. Metab.*, vol. 14, pp. 95–103.

Otis, C. L. *et al.* (1997), 'American College of *Sports Medicine* position stand. The Female Athlete Triad'. *Med. Sci. Sport Exerc.*, vol. 29, pp. i–ix.

Owens, B. M. (2007), 'The potential effects of pH and buffering capacity on dental erosion'. *Gen. Dent.*, vol. 55(6), pp. 527–31.

Paddon-Jones, D. *et al.* (2001), 'Short term HMB supplementation does not reduce symptoms of eccentric muscle damage'. *Int. J. Sport Nutr.*, vol. 11, pp. 442–50.

Pagoto S. L. and Appelhans B. M. (2013), 'A call for an end to the diet debates'. *JAMA*, vol 310(7), pp. 687–688.

Pannemans, D. L. *et al.* (1997), 'Calcium excretion, apparent calcium absorption and calcium balance in young and elderly subjects: influence of protein intake'. *Brit. J. Nutr.*, vol. 77(5), pp. 721–9.

Parry-Billings, M. *et al.* (1992), 'Plasma amino acid concentrations in over-training syndrome: possible effects on the immune system'. *Med. Sci. Sport Ex.*, vol. 24, pp. 1353–8.

Pasiakos, S. M, and McClung, J. P. (2011), 'Supplemental dietary leucine and the skeletal muscle anabolic response to essential amino acids'. *Nutr. Rev.*, vol. 69(9), pp. 550–57.

Pasiakos, S. M., McClung, H. L., McClung, J. P. (2011), 'Leucine-enriched essential amino acid supplementation during moderate steady state exercise enhances post-exercise muscle protein synthesis'. *Am. J. Clin. Nutr.*, vol. 94(3), pp. 809–18.

Pasiakos S. M. *et al.* (2013), 'Effects of high-protein diets on fat-free mass and muscle protein synthesis following weight loss: a randomized controlled trial'. *FASEB J.*, vol 27(9), pp.3837–47.

Pasricha, S. R. *et al.* (2014), 'Iron Supplementation Benefits Physical Performance in Women of

Reproductive Age: A Systematic Review and Meta-Analysis'. *J. Nutr. 2014* jn.113.189589; first published online April 9, 2014.

Passe, D. H. *et al.* (2004), 'Palatability and voluntary intake of sports beverages, diluted orange juice and water during exercise'. *Int. J. Sport Nutr. Exerc. Metab.*, vol. 14, pp. 272–84.

Patterson, S. D. and Gray, S. C. (2007), 'Carbohydrate-gel supplementation and endurance performance during intermittent high-intensity shuttle running'. *Int. J. Sports Nutr. Exerc. Metab.*, vol. 17, pp. 445–55.

Paulsen, G., Cumming, K. T. *et al.* (2013), 'Vitamin C and E supplementation hampers cellular adaptation to endurance training in humans: a double-blind randomized controlled trial'. *J. Physiol.* 2013.267419

Pennings, B. *et al.* (2011), 'Exercising before protein intake allows for greater use of dietary protein-derived amino acids for de novo muscle protein synthesis in both young and elderly men'. *Am. J. Clin. Nutr.*, vol. 93, pp. 322–31.

Pennings, B. *et al.* (2012), 'Amino acid absorption and subsequent muscle protein accretion following graded intakes of whey protein in elderly men'. *Am. J. Physiol. Endocrinol. Metab.*, vol. 302, pp. E992–9.

Pereira, M. *et al.* (2004), 'Effects of a low glycaemic load diet on resting energy expenditure and heart disease risk factors during weight loss'. *JAMA*, vol. 292, pp. 2482–90.

Perkins, I. C. *et al.* (2015), 'New Zealand blackcurrant extract improves high-intensity intermittent running'. *Int. J. Sport Nutr. Exerc. Metab.*, vol. 25(5), pp. 487–93.

Peternelj, T. T. and Coombes, J. S. (2011), 'Antioxidant supplementation during exercise training: beneficial or detrimental?' *Sports Med.*, vol. 41(12), pp. 1043–69.

Peters, E. M. *et al.* (1993), 'Vitamin C supplementation reduces the incidence of post-race symptoms of upper-respiratory-tract infection in ultra-marathon runners'. *Am. J. Clin. Nutr.*, vol. 57, pp. 170–4.

Peters, E. M. *et al.* (2001), 'Vitamin C supplementation attenuates the increases in circulating cortisol, adrenaline and anti-inflammatory polypeptides following ultra-marathon running'. *Int. J. Sports Med.*, vol. 22(7), pp. 537–43.

Peterson, M. *et al.* (2011). 'Influence of resistance exercise on lean body mass in aging adults: a meta-analysis'. *Med. Sci. Sports Exerc.*, vol. 43, pp. 249–58.

Petrie, T. A. (1993), 'Disordered eating in female collegiate gymnasts'. *J. Sport Ex. Psych.*, vol. 15, pp. 434–6.

Pfeiffer, B. *et al.* (2010a), 'Oxidation of solid versus liquid CHO sources during exercise'. *Med. Sci. Sports Exerc.*, vol. 42(11), pp. 2030–7.

Pfeiffer, B. *et al.* (2010b), 'CHO oxidation from a CHO gel compared with a drink during exercise'. *Med. Sci. Sports Exerc.*, vol. 42(11), pp. 2038–45.

Phillips, P. A. *et al.* (1984), 'Reduced thirst after water deprivation in healthy elderly men'. *N. Engl. J. Med.*, vol. 311, pp. 753–59.

Phillips, S. M. (2012), 'Dietary protein requirements and adaptive advantages in athletes'. *Br. J. Nutr.*, vol. 108, Suppl. 2, pp. S158–67.

Phillips, S. M. *et al.* (1997), 'Mixed muscle protein synthesis and breakdown after resistance training in humans'. *Am. J. Physiol.*, vol. 273(1), pp. E99–E107.

Phillips, S. M. *et al.* (1999), 'Resistance training reduces acute exercise-induced increase in muscle protein turnover'. *Am. J. Physiol.*, vol. 276(1), pp. E118–24.

Phillips, S. M. *et al.* (2005), 'Dietary protein to support anabolism with resistance exercise in young men'. *J. Am. Coll. Nutr.*, vol. 24(2), pp. 134S–9S.

Phillips, S. M. *et al.* (2007), 'A critical examination of dietary protein requirements, benefits and excesses in athletes'. *Int. J. Sports Nutr. Exerc. Metab.*, vol. 17, pp. 58–78.

Phillips, S. M. and Van Loon, L. J. (2011), 'Dietary protein for athletes: from requirements to optimum adaptation'. *J. Sports Sci.*, vol. 29, Suppl. 1, pp. S29–38.

Phillips, S. M., *et al.* (2011), 'Nutrition for weight and resistance training'. In: Lanham-New, S. A. *et al.* (eds), *Sport and Exercise Nutrition* (Oxford: Wiley-Blackwell).

Phillips, T. *et al.* (2003), 'A dietary supplement attenuates IL-6 and CRP after eccentric exercise in untrained males'. *Med. Sci. Sports Exerc.*, vol. 35(12), pp. 2032–7.

Phinney, S. D. *et al.* (1983), 'The human metabolic response to chronic ketosis without caloric restriction: preservation of submaximal exercise capability with reduced carbohydrate oxidation'. *Metabolism*, vol. 32(8), pp. 69–76.

Pilegaard, H. *et al.* (2005), 'Substrate availability and transcriptional regulation of metabolic genes in human skeletal muscle during recovery from exercise'. *Metabolism*, vol. 54(8), pp. 1048–55.

Pöchmüller, M. et al (2016), 'A systematic review and meta-analysis of carbohydrate benefits associated with randomized controlled competition-based performance trials'. *J. Int. Soc. Sports Nutr.* Vol. 13, pp 27.

Pollock, M. L. and Jackson, A. S. (1984), 'Research progress invalidation of clinical methods of assessing body composition'. *Med. Sci. Sport Ex.*, vol. 16, pp. 606–13.

Poortmans, J. R. and Francaux, M. (1999), 'Longterm oral creatine supplementation does not impair renal function in healthy athletes'. *Med. Sci. Sports Ex.*, vol. 31(8), pp. 1103–10.

Pottier, A. et al. (2010), 'Mouth rinse but not ingestion of a carbohydrate solution improves 1-h cycle time trial performance', *Scand. J. Med. Sci. Sports*, vol. 20(1), pp. 105–11.

Powers, M. E. (2002), 'The safety and efficacy of anabolic steroid precursors: what is the scientific evidence?'. *J. Athol. Training*, vol. 37(3), pp. 300–5.

Powers, S. et al. (2011), 'Antioxidant and vitamin D supplements for athletes: sense or nonsense?' *J. Sports Sci.*, vol. 29, Suppl. 1, S47–55.

Quesnele, J. J. et al. (2014), 'The effects of Beta-alanine supplementation on performance: a systematic review of the literature'. *Int. J. Sport Nutr. Exerc. Metab.*, vol. 24(1), pp. 14–27.

Rawson, E. S. and Volek, J. S. (2003), 'Effects of creatine supplementation and resistance training on muscle strength and weightlifting performance'. *J. Strength Cond. Res.*, vol. 17, pp. 822–31.

Ready, S. L. et al. (1999), 'The effect of two sports drink formulations on muscle stress and performance'. *Med. Sci. Sports Exerc.*, vol. 31(5), p. S119.

Reidy, P. T. et al. (2013), 'Protein blend ingestion following resistance exercise promotes human muscle protein synthesis'. *J. Nutr.*, vol. 143(4), pp. 410–16.

Rennie, M. J. (2009), 'Anabolic resistance: the effects of aging, sexual dimorphism, and immobilization on human muscle protein turnover'. *Appl. Physiol. Nutr. Metab.*, vol. 34, pp. 377–81.

Res, P. T. et al. (2012), 'Protein ingestion prior to sleep improves post-exercise overnight recovery'. *Med. Sci. Sports Exerc.*, Feb 9 (Epub ahead of print).

Ribeiro, A. S. et al. (2016), 'Effect of conjugated linoleic acid associated with aerobic exercise on body fat and lipid profile in obese women: a randomized, double-blinded, and placebo-controlled trial'. *Int. J. Sport Nutr. Exerc. Metab.*, vol. 26(2), pp. 135–44.

Richter, E. A. et al. (1991), 'Immune parameters in male athletes after a lacto-ovo-vegetarian diet and a mixed Western diet'. *Med. Sci. Sports Exerc.*, vol. 23, pp. 517–21.

Rivera-Brown, A. M. et al. (1999), 'Drink composition, voluntary drinking and fluid balance in exercising trained heat-acclimatized boys'. *J. Appl. Physiol.*, vol. 86, pp. 78–84.

Rizkalla, S. et al. (2004), 'Improved plasma glucose control, whole body glucose utilisation and lipid profile on a low glycaemic index diet in type 2 diabetic men: a randomised controlled trial'. *Diab. Care*, vol. 27, pp. 1866–72.

Robertson, J. et al. (1991), 'Increased blood antioxidant systems of runners in response to training load'. *Clin. Sci.*, vol. 80, pp. 611–18.

Robinson. T. M. et al. (2000), 'Dietary creatine supplementation does not affect some haematological indices, or indices of muscle damage and hepatic and renal function'. *Brit. J. Sports Med.*, vol. 34, pp. 284–8.

Rodriguez, N. R., Di Marco, N. M., Langley, S., et al. (2009), 'American College of Sports Medicine position stand: Nutrition and athletic performance', *Med. Sci. Sports Exerc.*, vol. 41(3), pp. 709–31.

Rogers, J. et al. (2005), 'Gastric emptying and intestinal absorption of a low carbohydrate sport drink during exercise'. *Int. J. Sport Nutr. Exerc. Metab.*, vol. 15, pp. 220–35.

Rogerson, S. et al. (2007), 'The effect of five weeks of Tribulus terrestris supplementation on muscle strength and body composition during preseason training in elite rugby league players'. *J. Strength Cond. Res.*, vol. 21(2), pp. 348–53.

Rokitzki, L. et al. (1994), 'a-tocopherol supplementation in racing cyclists during extreme endurance training'. *Int. J. Sports Nutr.*, vol. 4, pp. 235–64.

Rollo, I. et al. (2008), 'The influence of carbohydrate mouth rinse on self-selected speeds during a 30-min treadmill run,' *Int. J. Sport Nutr. Exerc. Metab.*, vol 18(6), pp. 585–600.

Rolls, B. J. and Shide, D. J. (1992), 'The influence of fat on food intake and body weight'. *Nutr. Revs.*, vol. 50(10), pp. 283–90.

Romano-Ely, B. C. et al. (2006), 'Effects of an isocaloric carbohydrate-protein-antioxidant drink on cycling performance'. *Med. Sci. Sports Exerc.*, vol. 38, pp. 1608–16.

Rosen, L. W. *et al.* (1986), 'Pathogenic weightcontrol behavior in female athletes'. *Phys. Sports Med.*, vol. 14, pp. 79–86.

Rowbottom, D. G. *et al.* (1996), 'The energizing role of glutamine as an indicator of exercise stress and overtraining'. *Sports Med.*, vol. 21(2), pp. 80–97.

Rustad, P.I. *et al* (2016), 'Intake of Protein Plus Carbohydrate during the First Two Hours after Exhaustive Cycling Improves Performance the following Day'. *PLoS One*, vol. 11(4) e0153229.

SACN (2015), 'Carbohydrates and Health'. www.gov.uk/government/publications/sacn-carbohydrates-and-health-report. Accessed March 2016.

Santos, V. C. *et al.* (2013), 'Effects of DHA-rich fish oil supplementation on lymphocyte function before and after a marathon race'. *Int. J. Sport Nutr. Exerc. Metab.*, vol. 23(2), pp. 161–9.

Saunders, M. J. *et al.* (2004), 'Effects of a carbohydrate-protein-beverage on cycling endurance and muscle damage'. *Med. Sci. Sports Exerc.*, vol. 36, pp. 1233–8.

Saunders, M. J. (2007), 'Coingestion of carbohydrate-protein during endurance exercise: influence on performance and recovery'. *Int. J. Sports Nutr. Exerc. Metab.*, vol. 17, S87–S103.

Sawka, M. N. (1992), 'Physiological consequences of hypohydration: exercise performance and thermoregulation'. *Med. Sci. Sports Exerc.*, vol. 24, pp. 657–70.

Sawka, M. N. *et al.* (2007), 'American College of Sports Medicine Position stand. Exercise and fluid replacement'. *Med. Sci. Sports Exerc.*, vol. 39, pp. 377–90.

Schoenfeld, B. J. *et al.* (2013), 'The effect of protein timing on muscle strength and hypertrophy: a meta-analysis'. *J. Int. Soc. Sports Nutr.*, vol. 10(1), pp. 53.

Schoenfeld, B. J. *et al* (2017), 'Pre- versus post-exercise protein intake has similar effects on muscular adaptations'. *PeerJ.*, vol. 5, e2825.

Schokman, C. P. *et al.* (1999), 'Pre- and post game macronutrient intake of a group of elite Australian Football Players'. *Int. J. Sport Nutr.*, vol. 9, pp. 60–9.

Seebohar, B. (2014), 'Metabolic efficiency training: teaching the body to burn more fat'. (2nd edn), www.enrgperformance.com.

Seiler, D. *et al.* (1989), 'Effects of long-distance running on iron metabolism and hematological parameters'. *Int. J. Sports Med.*, vol. 10, pp. 357–62.

Seip, R. L. and Semenkovich, C. F. (1998), 'Skeletal muscle lipoprotein lipase: molecular regulation and physiological effects in relation to exercise'. *Exerc. Sport Sci. Rev.*, vol. 26, pp. 191–218.

Sherman, W. M. *et al.* (1981), 'Effect of exercise-diet manipulation on muscle glycogen and its subsequent utilisation during performance'. *Int. J. Sports Med.*, vol. 2, pp. 114–18.

Sherman, W. M. *et al.* (1991), 'Carbohydrate feedings 1 hour before exercise improve cycling performance'. *Am. J. Clin. Nutr.*, vol. 54, pp. 866–70.

Shimomura, Y. *et al.* (2006), 'Nutraceutical effects of branched chain amino acids on skeletal muscle'. *J. Nutr.*, vol. 136, pp. 529–32.

Shing, C. M., Hunter, D. C., Stevenson, L. M. (2009), 'Bovine colostrum supplementation and exercise performance: potential mechanisms'. *Sports Med.*, vol. 39(12), pp. 1033–54.

Shing, C.M. *et al.* (2007), 'Effects of bovine colostrum supplementation on immune variables in highly trained cyclists'. *J. Appl. Physiol.*, vol. 102, pp. 1113–22.

Shirreffs, S. M., *et al.* (1996), 'Post-exercise rehydration in man: effects of volume consumed. and drink sodium content'. *Med. Sci. Sports Ex.*, vol. 28, pp. 1260–71.

Shirreffs S. M. *et al.* (2004), 'Fluid and electrolyte needs for preparation and recovery from training and competition'. *J. Sports Sci.*, vol. 22(1), pp. 57–63.

Shirreffs, S. M. *et al.* (2007), 'Milk as an effective post-exercise rehydration drink'. *Br. J. Nutr.*, vol. 98, pp. 173–180.

Shirreffs, S. M. and Sawka, M. N. (2011), 'Fluid and electrolyte needs for training, competition, and recovery'. *J. Sports Sci.*, vol. 29, suppl 1, pp. S39–46.

Short, S. H. and Short, W. R. (1983), 'Four-year study of university athletes' dietary intake'. *J. Am. Diet. Assoc.*, vol. 82, p. 632.

Silva-Cavalcante, M. D. *et al.* (2013), 'Caffeine increases anaerobic work and restores cycling performance following a protocol designed to lower endogenous carbohydrate availability'. PLoS One, vol. 8(8), e72025.

Simopoulos, A. P. and Robinson, J. (1998). *The Omega Plan* (New York, HarperCollins).

Sinning, W. E. (1998), 'Body composition in athletes'. In Roche, A. F. *et al.* (eds.) *Human Body Composition*, (Champaign, IL: Human Kinetics), pp. 257–73.

Skaug, A., Sveen, O., and Raastad, T. (2014), 'An antioxidant and multivitamin supplement reduced improvements in VO²max'. *J. Sports Med. Phys. Fitness.*, vol. 54(1), pp. 63–9.

Slater, G. *et al.* (2001), 'HMB supplementation does not affect changes in strength or body composition during resistance training in trained men'. *Int. J. Sport Nutr.*, vol. 11, pp. 383–96.

Sloth, B. *et al.* (2004), 'No difference in body weight decrease between a low GI and high GI diet but reduced LDL cholesterol after 10 wk ad libitum intake of the low GI diet'. *Am. J. Clin Nutr.*, vol. 80, pp. 337–47.

Snijders, T. *et al.* (2015), 'Protein ingestion before sleep increases muscle mass and strength gains during prolonged resistance-type exercise training in healthy young men'. *J. Nutr.* In press, Apr 29, 2015.

Snyder, A. C. *et al.* (1989), 'Influence of dietary iron source on measures of iron status among female runners'. *Med. Sci. Sports Exerc.*; vol. 21, pp. 7–10.

Spector, T. (2015), *The Diet Myth: The real science behind what we eat* (WBH).

Speedy, D. B. *et al.* (1999), 'Hyponatremia in ultra-distance triathletes'. *Med. Sci. Sports Exerc.*, vol. 31, pp. 809–15.

Spencer, E. A. *et al.* (2003), 'Weight gain over 5 years in 21,966 meat-eating, fish-eating, vegetarian, and vegan men and women in EPIC-Oxford'. *Int. J. Obes. Relat. Metab. Disord.* Jun; 27(6), pp. 728–34.

Spriet, L. (1995), 'Caffeine and performance'. *Int. J. Sport Nutr.*, vol. 5, pp. S84–S99.

Steen, S. N. and McKinney, S. (1986), 'Nutrition assessment of college wrestlers'. *Phys. Sports Med.*, vol. 14, pp. 100–6.

Steenge, G. R. *et al.* (1998), 'The stimulatory effect of insulin on creatine accummulation in human skeletal muscle'. *Am. J. Physiol.*, vol. 275, pp. E974–9.

Stegen, S. *et al.* (2014), 'The beta-alanine dose for maintaining moderately elevated muscle carnosine levels'. *Med. Sci. Sports Exerc.*, 1 (Epub ahead of print).

Stellingwerff, T. *et al.* (2006), 'Decreased PDH activation and glycogenolysis during exercise following fat adaptation with carbohydrate restoration'. *Am. J. Physiol. Endocrinol. Metab.*, vol. 290(2), pp. 380–8.

Stevenson, E. *et al.* (2005), 'Improved recovery from prolonged exercise following the consumption of low glycaemic index carbohydrate meals'. *Int. J. Sport Nutr. Exerc. Metab.*, vol. 15, pp. 333–49.

Sun, G. *et al.* (2005), 'Comparison of multifrequency bioelectrical impedance analysis with dual-energy X-ray absorptiometry for assessment of percentage body fat in a large, healthy population'. *Am. J. Clin Nutr.*, vol. 81, pp. 74–8.

Sundgot-Borgen, J. (1994a), 'Eating disorders in female athletes'. *Sports Med.*, vol. 17(3), pp. 176–88.

Sundgot-Borgen, J. (1994b), 'Risk and trigger factors for the development of eating disorders in female elite athletes'. *Med. Sci. Sports Ex.*, vol. 26, pp. 414–19.

Sundgot-Borgen, J. and Larsen, S. (1993), 'Nutrient intake and eating behaviour in elite female athletes suffering from anorexia nervosa, anorexia athletica and bulimia nervosa'. *Int. J. Sport Nutr.*, vol. 3, pp. 431–42.

Sundgot-Borgen, J. and Torstveit M. K. (2004), 'Prevalence of eating disorders in elite athletes is higher than in the general population'. *Clin. J. Sport Nutr.*, vol. 14, pp. 25–32.

Sundgot-Borgen, J. and Torstveit, M. K. (2010), 'Aspects of disordered eating continuum in elite high-intensity sports'. *Scand. J. Med. Sci. Sports.*, vol. 20 (Suppl 2), pp. 112–21.

Swaminathan, R. *et al.* (1985), 'Thermic effect of feeding carbohydrate, fat, protein and mixed meal in lean and obese subjects'. *Am. J. Clin. Nutr.*, vol. 42, pp. 177–81.

Tanaka, H. and Seals, D.R (2008) 'Endurance exercise performance in Masters athletes: age-associated changes and underlying physiological mechanisms.' J Physiol. Vol. 586(1), p.55–63.

Tang, J. E. *et al.* (2009), 'Ingestion of whey hydrolysate, casein, or soy protein isolate: effects on mixed muscle protein synthesis at rest and following resistance exercise in young men'. *J. Appl. Physiol.*, vol. 107(3), pp. 987–92.

Tarnopolsky, M. and MacLennan, D. P. (1988), 'Influence of protein intake and training status in nitrogen balance and lean body mass'. *J. Appl. Physiol*, vol. 64, pp. 187–93.

Tarnopolsky, M. and MacLennan, D. P. (1992), 'Evaluation of protein requirements for trained strength athletes'. *J. Appl. Physiol*, vol. 73, pp. 1986–95.

Tarnopolsky, M. and MacLennan, D. P. (1997), 'Post exercise protein–carbohydrate and carbohydrate supplements increase muscle glycogen in males and females'. *J. Appl. Physiol.*, Abstracts, vol. 4, p. 332A.

Tarnopolsky, M. and MacLennan, D. P. (2000), 'Creatine monohydrate supplementation enhances high-intensity exercise performance in males and females'. *Int. J. Sport Nutr.*, vol. 10, pp. 452–63.

Theodorou, A.A. *et al.* (2011), 'No effect of antioxidant supplementation on muscle performance and blood redox status adaptations to eccentric training'. *Am. J. Clin. Nutr.*, vol. 93(6), pp. 1373–83.

Thomas, D. E. *et al.* (1991), 'Carbohydrate feeding before exercise: effect of glycaemic index'. *Int. J. Sports Med.*, vol. 12, pp. 180–6.

Thomas, D. E. *et al.* (1994), 'Plasma glucose levels after prolonged strenuous exercise correlate inversely with glycaemic response to food consuMed. before exercise'. *Int. J. Sports Nutr.*, vol. 4, pp. 261–73.

Thompson, C. *et al* (2016), 'Dietary nitrate supplementation improves sprint and high-intensity intermittent running performance'. *Nitric Oxide*, vol. 61, pp. 55-61.

Tipton, C. M. (1987), 'Commentary: physicians should advise wrestlers about weight loss'. *Phys. Sports Med.*, vol. 15, pp. 160–5.

Tipton, K. D. and Witard, O. C. (2007), 'Protein requirements and recommendations for athletes: relevance of ivory tower arguments for practical recommendations'. *Clin. Sports Med.*, vol. 26(1), pp. 17–36.

Tipton, K. D. and Wolfe, R. (2007), 'Protein needs and amino acids for athletes'. *J. Sports Sci.*, vol 22(1), pp. 65–79.

Tipton K. D. *et al.* (2001), 'Timing of amino acid–carbohydrate ingestion alters anabolic response of muscle to resistance exercise'. *Am. J. Physiol.*, vol. 281(2), pp. E197–206.

Tipton, K. D. *et al.* (2004), 'Ingestion of casein and whey proteins result in muscle analbolism after resistance exercise'. *Med. Sci. Sports Exerc.*, vol. 36 (12), pp. 2073–81.

Tipton, K. D *et al.* (2007), 'Stimulation of net protein sythesis by whey protein ingestion before and after exercise'. *Am. J. Physiol. Endocrinol. Metab.*, vol. 292(1), pp. E71–6.

Tobias, Deirdre K. *et al.* (2015), 'Effect of low-fat diet interventions versus other diet interventions on long-term weight change in adults: a systematic review and meta-analysis'. *The Lancet Diabetes & Endocrinology*, vol. 3(12), pp. 968–79.

Torstveit, M. K. and J. Sundgot-Borgen (2005), 'Participation in leanness sports but not training volume is associated with menstrual dysfunction: a national survey of 1276 athletes and controls'. *Br. J. Sports Med.*, vol. 39, pp. 141–7.

Toth, P. P. (2005), 'The "good cholesterol": High-density lipoprotein', *Circulation*, vol. 111(5), pp. 89–91.

Truby, H. *et al.* (2008), 'Commercial weight loss diets meet nutrient requirements in free living adults over 8 weeks: a randomised controlled weight loss trial'. *Nutrition Journal* 2008, vol. 7, p. 25.

Tsintzas, O. K. *et al.* (1995), 'Influence of carbohydrate electrolyte drinks on marathon running performance'. *Eur. J. Appl. Physiol.*, vol. 70, pp. 154–60.

Uauy, R. *et al.* (2009), 'WHO Scientific Update on trans fatty acids: summary and conclusions'. *Eur. J. Clin. Nutr.*, vol. 63, pp. S68–S75.

Unnithan, V. B. *et al.* (2001), 'Is there a physiologic basis for creatine use in children and adolescents?' *J. Strength Cond. Res.*, vol. 15(4), pp. 524–8.

Vahedi, K. (2000), 'Ischaemic stroke in a sportsman who consumed mahuang extract and creatine monohydrate for bodybuilding'. *J. Neur., Neurosurgery and Psych.*, vol. 68, pp. 112–13.

Vandenbogaerde, T. J. and Hopkins, W. G. (2011), 'Effects of acute carbohydrate supplementation on endurance performance: a meta-analysis'. *Sports Med.*, vol. 41(9), pp. 773–92.

Van Essen M. and Gibala, M. J. (2006), 'Failure of protein to improve time trial performance when added to a sports drink'. *Med. Sci. Sports Exerc.*, vol. 38(8), pp. 1476–83.

Van Loon, L. J. C. (2007), 'Application of protein or protein hydrolysates to improve postexercise recovery'. *Int. J. Sports Nutr. Exerc. Metab.*, vol. 17, S104–17.

Van Loon, L. J. C. (2014), 'Is there a need for protein ingestion during exercise?' *Sports Med.*, vol. 44 (Suppl. 1), pp. 105–11.

Van Proeyen, K. *et al.* (2011), 'Beneficial metabolic adaptations due to endurance exercise training in the fasted state'. *J. Appl. Physiol.*, vol. 110(1), pp. 236–45.

Van Someren, K. A. *et al.* (2005), 'Supplementation with HMB and KIC reduces signs and symptoms of exercise-induced muscle damage in man'. *Int. J. Sport Nutr. Exerc. Metab.*, vol. 15, pp. 413–24.

Van Thienen, R. *et al.* (2009), 'Beta-alanine improves sprint performance in endurance cycling'. *Med. Sci. Sports Exerc.*, vol. 41, pp. 898–903.

Venables, M. *et al.* (2005), 'Erosive effect of a new sports drink on dental enamel during exercise'. *Med. Sci. Sports Exerc.*, vol. 37(1), pp. 39–44.

Volek, J. S. (1997), 'Response of testosterone and cortisol concentrations to high-intensity resistance training following creatine supplementation'. *J. Strength Cond. Res.*, vol. 11, pp. 182–7.

Volek, J. S. *et al.* (1999), 'Performance and muscle fibre adaptations to creatine supplementation and heavy resistance training'. *Med. Sci. Sports Ex.*, vol. 31(8), pp. 1147–56.

Volek, J. S. *et al.* (2013), 'Whey protein supplementation during resistance training augments lean body mass'. *J. Am. Coll. Nutr.*, vol. 32(2), pp. 122–35.

Walser, B., Giordano, R. M. and Stebbins, C. L. (2006), 'Supplementation with omega-3 polyunsaturated fatty acids augments brachial artery dilation and blood flow during forearm contraction'. *Eur. J. Appl. Physiol.* Jun; 97(3), pp. 347–54.

Wang, Y. *et al.* (2005), 'Comparison of abdominal adiposity and overall obesity in predicting risk of type 2 diabetes among men'. *Am. J. Clin. Nutr.*, vol. 8, pp. 555–63.

Wansink, B. (2005), 'Bad popcorn in big buckets: portion size can influence intake as much as taste'. *J. Nutr. Educ. Behav.*, vol. 37(5), pp. 42–5.

Wansink, B. *et al.* (2005), 'Bottomless bowls: why visual cues of portion size may influence intake'. *Obes. Res.*, vol. 13(1), pp. 93–100.

Warburton, D. E., Nicol, C. W. and Bredin, S. S. (2006), 'Health benefits of physical activity: the evidence'. *CMAJ*, vol. 174(6), pp. 801–9.

Warren, J. *et al.* (2003), 'Low glycaemic index breakfasts and reduced food intake in preadolescent children'. *Paediatrics*, vol. 112, pp. 414–19.

Watt, K. K. O. *et al.* (2004), 'Skeletal muscle total creatine content and creatine transporter gene expression in vegetarians prior to and following creatine supplementation'. *Int. J. Sport Nutr. Exerc. Metab.*, vol. 14, pp. 517–31.

WCRF/AICR (2007), 'Food, Nutrition, Physical Activity, and the Prevention of Cancer: a Global Perspective'.

Weisgarber, K. D., Candow, D. G. and Vogt, E. S. M. (2012), 'Whey protein before and during resistance exercise has no effect on muscle mass and strength in untrained young adults'. *Int. J. Sport Nutr. Exerc. Metab.*, vol. 22(6), pp. 463–9.

Wemple, R. D. *et al.* (1997), 'Caffeine vs. caffeine-free sports drinks: effects on urine production at rest and during prolonged exercise'. *Int. J. Sports Med.*, vol. 18(1), pp. 40–6.

West, N. P. *et al.* (2011), 'Supplementation with Lactobacillus fermentum VRI (PCC) reduces lower respiratory illness in athletes and moderate exercise-induced immune perturbations'. *Nutrition Journal*, vol. 10, p. 30.

Westerterp-Plantenga, M. S. *et al.* (2012), 'Dietary protein – its role in satiety, energetics, weight loss and health'. *Br. J. Nutr.*, vol. 108, Suppl 2, pp. S105–12.

Wilborn, C. D. *et al.* (2004), 'Effects of zinc magnesium aspartate (ZMA) supplementation on training adaptations and markers of anabolism and catabolism'. *J. Int. Soc. Sports Nutr.*, vol. 1(2), pp. 12–20.

Wilk, B. and Bar-Or, O. (1996), 'Effect of drink flavour and NaCl on voluntary drinking and rehydration in boys exercising in the heat'. *J. Appl. Physiol.*, vol. 80, pp. 1112–17.

Wilkinson, S. B. *et al.* (2007), 'Consumption of fluid skim milk promotes greater protein accretion after resuistece exercise than does consumption of an isonitrogenous and isoenergetic soy-protein beverage'. *Am. J. Clin. Nutr.*, vol. 85(4), pp. 1031–40.

Willems, M. E. T. *et al.* (2014), 'CurraNZ blackcurrant improves cycling performance and recovery in trained endurance athletes'. *J. Int. Soc. Sports Nutr.*, vol. 11 (Suppl 1), p. 14.

Williams, M. H. (1985), *Nutritional Aspects of Human Physical and Athletic Performance*, (Springfield, IL: Charles C Thomas Publisher).

Williams, C. and Devlin, J. T. (eds) (1992), *Foods, Nutrition and Performance: An International Scientific Consensus* (London: Chapman and Hall). Williams, M. H. (1992), *Nutrition for Fitness and Sport* (Dubuque, IO: WilliAm. C. Brown).

Williams, M. H. (1999), *Nutrition for Health, Fitness and Sport*, 5th ed. (New York: McGraw-Hill). Williams, M. H. *et al.* (1999), *Creatine: The Power Supplement* (Champaign, IL: Human Kinetics).

Williams, M. H. (1998), *The Ergogenics Edge* (Champaign, IL: Human Kinetics).

Williamson, D. A. *et al.* (1995), 'Structured equation modeling of risk factors for the development of eating disorder symptoms in female athletes'. *Int. J. Eating Disorders*, vol. 17(4), 387–93.

Willis, L. H. *et al.* (2012), 'Effects of aerobic and/or resistance training on body mass and fat mass in overweight or obese adults'. *J. Appl. Physiol.* Dec, 113(12), pp. 1831–7. http://www.ncbi.nlm.nih.gov/pubmed/23019316

Wilmore, J. H. (1983), 'Body composition in sport and exercise'. *Med. Sci. Sports Ex.*, vol. 15, pp. 21–31.

Witard, O. C. *et al.* (2011), 'Effect of increased dietary protein on tolerance to intensified training'. *Med. Sci. Sports Exerc.*, vol. 43(4), pp. 598–607.

Witard, O. C. *et al.* (2014), 'High dietary protein restores overreaching induced impairments in leukocyte trafficking and reduces the incidence of upper respiratory tract infection in elite cyclists'. *Brain Behav. Immun.*, vol. 39, pp. 211–9.

Witard, O. C. *et al.* (2014), 'Myofibrillar muscle protein synthesis rates subsequent to a meal in response to increasing doses of whey protein at rest and after resistance exercise'. *Am. J. Clin. Nutr.*, vol. 99(1), pp. 86–95.

Witard O.C, et al (2016), 'Protein Considerations for Optimising Skeletal Muscle Mass in Healthy Young and Older Adults.' Nutrients. Vol 8 (4), p.181.

Wright, D. W. *et al.* (1991), 'Carbohydrate feedings before, during or in combination improve cycling endurance performance'. *J. Appl. Physiol.*, vol. 71, pp. 1082–88.

Wu, C. L. and Williams, C. (2006), 'A low glycaemic index meal before exercise improves endurance running capacity in men'. *Int. J. Sports Nutr. Exerc. Metab.*, vol 16, pp. 510–27.

Wu, C. L. *et al.* (2003), 'The influence of high carbohydrate meals with different glycaemic indices on substrate utilisation during subsequent exercise'. *Br. J. Nutr.*, vol. 90(6), pp. 1049–56.

Wylie, L. J. *et al.* (2013), 'Beetroot juice and exercise: pharmacodynamic and dose-response relationships'. *J. Appl. Physiol*, vol 115(3), pp. 325–36.

Yaspelkis, B. B., *et al.* (1993), 'Carbohydrate supplementation spares muscle glycogen during variable-intensity exercise'. *J. Appl. Physiol.* Oct, 75(4), pp. 1477–85.

Yeo, W. K. *et al.* (2008), 'Skeletal muscle adaptation and performance responses to once a day versus twice-every-second-day endurance training regimens'. *J. Appl. Physiol.*, vol. 105, pp. 1462–70.

Yfanti, C. *et al.* (2010), 'Antioxidant supplementation does not alter endurance training adaptation'. *Med. Sci. Sports Exerc.*, vol. 42(7), pp. 1388–95.

Zajac, A. *et al.* (2014), 'The effects of a ketogenic diet on exercise metabolism and physical performance in off-road cyclists'. *Nutrients,* vol. 6(7), pp. 2493–508.

Zawadzki, K. M. *et al.* (1992), 'Carbohydrate-protein complex increases the rate of muscle glycogen storage after exercise'. *J. Appl. Physiol.*, vol. 72, pp. 1854–9.

Ziberna, L. *et al.* (2013), 'The endothelial plasma membrane transporter bilitranslocase mediates rat aortic vasodilation induced by anthocyanins'. *Nutr. Metab. Cardiovasc. Dis.*, vol. 23(1), pp. 68–74.

Ziegenfuss, T. *et al.* (1997), 'Acute creatine ingestion: effects on muscle volume, anaerobic power, fluid volumes and protein turnover'. *Med. Sci. Sports Ex.*, vol. 29, supp. 127.

Ziegler, P. J. *et al.* (1999), 'Nutritional and physiological status of US National Figure Skaters'. *Int. J. Sport Nutr.*, vol. 9, pp. 345–60.

Ziegler, P. J. *et al.* (1998), 'Nutritional status of nationally ranked junior US figure skaters'. *J. Am. Diet. Assoc.*, vol. 98, pp. 809–11.

Zucker, N. L. *et al.* (1999), 'Protective factors for eating disorders in female college athletes'. *Eating Disord.*, vol. 7, pp. 207–18.

NUTRITION ANALYSIS

Dietplan7: http://www.foresoft.co.uk/
Nutritics: www.nutritics.com
Nutrachek: www.nutracheck.co.uk

ONLINE RESOURCES

British Nutrition Foundation

www.nutrition.org.uk

The website of the British Nutrition Foundation, contains information, fact sheets and educational resources on nutrition and health.

Academy of Nutrition and Dietetics

www.eatright.org

The website of the US Academy of Nutrition and Dietetics, provides nutrition articles, news, tips and resources.

British Dietetic Association

www.bda.uk.com

The website of the British Dietetic Association includes fact sheets and information on healthy eating for children. It also provides details of Registered Dietitians working in private practice.

Gatorade Sports Science Institute

www.gssiweb.com

This website provides a good database of articles and consensus papers on nutritional topics written by experts.

Runner's World

www.runnersworld.co.uk

The website of the UK edition of *Runner's World* magazine provides an extensive library of excellent articles on nutrition, training and sports injuries, and sports nutrition product reviews.

Vegetarian Society

www.vegsoc.org

This website provides comprehensive information and fact sheets on vegetarian nutrition and health, as well as recipes.

Weight Concern

www.weightconcern.org.uk

Excellent information on obesity issues, including a section on children's health and a BMI calculator.

Health Supplements Information Service

www.hsis.org

This website provides balanced information on vitamins, minerals and supplements.

Weight Loss Resources

www.weightlossresources.co.uk

This UK website provides excellent information on weight loss, fitness and healthy eating as well as a comprehensive calorie database and a personalised weight loss programme.

Diabetes UK

www.diabetes.org.uk

Diabetes UK is the leading charity for people with diabetes and this website provides authoritative information on living with diabetes, as well as sections for children, teenagers and young adults.

The Mayo Clinic

www.mayoclinic.com

Written by medical experts, this US site offers good nutrition and health information, as well as advice on medical conditions in a user-friendly format.

WebMD

www.webmd.com

This comprehensive US website has an A–Z dictionary of health topics and advice on many aspects of nutrition and fitness.

Health Status

www.healthstatus.com

This US website provides useful health calculators and assessments that help you work out your body mass index, body fat percentage, number of calories burned during exercise and daily calorie intake.

Nutrition Data

http://nutritiondata.self.com

This US website provides a detailed nutrition database together with nutritional information from food manufacturers and restaurants.

Net Doctor

www.netdoctor.co.uk/dietandnutrition

This UK website provides excellent advice on healthy eating, weight loss, health conditions, weight problems and lifestyle management.

Beat (Beat Eating Disorders)

www.b-eat.co.uk

The website of Beat (the working name of the Eating Disorders Association) provides helplines, online support and a network of UK-wide self-help groups as well as information sheets and booklets, which can be downloaded free.

Australian Institute of Sport

www.ausport.gov.au/ais/nutrition

The website of AIS provides excellent and up-to-date fact sheets on sports nutrition written by sports dietitians.

Sports Dietitians Australia

www.sportsdietitians.com.au

The SDA website provides excellent fact sheets on a wide range of sports nutrition topics.

TO FIND A SPORT AND EXERCISE NUTRITIONIST:

www.associationfornutrition.org (the UK Voluntary Register of Nutritionists)

www.senr.org.uk (the voluntary competency-based register for Sport and Exercise Nutritionists)

www.scandpg.org (a register for dietitians specialising in sport nutrition in the US)

INDEX

Recipe Index